SPORTS MEDICINE
FOR THE
ATHLETIC FEMALE

Edited by Christine E. Haycock, M.D.

Medical Economics Company 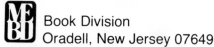 Book Division
Oradell, New Jersey 07649

Library of Congress Cataloging in Publication Data

Main entry under title:

Sports medicine for the athletic female.

Includes bibliographical references.
1. Sports medicine.   2.   Sports for women.
3.   Women—Health and hygiene.   I.   Haycock,
Christine E.   [DNLM: 1.   Sports medicine.   2.   Women.
QT260 S7704]
RC1210.S69   617'.1027   80-14228
ISBN 0-87489-212-0

Design by James M. Walsh

ISBN 0-87489-212-0

Medical Economics Company
Oradell, New Jersey 07649

Printed in the United States of America

Contents

Contributors

Marlene J. Adrian, D.P.E.
Professor of Physical Education
Washington State University
Pullman, Washington

Leslie M. Bodnar, M.D.
Coordinator of Sports Medicine
University of Notre Dame
Notre Dame, Indiana

Thomas L. Bodnar, J.D.
Private Practice of Law
South Bend, Indiana

Roger H. Brodkin, M.D.
Clinical Professor of Medicine
College of Medicine and Dentistry of New Jersey,
  N.J. Medical School
Newark, New Jersey

John W. Cavo Jr., M.D.
Clinical Instructor
University of Connecticut School of Medicine
Farmington, Connecticut
Private Practice of Otolaryngology
New Britain, Connecticut

Alfonse A. Cinotti, M.D.
Professor of Ophthalmology
College of Medicine and Dentistry of New Jersey,
  N.J. Medical School
Newark, New Jersey

Roger W. Countee, M.D.
Associate Professor of Neurosurgery
College of Medicine and Dentistry of New Jersey,
  N.J. Medical School
Newark, New Jersey

John A. Feagin, M.D.
Private Practice of Orthopedic Surgery
Jackson, Wyoming
Formerly Team Physician and
Professor of Military Hygiene
United States Military Academy
West Point, New York

William F. Grant, M.D.
Assistant Professor of Ophthalmology
College of Medicine and Dentistry of New Jersey,
  N.J. Medical School
Newark, New Jersey

Ralph W. Hale, M.D.
Professor of Obstetrics and Gynecology
University of Hawaii John A. Burns School of
  Medicine
Honolulu, Hawaii

Mervyn B. Haycock, M.S.
Head Football Coach
Bergan High School
Peoria, Illinois

Harry A. Kaplan, M.D.
Professor of Neurosurgery
College of Medicine and Dentistry of New Jersey,
  N.J. Medical School
Newark, New Jersey

Walter J. Kennedy, M.D.
Private Practice of Pediatrics
Yakima, Washington

Kristen J. Kuehnle, Ed.D.
Clinical Fellow in Psychiatry
Massachusetts General Hospital
Boston, Massachusetts

Arthur S. Leon, M.D.
Professor of Physiological Hygiene
University of Minnesota School of Public Health
Professor of Medicine
University of Minnesota School of Medicine
Minneapolis, Minnesota

Allan M. Levy, M.D.
Director of Sports Medicine
Pascack Valley Hospital
Westwood, New Jersey

John C. Loomis, D.D.S.
Private Practice of Dental Surgery
Orland, Maine

Meredith Melvin, M.Ed., A.T.C.
Research Assistant
Institute of Sports Medicine and Athletic Trauma
Lenox Hill Hospital
Athletic Trainer
New York City Ballet
New York, New York

Louis R. Munch, D.P.E.
Associate Professor of Health, Physical Education,
  and Recreation
Ithaca College
Ithaca, New York

Elizabeth D. Munves, Ph.D.
Professor of Medicine
College of Medicine and Dentistry of New Jersey,
 N.J. Medical School
Newark, New Jersey

Chester M. Pierce, M.D.
Professor of Education and Psychiatry
Harvard University
Cambridge, Massachusetts

Allen B. Richardson, M.D.
Chairman, Competitive Swimming
Sports Medicine Committee
Amateur Athletic Union
Private Practice of Orthopedic Surgery
Honolulu, Hawaii

Mona M. Shangold, M.D.
Assistant Professor of Obstetrics and Gynecology
The Albert Einstein College of Medicine
Bronx, New York

Gail Shierman, Ph.D.
Assistant Professor of Health, Physical Education,
 and Recreation
University of Oklahoma
Norman, Oklahoma

William F. Straub, Ph.D.
Professor of Health, Physical Education,
 and Recreation
Ithaca College
Ithaca, New York

Irving Strauchler, M.D.
Assistant Professor of Orthopedic Surgery
College of Medicine and Dentistry of New Jersey,
 N.J. Medical School
Newark, New Jersey

Steven I. Subotnick, D.P.M.
Associate Professor of Biomechanics and Surgery
California College of Podiatric Medicine
Professor of Kinesiology
California State University
Hayward, California

Joan Gillette Tannenbaum, M.A., A.T.C.
Certified Athletic Trainer
Las Vegas, Nevada

Melody E. Toth, A.T.C.
Certified Athletic Trainer
University of Hawaii
Honolulu, Hawaii

Andrew Weiss, M.D.
Professor of Orthopedic Surgery
College of Medicine and Dentistry of New Jersey,
 N.J. Medical School
Newark, New Jersey

Holly Wilson, M.S., A.T.C.
Assistant Athletic Trainer
University of Iowa
Iowa City, Iowa

Foreword

Walter J. Kennedy, M.D.

In the past 30 years, athletics for women has changed greatly. A comparison of present attitudes with those prevailing during the '40s toward physical activity for the growing female makes this evident. During the years immediately after World War II, only a handful of sports was available to the adolescent female. Today, she is encouraged to be physically active, and the opportunities provided her in organized sports have multiplied tremendously.

From 1970 to 1978, the number of females participating in interscholastic sports has increased more than seven times, according to a survey compiled by the National Federation of State High School Associations. In the school year of 1970-71, 294,000 participated in high-school sports. In 1977-78, there were 2,083,000 participants. During this same period, the number of interscholastic sports available to females increased from 14 to 27. In order of popularity, these sports are track and field, basketball, volleyball, softball, tennis, swimming, diving, gymnastics, field hockey, golf, and cross-country. Females also compete in archery, badminton, baseball, bowling, curling, drill team, fencing, ice hockey, lacrosse, the pentathlon, riflery, skiing, soccer, table tennis, water polo, and weight lifting.

The increasing emphasis on sports for school-age and adult women is partly due to recognition of a need for increased physical activity and exercise to compensate for changes in the character of work, whereby brain power and sedentary occupations have replaced muscle power. More precisely, it is a result of the passage of the Education Amendments Act of 1972, mandating equal opportunities and facilities for girls and boys in organized school sports, and the increasing awareness in girls and women of sports and recreation. This has probably been prompted in part by the television exposure given to successful women athletes.

Perhaps this broadening of the variety of sports available to both girls and boys on the interscholastic level and in the community represents a maturation. Although there continues to be considerable interest in traditional sports, new favorites have emerged. Many sports are highly competitive, but some of the newer ones have become popular purely for their recreational benefits and as an aid in maintaining physical fitness. A number of the new sports can be played jointly by women and men without the usual highly competitive atmosphere. Also, many of the activities—tennis, golf, recreational swimming, skiing, and bowling—can be enjoyed throughout life.

Nevertheless, adults and youngsters of both sexes continue to recognize the value of competition, and women still want to play strenuous contact sports. Because many of these carry a certain risk of injury, despite continuing efforts directed toward prevention, services of physicians and other members of the health-care team are required, as they always have been. Moreover, the recent surge of interest in all physical activity, in particular the increased emphasis on sports for the preadolescent and adolescent female, leads to many new challenges for the health professionals who care for these athletes. It also affords them many opportunities to provide more comprehensive health care, including both preventive and treatment aspects. Today, many girls are receiving much better medical care because of disorders that were discovered during the required preparticipation physical examination. Because of their new and active role in sports, women now seek out physicians for medical advice about nutrition, methods to improve athletic performance, and how to prevent sports injuries.

In this respect, then, sports medicine is not only a means of providing treatment for illnesses and injuries; it can also be a vehicle for delivering preventive health care and introducing good health practices to women athletes. We hope these practices will be continued throughout life.

Preface

It is only in the past decade that the medical profession has recognized sports medicine as a subspecialty. The number of publications in the field has grown within the past several years, yet no book devoted directly and specifically to the female athlete and the broad range of her medical problems has been available until now.

I hope that this text will fill the void, particularly for the family practitioner. And I hope that the coach, trainer, athletic director, and the athlete herself will also find the book a valuable asset.

I owe a debt of gratitude to each of the contributing authors whose efforts have made this book possible.

I also wish to extend thanks to my secretary, Gene Grayson, who helped me prepare the book; to my husband, an editor and publisher himself, who gave me technical advice; and to my colleagues who encouraged me. A special word of thanks is due to Dr. Walter Kennedy, a fellow member of the A.M.A. Ad Hoc Committee on Sports Medicine, for his Foreword.

Christine E. Haycock, M.D.

Publisher's Notes

Christine E. Haycock, M.D., is associate professor of surgery at the College of Medicine and Dentistry of New Jersey, New Jersey Medical School, and a registered nurse. Also an athlete, Dr. Haycock has fenced competitively. In 1949-50, she was New Jersey State fencing champion, and for 30 years has pitched softball.

Dr. Haycock has written articles on sports medicine for many periodicals including *Women Coach, Jogger, American Medical Woman's Association Journal*, and the *Journal of the American Medical Association*. She and Dr. Gail Shierman, one of the contributors to this book, are the authors of *Total Woman's Fitness Guide* (World Publications, 1979).

FAMOUS
WOMEN
IN
SPORTS

Joan Gillette Tannenbaum, M.A., A.T.C.

CHAPTER

1

H istorians tell us that women participated in sports more than a millennium and a half before the Christian era. In ancient Sparta, women were given the opportunity of learning gymnastics, calisthenics, and competitive games. Eventually, however, the popularity of this co-ed Spartan doctrine waned, and by the time of the Golden Age of Greece, women were not allowed to attend Olympic events.

Not until 1896 was the first modern Olympiad held, thanks to Baron Pierre de Coubertin's efforts and the founding of the International Olympic Committee. But women's participation was minimal. The 1948 Olympic games had 385 female participants; in 1952 there were more than 500 in Helsinki. From 1972 on, the total of women competing reached capacity.

Changing times and mores allowed women to enter the male-dominated world of sports more easily. But at the turn of the century, women still had to turn their backs on society if they wanted to become great athletes. They had to be filled with a kind of missionary zeal.

Annie Oakley, for example, was 8 years old when she offered shooting competitions at a country store. When she was 15, she beat Frank Butler, a recognized champion shot. They subsequently married and joined Buffalo Bill's Wild West Show. Annie Oakley became a household name during 17 years of touring as the show's featured attraction.

Illnesses and accidents took her out of the limelight from time to time. Nevertheless, at the age of 65, she scored 97 out of 100 targets at the 1925 Grand American shooting competition. Perhaps she's best remembered for her trick shots: blasting the center spot out of a five of spades as it fell from a flagpole, splitting a playing card held edgewise from 50 paces, shooting balls out of the air while lying on the back of a galloping pony.

Other women have made their athletic marks:

• Beatrix Hoyt who, in 1896 at the tender age of 16, won the second U.S. Golf Association women's amateur tournament, the youngest player ever to win it.

• Eleanora Sears, born in 1881, who was the first woman to race a car, fly an airplane, swim the 4½ miles along Newport Shore; who wore untraditional and "shocking" attire for swimming, sailing, figure skating, squash, and tennis; who, in her 40s, took up long-distance walking and completed the 73 miles from Newport to Boston in 17 hours.

• Marion Hollins, golf champion in 1921, first woman to enter an automobile in the Vanderbilt Cup Road Races on Long Island.

• Helen Wills, known as "Little Miss Poker Face," who won eight Wimbledon singles championships between 1927 and 1938, and played on 10 U.S. Wightman Cup teams.

• Gertrude Ederle, an Olympic gold medalist, who in 1926 swam the 26-mile English Channel in 14 hours and 31 minutes.

• Helen Hull Jacobs, who challenged Helen Wills, eventually capturing the Wimbledon crown in 1936, and who is known to this day as "Helen the Second" or the most famous runner-up in the history of tennis.

• Eleanor Holm, who made her Olympic debut at the age of 14 with a fifth-place finish in the 100-meter backstroke, won a gold medal in the 1932 Olympics, and held national swimming titles more than a dozen times.

Babe Didrikson deserves very special mention. She was the Associated Press's Woman Athlete of the Year in 1932, 1945, 1946, 1947, 1950, and 1954. She had a spectacular career as a basketball star, an Olympic gold medalist in track and field, and a champion in amateur and professional golf.

Although she won Olympic gold medals in 1932 for the javelin throw and the 80-meter hurdles, her final high jump, which could have been a record, was voided because of her jumping style. To assuage her disappointment, Grantland Rice, the famous sportswriter, invited Babe to golf with him. In that game, Babe hit several 250-yard drives and finished with a score under 100—a respectable showing for someone who had previously played little golf. A story began to circulate that she had never played a complete round of golf before this game, but this was a myth that Babe later denied.

After two years of professional basketball, tennis, and baseball (she was the only woman on the House of David baseball team), she decided to concentrate on golf. The public's desire to see this athletic marvel was satisfied once more when she joined pro golfer Gene Sarazen for a series of exhibition matches. In 1938, when she was 23, she entered the Los Angeles Open in which women rarely competed. She won the American Women's Amateur golf title in 1946 and 1950, the 1947 British Women's Amateur golf title—a first for an American—and the 1948 National Open. Over the 1946 and 1947 seasons, she set an all-time record by winning 17 straight golf championships.

In 1953, Babe discovered she had cancer. Yet, 3½ months after surgery, with the support of her husband, wrestler George Zaharias, she was competing once more. She was awarded the Ben Hogan Trophy for the greatest comeback of the year and also won the 1954 U.S. Women's Open and the All-American Open. Her cancer recurred, and she died in 1956. Her greatest tribute is that she'll always be considered American's finest woman athlete of the first half of the 20th century.

Patty Berg reached the finals of the national amateur golf tournament at the age of 17. By 1938, she had eclipsed women stars of the '30s. Called the best woman golfer in history, she also was named Woman Athlete of the Year in three different decades—in 1938, 1943, and 1955. She founded the Ladies' Professional Golf Association in 1948 and became, in 1972, one of the 13 charter members in the golf hall of fame. Eleven are men.

Florence Chadwick lived by the motto, "Winners never quit, quitters never win." Her goal was to swim the English Channel. She did it in 1950, beating Gertrude Ederle's time by one hour, 11 minutes. But her next goal was to reverse the trip, going from England to France against tides and winds. She did that, too.

After 16 hours and 22 minutes, Florence climbed out of the water to shake hands with the mayor of Songatte, France.

Dot Wilkinson was to softball what Babe Didrikson was to golf. As members of the Phoenix (Arizona) Ramblers softball team, Dot and her friends became, in 1938, the first American women's club to play in Madison Square Garden. They won world championships in 1940, 1948, and 1949.

In 1950, Althea Gibson became the first black athlete to compete in the Forest Hills tennis championship. She was eventually to become the Jackie Robinson of tennis. Despite setbacks and the color barrier that still existed, Althea earned recognition and won the Wimbledon and the National Clay Court Championships.

Denise McCluggage opened doors for women. As the first female sports reporter for the *San Francisco Chronicle* and *New York Herald Tribune,* she was thrown out of press boxes long before anyone thought it was against the Constitution. More than that, she was the first reporter to become a genuine contender in a sport she covered—car racing.

Maureen Connolly made headlines by being the youngest woman (14) to win the National Junior title in tennis, the youngest winner of the Women's National Tennis Championship in nearly 50 years, and the youngest member of the U.S. Wightman Cup team. In 1953, she became the first—and still only—woman to score a grand slam: the Australian, French, British, and U.S. titles in one year.

Tenley Albright, the daughter of a Boston surgeon, won a silver medal as a member of the 1952 U.S. Olympic skating team. A year later, she took the world crown in Switzerland—an American first. Because of college study pressures, she lost her crown in 1954. That stirred her competitive spirit and, in 1956, she became the first American woman to win an Olympic gold medal in figure skating. She's now a successful surgeon, wife, home manager, and member of the Olympic committee for figure skating.

The athletic achievements of Wilma Rudolph are especially remarkable in light of the poor health and physical handicaps that dominated her early life. She had partial paralysis of the left leg but was able to walk—with a limp. Ignoring the heavy orthopedic shoe the doctors provided, she began to play basketball with her brothers. By the age of 11, she threw her special shoe away. Within a few years, she became an all-state basketball player, breaking the Tennessee State High School record by scoring 803 points in 25 games. Wilma started her track career in 1955 and won a bronze medal at the 1956 Olympics. Her performance at the Rome Olympics won her the title of "world's fastest woman." In 1960, she was tops in the United Press Athlete of the Year sports poll and named Associated Press Athlete of the Year, an honor she received also in 1961. She was the third woman in history to receive the A.A.U.'s James E. Sullivan Memorial Trophy.

Billie Jean King knew when she was 16 that she wanted to be a tennis champ. With Alice Marble as her coach, Billie Jean managed to raise her 19th-place rating to fourth, in six months. She established her reputation in 1962 at the age of 18 by beating top-seeded Margaret Court Smith in the second round of the Wimbledon Championships. Billie Jean turned pro in 1968. Among her titles are numerous Wimbledons, U.S. singles, and other tournament wins all over the world. Two of her awards are Associated Press Athlete of the Year and Woman Athlete of the Year.

One of her most significant achievements was to lead the fight against sexism in tennis. The unforgettable match between her and Bobby Riggs helped give women the recognition they deserve.

The fawnlike Peggy Fleming symbolizes the grace and beauty of the world of figure skating. In 1964, she won the first of her five national championships. In 1966, 1967, and 1968, she captured the World Ladies' Title and in 1968 an Olympic gold medal, as well. She's a pro today, skating with the Ice Follies and on TV specials.

Christine Marie Evert was nationally ranked in tennis at the age of 15 and soon became the darling of the galleries. Her victories are impressive: winner at Wimbledon, Forest Hills, France, South Africa, Canada, Italy, and elsewhere on the women's professional tour. She broke the record for earnings in a single season by a woman and topped all women players in the 1974 and 1975 seasons. She was elected Associated Press Athlete of the Year and Woman Athlete of the Year.

The champions of yesterday played for fun, adventure, and competition. Today's champions play for those reasons and for money as well. They have made a way of life for themselves and for the women who choose to follow them.

PSYCHOLOGY OF THE ATHLETE

William F. Straub, Ph.D.

CHAPTER

2

Although much has been said about the physical aspects of women's participation in sport, the psychology of the female athlete has been largely ignored. Therefore, women often fail to understand the diverse psychological factors that influence their athletic involvement. Usually, increased knowledge brings improved performance and greater personal satisfaction.

Personality of the female athlete

Since the early 1960s, when the modern era of sport psychology began, there have been many studies of the personality characteristics of male athletes. Few studies, however, have been completed on female performers. In his review of this limited literature, John Kane, British sport psychologist, found support for the generalization that women athletes are lower in dominance and confidence than men, and higher in impulsiveness, tension, and general anxiety.[1] The fact that women, until recently, have had limited opportunities to participate in interscholastic and intercollegiate sports may be responsible, in part, for these sex differences. Margaret Mead believed that feminine and masculine roles and their associated personality and character are more a product of culture than of biology.

Jean Williams agreed, pointing out that American culture has traditionally advocated that females be nonaggressive, passive, dependent, and social, rather than achievement-oriented.[2] It is Williams's belief that sex-role stereotyping strongly influences women's participation or lack of participation in sport.

I feel that male/female differences in personality result from an interaction of genetic and environmental forces. Although the environment may have a profound effect on behavior, genetic factors serve as a blueprint for personality development.

However, personality differences do not suggest that either sex should not participate in sport. They do indicate that sport involvement may serve different purposes for men and women. It is commonly known, for example, that males are more concerned with the competitive aspect of winning, whereas females participate because they enjoy interacting and socializing with other players.[3] Because success is more important for men, it has greater effect on their concept of self.

Knowing oneself

One of the most important and neglected personality fundamentals is knowing oneself. Gaining insight into one's personal make-up may lead to better interpersonal relations, improved performance, and improved concept of self. For coaches, knowing the athlete is the first step in coaching her successfully. But how do you acquire this information? And more important, how do you utilize it to good advantage? These are difficult questions.

Knowledge of one's personality may be acquired in a number of ways. During the 1960s, for example, paper-and-pencil tests were used by coaches to assess the personality traits of their players. Although this method has been criticized, it does, in a general way, provide useful information. If the athlete is sincere and honest in her responses, tests such as the Sixteen Personality Factor Test, the Minnesota Multiphasic Personality Inventory, and the California Psychological Inventory reveal broad measures of personality—dominance, extroversion, introversion, and the like. It is, of course, necessary to have these tests administered, scored, and interpreted by qualified persons.

Another source of information is feedback from parents, friends, and teachers. This information helps us formulate an impression of ourselves and shapes our overt and covert behavior. From the way people interact with us, we obtain a good idea of how well they accept us. If people give us the cold shoulder, we become aware that there is something about us that they don't like. Then, if we wish to be accepted, we must change our behavior. Or, if we are not in agreement with the other person's values and life-style, we may choose to continue as we are. After all, few persons are accepted by everyone.

Behaviorist B.F. Skinner contends that people are different in different places and probably because of those places. Skinner points out the role that the environment plays in shaping our behavior. He would say that the athlete learns to behave in many different ways, depending on situational factors. Thus, there are in-church, in-classroom, at-home, with-peers, on-field, and other situation-specific personalities. On the other hand, trait theorists such as R.B. Cattell believe that behavior is stable across the board. For example, Cattell would say that an aggressive person is aggressive in everything.

Personality may influence not only the kind of sports we want to play—distance runners, for example, tend to be introverted—but

FIGURE 2-1

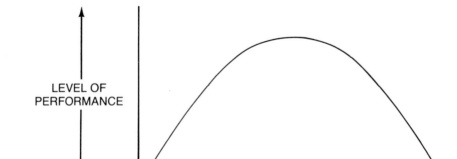

Diagrammatic presentation of Yerkes-Dodson law regarding the relationship between performance and arousal.

also the position we play within a team. Baseball and softball coaches, for instance, usually select as catchers players who are extroverted. They contend that the catcher's position takes advantage of their inclination to take charge and stimulate the team to play well. Introverted players generally play outfield positions that require less interactions with teammates.

Thus, personality may be thought of as the individual's most striking or dominant characteristic or trait.[4] And although there is no universal definition, personality is often equated with the ability to elicit positive reactions from other people. Allport presented a more formal definition when he called personality "the dynamic organization within the individual of those psychophysical systems that determine his characteristic behavior and thought."[5]

Motivation and performance

One of the most important and interesting aspects of the psychology of sport is the motivation of the individual athlete and team. Because performance is a function of skill plus motivation, even the very talented athlete does not play well if she isn't motivated.

Motivation has a direct relationship to one's level of arousal or activation. The Yerkes-Dodson law, formulated in the early 1920s, states that there is an inverted-U relationship between arousal and performance (see Figure 2-1). That is, as arousal or level of excitation increases, so does performance—until a person becomes too highly aroused, when performance deteriorates. The modern interpretation of this law is that it is task- and individual-athlete specific. That is, there appears to be an optimum level of arousal for each task as well as for each athlete. Thus, putting in golf requires a lower level of excitation than does defensive line play in football. Additionally, each athlete must find the level of activation that is best for her. Some players apparently play better at low levels of activation, whereas others function better at high levels. The implication is that the coach must help players find the point on the activation-deactivation continuum that is best for each of them. Reaching this point each time she takes the field will help the athlete to play well.

What is the source of this activation or arousal? Butt suggests that the first source of motivation is biological in nature (see Figure 2-2).[6] That is, drawing from Freud's psychodynamic theory, Butt proposes that libido or the life instinct provides the energy for human movement. The energy source, derived from the id, manifests itself in aggression, neurotic conflict, and competency motives. Butt presents excellent examples of athletes who played sport primarily to satisfy these three drives.

The second source of motivation, Butt suggests, comes from rewards found in the environment. These rewards may be internal or external—jogging may give participants an elated sense of body awareness, whereas crowd approval may provide reinforcement for players who participate primarily to achieve recognition and

FIGURE 2-2

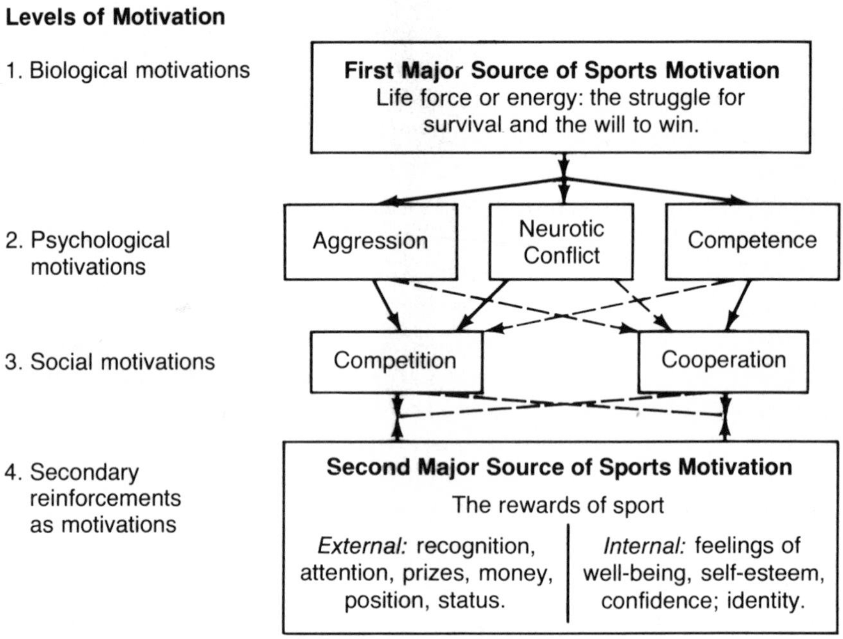

Levels of Motivation

1. Biological motivations

2. Psychological motivations

3. Social motivations

4. Secondary reinforcements as motivations

Butt's model of athletic motivation. (From *Psychology of Sport* by Dorcas Susan Butt © 1976 by Litton Educational Publishing Inc. Reprinted by permission of Van Nostrand Reinhold Company.)

prestige. Although players may at first be attracted to sport because of the extrinsic rewards, Butt contends that those who participate for long periods of time do so for intrinsic reasons.

Aggression in sport

Although aggression in its strict psychological definition (the intent to inflict harm on another individual) is not usually applied to women in sport, it has become of great concern in men's athletics, particularly at professional levels of competition. Winning at all costs too often characterizes sport involvement from Little League to professional levels, and humanistic approaches to sport have been talked about but seldom implemented.

George Sage provided a framework for a humanistic psychology of sport.[7] One of the first tenets, Sage contends, is to reject the traditional sex-role stereotypes and regard sport as being neither a masculine nor feminine activity. Sport involvement, according to the human-potential movement, is an effective way to achieve self-actualization.

Finn reported on the perception of violence among women exposed to sport films.[8] The 120 women, aged 17 to 22 years, were undergraduates at Springfield College. Following the administration of the Buss-Durkee Inventory of Hostility, the women were divided into high-hostile and low-hostile groups. Four subgroups were formed to produce 30 high-hostile athletes, 30 low-hostile athletes, 30 high-hostile nonathletes, and 30 low-hostile nonathletes. The subgroups were then randomly divided and assigned to view a violent or nonviolent sport film. A binocular rivalry technique was used to determine perception-of-violence scores for each subject.

Finn found no difference in perception of violence among athletic and nonathletic subjects. Thus, from the data she collected, it doesn't appear that sport participation by women affects their perception of violence.

Konrad Lorenz, the Nobel prizewinning ethologist, is of the opinion that aggression is innate and may be reduced through participation in vigorous physical activity.[9] There is, however, little evidence to support this view. Lorenz's beliefs are obviously linked to Freud's conceptualization of a buildup of libido that may be released in undesirable ways if other, more appropriate outlets are not found.

One of the more popular conceptualizations of aggression is found in the belief that frustration leads to aggression, a view expressed in the 1920s. A more recent interpretation is that frustration does not always lead to aggression. The person who is frustrated may not express her aggression if there are powerful objects within the environment that are opposed to it.

Behavior modification

In behavior modification, sport psychologists determine the baseline rate at which a particular behavior is occurring and then develop intervention procedures designed to alter that behavior. For example, a player may be having difficulty making free-throw shots in pressure-packed road basketball games. Let's say that she is shooting 55 per cent on the road and 75 per cent at home. After observing this player during several games at home and away, the sport psychologist postulates that the primary reason for her poor free-throw shooting during road games is the hostile reactions of the opposing team's fans. Therefore, an intervention program is designed to try and alter her road-game free-throw shooting behavior. Attention-control training (ACT) may be used to teach the player to block out external stimuli. Robert Nideffer's ACT program and his Test of Attentional and Interpersonal Style may be used for this purpose.[10] At the end of several weeks, the player's free-throw shooting average for road games will again be calculated to see if there is significant improvement. If not, the intervention procedures will have to be altered.

Although behavior modification has been used in a wide variety of clinical and educational settings, its application to sport has not been fully explored.

Maximizing and improving performance

One of the tasks of sport psychologists is helping athletes maximize and improve their performances. In Europe, sport psychologists, biomechanics of sport persons, sport physiologists, and other professionals are working with coaches to bring about better performances. Abroad, blood analyses play a large part in management of national and world-class athletes. It appears that these blood samples do afford quite good predictions of performance in sports such as swimming.

One of the more important variables influencing performance is knowledge of results, or what is commonly called feedback. Following practice and games, athletes should be given information about the good and bad aspects of their play. The use of film, videotape, and other devices to record observations is essential if observations are to be objective. Each player should sit down with her coach and carefully review the film. Practice plans should then be formulated to help each player perfect the plays that were executed poorly. Game statistics should be kept and presented to the athlete to reinforce various aspects of her play.

Butt, a former Canadian tennis champion and a clinical psychologist, has written about some of the misconceptions concerned with maximizing performance.[6] The first misconception is that minor changes in equipment will alter the level of performance. A steel racquet or high-quality pair of sneakers, for example, may improve play, but once equipment reaches a certain quality level, minor changes have little effect. Skill is what counts.

Another misconception is that lessons bring vast improvement in performance. Butt suggests that lessons usually impart only the rudiments of technique, and that timing, coordination, and skill are produced only by practice.

Morehouse and Gross list four basic principles for learning a new skill.[11] First, the athlete should have a clear and vivid image of what she is going to do. If this image is faulty, she won't improve her game. In softball, for example, if the batter pictures the perfect swing as an upper-cut action, she will probably hit a lot of fly balls, but she won't bat for a high percentage. Second, Morehouse and Gross believe that the athlete must determine how far her present skills can take her. This principle implies that new skills should be built on existing skills. Third, skills should be divided into their component parts—the athlete should start with components already mastered. For example, she should learn the correct toss in tennis before the entire service is practiced. Fourth, the speed at which the movement is practiced should gradually approach the speed of execution required in games.

Practice does not necessarily make perfect. It won't help if the athlete practices a movement incorrectly. What really matters is how well she practices, not how much.

Team cohesiveness

Team cohesiveness refers to the amount of interpersonal attraction among members of sport teams. Although studies of team cohesiveness have produced conflicting findings, it is generally agreed that winning teams tend to be more cohesive than losing ones. My own work suggests that cohesiveness is a prerequisite for success in sports such as basketball and football.[12] In her review of the literature, Diane Gill called the data equivocal.[13] Some studies indicate that team cohesiveness is directly linked to the number of games won, whereas other investigations don't support this generalization.

In a classic study, Hans Lenk found that the German Rowing Eight of 1960 were able to become unbeaten Olympic champions despite sharp subgroup and leadership conflicts.[14] Lenk's work and the studies of others have led to the belief that cohesiveness is sport-specific—important in some sports but not in others.

Most of the studies of team cohesiveness have been done on men's teams. Behavioral observations of women's teams show that championship squads are usually very cohesive. I saw considerable peer reinforcement among members of a champion women's lacrosse team. When I asked the coach how she developed such great rapport she said: "It just happens, we don't really work at it." As with men's teams, however, jealousy and conflict can arise among women players and coaches. Unfortunately, it usually destroys team unity and performances suffer.

Although myths and stereotypes abound, sports involvement for women will increase. Not only will women use sport as a medium for self-expression, but they will experience improved physical and psychological health as a result of their play.

References

1. Kane JE: Psychological aspects of sport with special reference to the female. In *Women and Sport: A National Research Conference* (Harris DV, ed). University Park, Pa: College of Health, Physical Education, and Recreation, 1972

2. Williams JM: Personality characteristics of the successful female athlete. In *Sport Psychology: An Analysis of Athlete Behavior* (Straub WF, ed). Ithaca, NY: Mouvement Publications, 1978

3. Reis HT and Jelsma B: A social psychology of sex differences in sport. In *Sport Psychology: An Analysis of Athlete Behavior* (Straub WF, ed). Ithaca, NY: Mouvement Publications, 1978

4. Mischel W: *Introduction to Personality,* 2nd ed. New York: Holt, Rinehart and Winston, 1976

5. Allport GW: *Pattern and Growth in Personality.* New York: Holt, Rinehart and Winston, 1961

6. Butt DS: *Psychology of Sport.* New York: Van Nostrand Reinhold, 1976

7. Sage GH: Humanistic psychology and coaching. In *Sport Psychology: An Analysis of Athlete Behavior* (Straub WF, ed). Ithaca, NY: Mouvement Publications, 1978

8. Finn JA: Perception of violence among high-hostile and low-hostile women athletes and nonathletes before and after exposure to sport films. Doctoral dissertation, Springfield College, 1976

9. Lorenz K: *On Aggression.* New York: Harcourt, Brace & World, 1963

10. Nideffer RM: *Test of Attentional and Interpersonal Style.* Rochester, NY: Behavioral Research Applications Group, 1977

11. Morehouse LE and Gross L: *Maximum Performance.* New York: Simon and Schuster, 1977

12. Straub WF: Team cohesion in athletics. *Int J Sport Psych* 6:125, 1975

13. Gill DL: Cohesiveness and performance in sport groups. In *Exercise and Sport Sciences Reviews* (Hutton RS, ed). Santa Barbara: Journal Publishing Affiliates, 1977

14. Lenk H: Top performance despite internal conflict: An antithesis to a functionalistic proposition. In *Sport, Culture, and Society* (Loy JW Jr and Kenyon GS, eds). New York: Macmillan, 1969

HISTORY AND PHYSICAL EXAMINATION OF THE ADULT ATHLETE

**Ralph W. Hale, M.D., and
Melody E. Toth, A.T.C.**

CHAPTER

3

T he history and physical examination not only give the woman athlete information about her body limits and capacities, but also alert the physician and trainer to problems that may occur during the competitive season. This is important even though the woman may be only casually involved in sport—the weekend runner, for example. If muscular or ligamentous weaknesses in the body are identified, the physician/trainer can immediately begin a rehabilitative conditioning program designed to eliminate or, at least, mitigate the problem, thus decreasing the chance of injury.

The examination should include a complete evaluation of physical status with special emphasis on the body areas that are directly related to the specific sport in which she will be engaged. For example, a breast-stroke swimmer should have her knees carefully examined, and a tennis player should have her shoulder and elbow evaluated. However, the examination should never be restricted to the area involved in the sport.

Probably the most important laboratory tests for the female athlete are the hemoglobin and hematocrit. These determine if the athlete is receiving enough iron to meet her daily demands. Highly specific tests should be ordered only for definite reasons. Testing can be extremely valuable in the presence of problems, but the yield is low in the case of a healthy individual when testing is used for a general survey.

Taking the history

In our experience, taking a history from an athlete can best be accomplished by use of questionnaires. This method reduces the time it takes and can also prevent omission of key items. A sample of a simple one-page questionnaire is shown in Figure 3-1—it is not intended to be complete nor is it designed to go into great detail. The form should be filled out prior to the examination, and any positive items should be discussed by the physician/trainer at the time of the examination.

In addition to the general health form, we ask the athlete to complete a sports questionnaire. This form, shown in Figure 3-2, asks specific questions about athletic injuries, illnesses, or problems that are related to or affected by athletic participation. Here again, the trainer or physician should inquire in detail about any positive answers. These two forms allow gathering of all pertinent information with a minimum of time and effort. The history-taking process may need to be modified according to the age of the athlete, the level of performance, and the type of sport. No questionnaire can take into account all of the eventualities. For this reason, the interviewer should modify as necessary to obtain the desired information.

The physical examination

The female athlete should always have a complete physical examination. Variations in the examination depend upon factors such as the age of the patient and the type of sport. Athletes who have a history of trauma, injury, or other problems require a more complete evaluation of these areas. Specific evaluations are explained in detail in succeeding chapters. Here, we concentrate upon those aspects of the physical examination that should be common to all athletes.

A physical examination form that has been devised for us is most helpful in the completion of the examination (see Figure 3-3). We have adapted this form so that we can visualize a number of years at one time and, we hope, note any changes over the period.

General: Each athlete should have height, weight, blood pressure (sitting), and pulse recorded at the time she reports for ex-

FIGURE 3-1

Health Questionnaire

PLEASE PRINT

Date _____

NAME _____

           LAST   FIRST   MIDDLE/MAIDEN

AGE _____ Occupation _____

Marital Status   S   M   W   D   Sep   Remarried

MENSTRUATION:

Started at age: _____ Number of days from start of one period to start of next period _____

Number of days period lasts _____ Date of last normal menstrual period (1st day) _____

OBSTETRIC HISTORY:

How often have you been pregnant? _____ How many full-term babies? _____ Stillborns? _____

Prematures? _____ Miscarriages? _____ Abortions? _____ Operations? _____

Ages of Children _____

PLEASE CHECK BOX AFTER THE
FOLLOWING QUESTIONS

	YES	NO		YES	NO
Are your periods irregular?	☐	☐	Are you constipated?	☐	☐
Are they painful?	☐	☐	Do you often have diarrhea?	☐	☐
Do you pass clots with them?	☐	☐	Ever pass blood in the stools?	☐	☐
Do you bleed between periods?	☐	☐	Ever have black stools?	☐	☐
Do you bleed after douching or sexual relations?	☐	☐	Have painful bowel movements?	☐	☐
Do you get tense before periods?	☐	☐	Have you gained or lost weight?	☐	☐
Do you have any symptoms of pregnancy?	☐	☐	Is your appetite poor?	☐	☐
Are sexual relations uncomfortable?	☐	☐	Is your diet poor?	☐	☐
Are you troubled with a discharge (other than bloody)?	☐	☐	Do you vomit?	☐	☐
Does it itch or irritate?	☐	☐	Smoke more than a pack a day?	☐	☐
Have you ever had any other female trouble?	☐	☐	Do you use any contraception? (I.U.D., Pills, Other)	☐	☐
Do you urinate too often?	☐	☐	Do your ankles swell?	☐	☐
Do you get up at night to urinate?	☐	☐	Do you have varicose veins?	☐	☐
Do you have to go "right now"?	☐	☐	Do you get short of breath?	☐	☐
Do you pass blood in the urine?	☐	☐	Do you faint easily?	☐	☐
Do you lose urine when you cough or laugh?	☐	☐	Do you get headaches?	☐	☐
Does it feel like anything is pushing out of your vagina?	☐	☐	Do you get hot flashes?	☐	☐
Do you have to push anything up to empty the bowels or bladder?	☐	☐	Do you sleep poorly?	☐	☐
			Do you wake up tired?	☐	☐
			Do you cry easily?	☐	☐
			Have you ever been treated for nerves?	☐	☐
			Have you had any serious injuries?	☐	☐
			Any blood transfusions?	☐	☐

List and date hospitalizations and operations (other than deliveries)

_____

List any allergies _____

Check any of these you have had:

☐ Allergies	☐ Convulsions	☐ High Blood Pressure	☐ Lung Trouble
☐ Anemia	☐ Diabetes	☐ Jaundice	☐ TB
☐ Arthritis	☐ German Measles	☐ Kidney Trouble	☐ VD
☐ Cancer	☐ Heart Trouble		

Check any of the following occurring in your family:

☐ Twins	☐ Cancer	☐ High Blood Pressure	☐ Strokes
☐ Birth Defects	☐ Diabetes	☐ Bleeding Tendency	☐ TB
☐ Heart Trouble		☐ Lung Disease	

FIGURE 3-2

Sports Questionnaire

(Please circle your answer. If yes, please list below under Explanation.)

1. Have you ever had any illness, condition, or injury that:
   a. Required you to be hospitalized overnight? — Yes   No
   b. Required you to go to an emergency room or physician's office for X-rays? — Yes   No
   c. Caused you to miss practice or competition? — Yes   No
   d. Required a minor operation? — Yes   No

2. Have you ever "passed out"? — Yes   No

3. Have you ever been "knocked out"? — Yes   No
   a. Have you been told you had a concussion? — Yes   No

4. Have you had any injury to the spine, neck, or back that incapacitated you for one or more days? — Yes   No

5. Have you ever had a broken bone or fracture or a dislocated joint? — Yes   No
   a. Have you injured a ligament or cartilage? — Yes   No

6. Have you ever had a severe strain, sprain, or muscle injury? — Yes   No

7. Have you ever had an injury to any nerve or part of the nervous system? — Yes   No

8. Do you have any dental plates, partial or complete, or bridges? — Yes   No

9. Have you had a vision check in the last year? — Yes   No
   a. Do you wear glasses? — Yes   No
   b. Do you wear contacts? — Yes   No

10. Have you ever been told you had:
    a. Rheumatic fever, scarlet fever, or heart murmur? — Yes   No
    b. Infectious mononucleosis? — Yes   No
    c. Asthma or lung disease? — Yes   No
    d. Epilepsy? — Yes   No
    e. Liver disease or hepatitis? — Yes   No
    f. Diabetes? — Yes   No
    g. Anemia or blood disease? — Yes   No
    h. Arthritis? — Yes   No
    i. Bladder or kidney infection? — Yes   No
    j. Allergy, hay fever, or sinus problems? — Yes   No

11. Are you currently taking any pills, shots, or other medications (include those you buy from the drug store without a prescription)? — Yes   No
    If yes, please list: _____
    _____
    _____
    _____

12. Are you allergic to any drug or medication, including nonprescription items? — Yes   No
    If yes, please list: _____
    _____
    _____

13. Have you ever been told not to participate in any sport? — Yes   No

Item #   Explanation

____   _____
____   _____
____   _____
____   _____
____   _____
____   _____
____   _____
____   _____

FIGURE 3-3

Health Examination Form
(To be completed by examining physician)

			Check if Positive
			1 2 3 4

Height   1_____ 2_____   3_____ 4_____   ☐ ☐ ☐ ☐

Weight   1_____ 2_____   3_____ 4_____   ☐ ☐ ☐ ☐

BP (sitting)   __/__   __/__   __/__   __/__   ☐ ☐ ☐ ☐

Vision   L 20/___ L 20/___   L 20/___ L 20/___   ☐ ☐ ☐ ☐
        R 20/___ R 20/___   R 20/___ R 20/___   ☐ ☐ ☐ ☐

Eyes/Ears   1_____   3_____
        2_____   4_____   ☐ ☐ ☐ ☐

Mouth/Nose/   1_____   3_____
Throat   2_____   4_____   ☐ ☐ ☐ ☐

Skin   1_____   3_____
    2_____   4_____   ☐ ☐ ☐ ☐

Chest/   1_____   3_____
Breast/Ribs   2_____   4_____   ☐ ☐ ☐ ☐

Heart   1_____   3_____
     2_____   4_____   ☐ ☐ ☐ ☐

Lungs   1_____   3_____
     2_____   4_____   ☐ ☐ ☐ ☐

Lymphatics:
Cervical   1_____   3_____
Axillary   2_____   4_____   ☐ ☐ ☐ ☐
Inguinal

Abdominal   1_____   3_____
Organs   2_____   4_____   ☐ ☐ ☐ ☐

Pelvic   1_____   3_____
Genitalia   2_____   4_____   ☐ ☐ ☐ ☐

Urinalysis   1_____   3_____
         2_____   4_____   ☐ ☐ ☐ ☐

Blood   1_____   3_____
     2_____   4_____   ☐ ☐ ☐ ☐

Other   1_____   3_____
     2_____   4_____   ☐ ☐ ☐ ☐

Orthopedic Evaluation/Neurological
(To be completed by examining physician)

**Check if
Positive**
1 2 3 4

Cervical Spine/Back	1 _____ 2 _____ 3 _____ 4 _____	☐ ☐ ☐ ☐
Shoulders	1 _____ 2 _____ 3 _____ 4 _____	☐ ☐ ☐ ☐
Arm/Elbow Wrist/Hand	1 _____ 2 _____ 3 _____ 4 _____	☐ ☐ ☐ ☐
Knees	1 _____ 2 _____ 3 _____ 4 _____	☐ ☐ ☐ ☐
Ankles/Feet	1 _____ 2 _____ 3 _____ 4 _____	☐ ☐ ☐ ☐

Disposition

No Participation _____ _____ _____ _____
Requires _____ _____ _____ _____
Full Participation _____ _____ _____ _____
Signed 1 _____ MD 3 _____ MD
  2 _____ MD 4 _____ MD

The numbers 1 to 4 refer to years of eligibility.

amination. Temperature reading is optional; it has been found to be of little value in most examinations.

Skin: A visual inspection of the skin should be made throughout the examination. Specific areas of concern include pustules, scars, dermatitis including athlete's foot, and other defects.

Eyes: A standard vision test should be performed, including an evaluation of color discrimination. Pupil equality and reaction should be noted.

Ears: Careful examination of the ear canal and status of the tympanic membrane is necessary. Hearing acuity should be noted. Some physicians recommend a periodic audiometric exam, but as a routine this has not been very valuable.

Mouth, nose, and throat: Examination should include the nasal septum and any deviations, dental hygiene, missing or damaged teeth, dental prosthesis, and any abnormality of the oropharynx, including congenital anomalies of the palate.

Chest and lungs: Examination should include evaluation of symmetry and expansion as well as auscultation for abnormal sounds. Rib structure and any abnormality, especially of the sternoclavicular joint, should be noted.

Breast: Careful palpation of the breasts is necessary. It is also important to inquire about—and if necessary, teach—breast self-examination.

Heart: Cardiac examination should specifically include rhythm and murmurs. Any positive findings must be charted. Peripheral pulses in the wrist and groin should be noted and any abnormality recorded.

Abdomen: Examination of the abdomen should include evaluation of the liver and spleen for enlargement and palpation for areas of tenderness or masses. A careful palpation of the groin should also be included, and any lymphadenopathy recorded.

Pelvis/genitalia: Most physicians consider the pelvic examination to be optional. However, any sexually active female or female over the age of 20 who has not had a pelvic examination within the previous year should have one performed at the time of the physical examination. Specific attention should be paid to the presence or absence of hemorrhoids, vaginal vault relaxation, or cervical prolapse. Rectal exam confirms the extent of hemorrhoids and any other abnormalities that might be present.

Orthopedic evaluation

This evaluation should be performed on all athletes and should be performed in a careful, systematic fashion to avoid missing any defects. Problems should be thoroughly investigated. In our experience, the simplest and most complete method of performing this examination is to have the athlete stand or sit facing the examiner and perform a variety of motions utilizing the extremities and joints. Following this, a specific evaluation is performed of each general area. Our method is as follows:

Cervical spine: The athlete stands or sits and is instructed to flex and extend the neck; this is followed by rotation to look over each shoulder and then to try to place each ear on the shoulder.

Shoulder: The athlete is instructed to shrug the shoulders against counterresistance; extend the arms and rotate internally and externally; bring the hands in front and as far posterior as possible; flex and extend the elbows; pronate and supinate the wrists; and open and close the fist. The evaluation of the shoulder, elbow, wrist, and fingers is then repeated passively by the examiner to specifically look for restricted or limited motion, crepitation, or deformity. Should weakness be suspected, the examiner applies downward resistance on the arms while the athlete tries to hold them horizontal.

Back: Symmetrical development and position of the spine are noted when the athlete stands with back to the examiner. (In the female, scoliosis should always be considered.) During flexion, the movement of the spine is noted and any abnormality of motion can be discovered by twisting the shoulders to the right and then left.

Hip: The athlete is asked to squat and stand; this is followed by standing on first one leg and then the other (this is also viewed from the rear); the athlete then bends forward at the hip and is then requested to squat.

Knees: Because women's knees are very susceptible to injury, extra care should be given to this area. First, with the athlete standing or sitting, observe the knees for bilateral symmetry or obvious abnormalities. Internal and external rotation, flexion, extension, and medial and lateral movement are then performed passively by the examiner. Specifically, the examiner is looking for restricted or limited motion, crepitation, or signs of torn cartilage.

Ankles: This examination is performed while the athlete is sitting. The ankles are flexed, extended, and rotated internally and externally by the athlete. The same motions are repeated passively by the examiner.

Neurological

A gross neurological examination can be performed simultaneously with the remainder of the physical exam. Sensation and nerve integrity are necessary for completion of most of the muscle movements. A deep tendon reflex can be obtained while evaluating the knee, and a Babinski evaluated while examining the ankle. It is rarely necessary to do a specific neurological exam if no abnormalities are noted in the remainder of the evaluation.

Laboratory tests

Prior to participation in a sport, every female should have minimum lab work, including a hemoglobin/hematocrit and a urinalysis for protein. Whenever possible, the athlete should also have a complete blood count and a complete urinalysis. Additional laboratory tests may or may not be necessary. An athlete with a history or physical findings suggestive of an abnormality should have appropriate laboratory tests. These should be requested only when there is a reason, and not as a routine. An SMA-6 or SMA-12 is usually of little value—and yet many doctors order this on all potential athletes.

An electrocardiogram may be indicated if there is a history of suspected cardiac problems or suspicious physical findings in a young woman. We believe a baseline ECG with stress test is highly desirable for the postmenopausal woman before she begins a strenuous athletic program. Very few studies justify this contention; but until such time as it is shown to be unnecessary, we feel it should be performed.

X-rays are not a part of the routine pre-examination of an athlete. They should be reserved for the specific evaluation of an injury or a problem. Although modern technology has reduced the potential risk from X-ray, unnecessary exposure is still to be avoided, especially in the female.

HISTORY AND PHYSICAL EXAMINATION OF THE SCHOOL-AGE ATHLETE

Walter J. Kennedy, M.D.

CHAPTER

4

Although its primary purpose is to determine the health status of the prospective athlete, the preparticipation medical exam has other important functions. The examining physician can best serve the welfare of the youngster by becoming familiar with the aims of the examination and understanding the purpose of the entire athletic program.

Before making any decision based on the results of the medical evaluation, the examiner should find a satisfactory answer to the following questions:

• What is the overall health status of the prospective athlete?
• Are there any medical disorders or physical handicaps that might prevent the youngster from participating in a sport?
• If a disorder or handicap is present, can the problem be corrected so that it would be safe for the child to compete?
• How does the individual's size and maturity level compare with those of her competitors?
• Would participation in a particular sport place her at great disadvantage because of her size or level of maturity?
• How well conditioned is the youngster?
• If, because of medical disability, physical handicap, size, or level of maturity, she really shouldn't be participating in a sport, what other sport or alternative can be found to satisfy the child's needs?

The medical evaluation should be scheduled several weeks before the start of the sport season. This allows ample time for appropriate diagnostic procedures, correction or treatment, or for providing alternatives to satisfy the youngster's needs.

The frequency of and the interval between each medical appraisal of the athlete is also an important consideration. At one time, physical examinations were required prior to participation in each sport. For some youngsters this meant three or four examinations a year. The appraisals were often done hurriedly, under noisy, crowded, bullpen conditions that girls would hardly tolerate today. Because many physicians and educators questioned the worth of these evaluations, we progressed to the concept of one annual medical examination for all sports. However, because more emphasis has been placed on the *quality* of the examination, many physicians familiar with interscholastic sports medicine believe that the medical evaluation need not be annual. An interval of three to four years has been suggested: The initial exam would take place when the youngster first enters sports, followed by subsequent examinations when she progresses into middle school or into high school.[1]

Increased attention is being given to the medical history, to laboratory evaluations, and to allowing time for discussion and recommendations. A standard health questionnaire form for sports candidates—as shown in Figure 3-1—can provide an adequate and informative screening history.

In my opinion, the minimum laboratory examination should include a hemoglobin or hematocrit test, a urinalysis, and a tuberculin skin test.

The athlete's initial examination should receive special emphasis to insure its completeness. Frequently, this will be the first examination since infancy for many youngsters. The opportunity for the physician to provide meaningful service is much greater at this time. Existing abnormalities can be found and more easily corrected now than later. Rapport and trust between the youngster and the physician can be easily developed particularly if the physician allows enough time for discussion with the examinee.

The preparticipation medical examination can be done either at the physician's office or in a carefully organized group examination, if adequate time can be provided for a complete evaluation, including history, physical examination, laboratory studies, and discussion.

Evaluating the medical examination

The results of the sports examination are very important to the aspiring young athlete. All youngsters look forward to competing with their peers, and girls, like boys, enjoy physical activity and strenuous sports. Disqualification can be devastating to them.

Only rarely is exclusion or restriction from sport necessary. Before deciding on disqualification, every effort should be made to provide a more satisfactory alternative. The physician should be familiar with the classification of sports (see Table 4-1) and understand the physical demands of each sport. Usually, in female competition, the force of contact and the intensity of the activity are not as great as in male sports.

When possible, the disqualifying condition should be corrected. If correction is not feasible, another less strenuous sport can usual-

---

TABLE 4-1

Classification of Girls' Sports

CONTACT, STRENUOUS	CONTACT, MODERATELY STRENUOUS
Basketball	Baseball
Field hockey	Softball
Ice hockey	Volleyball
Lacrosse	
Soccer	
Water polo	NONCONTACT, MODERATELY STRENUOUS
	Badminton
NONCONTACT, STRENUOUS	Drill team
Cross-country	Golf
Fencing	Table tennis
Gymnastics	
Pentathlon	
Skiing	NONCONTACT, NONSTRENUOUS
Swimming and diving	Archery
Tennis	Bowling
Track and field	Curling
Weight lifting	Riflery

ly be found. Occasionally, a finding in either the history or the examination will have questionable significance; further evaluation or consultation is recommended.

Evaluation of disqualifying conditions can be difficult. Many conditions are only temporary, and if given time, correct themselves. Some require medical treatment or surgical correction.

Disqualifying conditions

Acute infections are usually self-limiting and require only temporary exclusion. However, exclusion *is* necessary to protect the ill youngster and those to whom she might pass on the infection. For this reason, the athlete with an acute respiratory infection should not be allowed to compete during the infectious stage. A contagious youngster and a common towel can cause more havoc to a sport team than all the injuries during a season. Acute pyogenic skin infections can also be transmitted from player to player, particularly in the contact sports.

Infectious mononucleosis and *hepatitis* are also causes for exclusion during the acute symptomatic phase. Youngsters with either of these conditions should not be allowed to return to contact sports until there is no longer evidence of splenic enlargement or liver involvement—because of the possibility of rupture of either organ.

Youngsters with *hemorrhagic diseases* should be referred for further evaluation. Classic *hemophilia* occurs only in boys; however, girls are subject to some of the less severe types of hemophilia. The tendency now is to treat these youngsters prophylactically with blood factors and allow them to compete in all noncontact sports. Swimming is considered to be the sport of choice for the youngster with hemophilia. *Leukemia* in remission is not a contraindication to full participation even in contact sports, but authorization should be obtained from the youngster's attending hematologist or oncologist.

The cardiovascular evaluation can be accomplished with little effort so that significant abnormalities can be differentiated from functional murmurs and benign arrhythmias. The essential components of the evaluation are observation of the youngster for color and for clubbing; blood pressure readings; palpation of the peripheral pulse and the chest, including the suprasternal notch; plus careful auscultation for murmurs, abnormal sounds, and arrhythmias. This can be followed, if necessary, by simple exercise stress tests.

Abnormal findings—systolic pressure over 140, diastolic pressure over 90, any evidence of cardiac enlargement, any diastolic murmur, any systolic murmur grade III/VI or greater, or any arrhythmia that doesn't disappear with exercise—are reasons for referral to a cardiologist.

Venous "hums" are normal sounds sometimes heard in young people and may be confused with murmurs, especially patent ductus murmurs. The hum, which is a continuous low-pitched sound heard over the upper chest, is produced by high-velocity flow through the great veins in the upper thorax. These sounds can be made to disappear by compressing the return flow in the neck. A thrill at the suprasternal notch is suggestive of aortic stenosis. Most arrhythmias in the young female are either ectopic beats or exaggerated sinus arrhythmias. Both disappear when the heart rate is increased over 140.

The examiner should also be aware of the significance of mid- to late systolic clicks and murmurs, as they might indicate a prolapsing mitral valve. This entity, present in a small per cent of young females and less common in boys, is being recognized more frequently, largely because of echocardiography. It usually has no clinical significance, but rarely it may be the cause of pathological arrhythmias. On very rare occasions, it may cause cardiac arrest.

Proteinuria is a frequent finding. Usually, it is transient and not detected in morning specimen. The most common form of transient proteinuria is orthostatic, especially in thin, adolescent girls. Young athletes also show temporary albuminuria after vigorous physical exertion. Although a persistent finding of proteinuria is not a reason for restriction or exclusion, it should be investigated to rule out renal disease.

The musculoskeletal examination of the young female athlete should include a very careful screening examination for scoliosis, as the disorder is approximately seven times more frequent in females. Idiopathic scoliosis accounts for 70 per cent of all cases of the disease, and approximately 90 per cent of the time it is hereditary, occurring as a sex-linked trait. When signs of scoliosis are detected, referral should be made to an orthopedist for examination and possible treatment with both the Milwaukee Brace and exercises.[2]

The knee of the adolescent girl deserves special consideration. In both girls and boys, this joint is the most frequently injured. Girls are more prone to subluxation resulting from instability of the patello-femoral joint. Resulting injuries can be reduced by strengthening exercises for the vastus medialis. *Osgood-Schlatter's* disease is rarely disabling, and is usually more mild in girls than in boys. It is not uncommon for an adolescent (boys more than girls) to complain of knee pain and have joint tenderness at the lower pole of the patella. This condition, called *Sinding-Larsen-Johansson disease* or "jumper's knee," apparently is a traction tendinitis of the tendon at its attachment to the patella. It is also self-limited and benign, but occasionally can be disabling for a short period.[3]

The paired organ controversy continues. The traditional stand has been firm against allowing participation in contact sports whenever there is absence of a paired organ, particularly the eye or kidney. On the other hand, those in favor of allowing participation in contact sports cite the lack of evidence of injury to the remaining organ during contact and point to examples of affected athletes who have successfully competed without injury. When the effect of the loss of either a remaining eye or kidney is weighed against any possible benefits of participation in a contact sport, especially when so many other satisfying sports are available, there seems to be little contest. Concern over injury to a remaining ovary has not been nearly as great, because this organ is so well protected.

References

1. Shaffer TE: The health examination for participation in sports. *Pediat Ann* 7:27, 1978

2. Keim HA: Scoliosis. *Clinical Symposia* 30:2, 1978

3. Medlar RC and Lyne ED: Sinding-Larsen-Johansson Disease: Its etiology and natural history. *J Bone Joint Surg* 60:1113, 1978

THE PHYSIOLOGY OF EXERCISE

Gail Shierman, Ph.D.

CHAPTER

5

Energy, which is required by the body to accomplish its work, is derived from food. The food is changed in the body from chemical energy into heat and mechanical energy so that the muscles can work. It is here that the law of conservation of energy comes into effect. This law states that energy cannot be created or destroyed. There is potential energy or stored energy, and kinetic energy or energy that produces work. An athlete should use her energy capabilities wisely and maintain a good performance weight by balancing her intake (food) with her outgo (energy expenditure).

Energy is measured in units called calories. A calorie (kilocalorie or kcal) is defined as the amount of heat necessary to raise the temperature of one kilogram of water one degree centigrade. When an athlete participates in an activity, she is converting stored energy into kinetic energy; not only does she accomplish her activity, but she produces heat as well. We are generally about 25 per cent efficient in energy production; the rest is not lost but is converted to heat.

Metabolism

Metabolism is the energy produced by the body from food. Everyone requires a certain minimum level of energy to exist in the waking state. This is called the basal metabolism rate (BMR). It is best determined in a laboratory where an individual's oxygen consumption can be measured under rigid guidelines. The BMR varies according to the amount of surface area and body fat a person has. In an athlete who is extremely active on a daily basis, the amount of oxygen consumed is far greater than the BMR. Hence, an increased amount of energy is derived from food.

Food is utilized as fuel in the form of proteins, carbohydrates, and fats. Oxidation of one gram of fat produces about 9.5 kcal of energy, whereas one gram of protein produces about 5.5 kcal, and carbohydrate produces about 4.5 kcal of energy when metabolized. The body uses carbohydrates preferentially in heavy work.

Food ingested into the stomach is acted upon initially by hydrochloric acid and then by a series of enzymes as it passes through the gastrointestinal tract. These enzymes act as catalysts and speed up the chemical reaction of the food. Each enzyme has a specific function, working on proteins, carbohydrates, or fats and breaking these compounds down into simpler compounds so they can be absorbed into the bloodstream.

When energy is required, a compound called adenosine triphosphate (ATP) serves as the energy source for work or muscle contraction. During muscle contraction, the ATP is quickly broken down, providing the needed energy. The resulting adenosine diphosphate (ADP) must combine with phosphate (P) and energy from the reserve fuel stored in the muscles to produce more ATP for continued muscle contraction. The reserve fuel used in this process is part of the energy stored in the chemical bonds of fats and carbohydrates.

Ingested carbohydrates are broken down into simple sugars, with glucose being the most abundant. Through the metabolic process, these carbohydrates produce ATP and, with the help of insulin, are transported through the cell membranes. The sugar molecule is then in the cell and is available as energy. If the glucose is not utilized immediately, it is stored as glycogen in the liver and muscles.

Fats, too, are important in the production of ATP. During submaximal endurance activities, fat is preferred over carbohydrates for ATP production. Carbohydrates, on the other hand, become the dominant fuel source during very heavy exercise.

Protein is a poor source of energy only because the body prefers

FIGURE 5-1

Energy Pathways

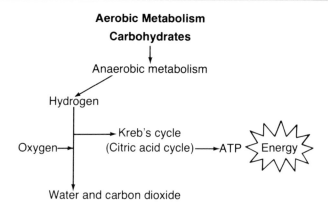

Aerobic Metabolism
Carbohydrates

Anaerobic metabolism

Hydrogen

Oxygen→

Kreb's cycle
(Citric acid cycle)——→ATP ⟨ Energy ⟩

Water and carbon dioxide

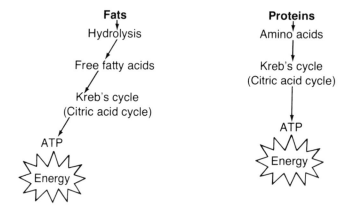

Fats
Hydrolysis

Free fatty acids

Kreb's cycle
(Citric acid cycle)

ATP
⟨ Energy ⟩

Proteins
Amino acids

Kreb's cycle
(Citric acid cycle)

ATP
⟨ Energy ⟩

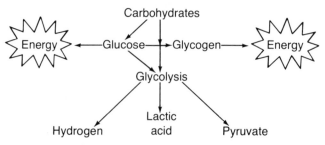

Anaerobic Metabolism
Carbohydrates

⟨ Energy ⟩ ←——Glucose——→Glycogen——→ ⟨ Energy ⟩

Glycolysis

Hydrogen   Lactic
              acid   Pyruvate

to use carbohydrates and fats. The only time it is used for energy is when there is an insufficient amount of fats and carbohydrates to meet the demands placed on the body.

The two pathways for energy production (see Figure 5-1) are aerobic (with oxygen) and anaerobic (without oxygen).

Aerobic pathway: All tissues in the body need oxygen to produce energy. This oxygen is brought to the tissues by a rather complex, but functionally efficient process. Air, which has oxygen, is brought into the lungs, where the oxygen is exchanged for carbon dioxide through the cell membranes and capillaries. The hemoglobin in the red cells of the blood carries this oxygen through the circulatory system to the tissues of the body. Again, oxygen is exchanged with carbon dioxide in the tissue fluids, and the carbon dioxide is carried back to the lungs and expired. The more work that is done by the athlete, the more oxygen is needed. Hence, the athlete breathes faster than the rate at which this oxygen-carbon dioxide exchange occurs. As breathing increases, so does the heart rate. In fact, there is a linear relationship between heart rate and oxygen consumption. The more work the athlete does, the higher her heart rate, and the more oxygen is consumed. Sports activities that are engaged in continuously for more than two minutes— for example a one-mile run—are said to be primarily aerobic.

Conditioning and training programs should be designed so that an athlete uses her oxygen more efficiently. In other words, the better-trained athlete does not breathe as hard or have as high a heart rate when performing the same sport as does an untrained athlete. She is more efficient and thus can do more for a longer period of time before getting fatigued.

In heavy exercise, a waste product called lactic acid accumulates in the muscles. This happens when the demand for oxygen exceeds the supply. Because of the problems associated with lactic-acid buildup, the concept of interval training arose. This type of training does not allow a large buildup of lactic acid because the workouts are interspersed with rest periods. As lactic-acid buildup contributes to fatigue, interval training allows for more work to be performed during a training workout.

Anaerobic pathway: When oxygen is not used to produce energy, the athlete is said to be in an anaerobic state. The glucose and glycogen in the muscles are producing energy, but only for a short

FIGURE 5-2

Structure of Muscles

LONGITUDINAL

1. Longitudinal—fibers longitudinal;
   gives range of motion but no strength

   example: sartorius

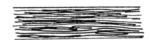

2. Quadrate—muscle slanted, fibers parallel

   example: pronator quadratus

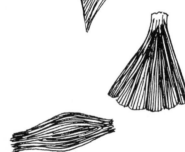

3. Triangular

   example: pectoralis major

4. Fusiform

   example: biceps

PENNIFORM

5. Single penniform—gives strength but no range of motion

   example: posterior tibialis

6. Bipenniform

   example: rectus femoris

7. Multipenniform

   example: deltoid

period of time. Lactic acid accumulates rapidly, and the body then must enter the aerobic state for continuous energy.

When the demand for oxygen in the muscles exceeds the supply of oxygen, the result is called oxygen debt. The circulatory and respiratory functions are not keeping up with the needs of the muscles. The oxygen debt must be repaid in a short period of time. When an athlete breathes fast, even after she has stopped her activity, she is repaying her oxygen debt. Short bursts of activity, such as the 100-yard dash, a fast break in basketball, or 100-meter freestyle swim, are considered primarily anaerobic activities; that is, an activity requiring less than 120 seconds. The more intense the activity, the greater the anaerobic energy contribution.

It is possible to improve the oxygen debt through training. A study conducted on two swimmers who were training for the 100-meter and the 200-meter freestyle events, respectively, showed that as their times improved for the distances, the oxygen debt capacity increased.[1] In other words, they were becoming more efficient in their use of oxygen.

Muscle contraction

Skeletal muscles have specific characteristics that are important for the athlete to know so that when she is training or conditioning she has a better idea of what is going on inside her. There are more than 400 muscles in the body. They are constructed in two general categories: longitudinal and penniform (see Figure 5-2). The longitudinal muscle group, with lengthwise fibers, includes the sartorius, biceps, rhomboids, and the pectoralis major. They favor range of motion rather than strength. In the penniform muscle group, the fibers are shaped much like a feather. An example is the tibialis anterior. A bipenniform muscle is the gastrocnemius, and a multipenniform muscle is the deltoid muscle. These muscles favor strength over range of motion.

When a muscle contracts, it does so in the direction of the muscle fibers. When a muscle contracts and a movement takes place that reduces the angle of the joint, it is said to be contracting concentrically. If the muscle contracts and the angle of the joint is increasing, it is said to be contracting eccentrically. For example, if you hold a five-pound barbell in your hand and bend your elbow, your

TABLE 5-2

Energy Expenditure in Sports Activities

Activity	Kg lb	50 110	53 117	56 123	59 130	62 137	65 143
Archery		3.3	3.4	3.6	3.8	4.0	4.2
Badminton		4.9	5.1	5.4	5.7	6.0	6.3
Basketball		6.9	7.3	7.7	8.1	8.6	9.0
Canoe: Racing		5.2	5.5	5.8	6.1	6.4	6.7
Climbing hills: No load		6.1	6.4	6.8	7.1	7.5	7.9
With 20-kg load		7.4	7.8	8.2	8.7	9.1	9.6
Cycling: Leisure (5.5 mph)		3.2	3.4	3.6	3.8	4.0	4.2
Racing		8.5	9.0	9.5	10.0	10.5	11.0
Dancing: Vigorous		8.4	8.9	9.4	9.9	10.4	10.9
Field hockey		6.7	7.1	7.5	7.9	8.3	8.7
Football		6.6	7.0	7.4	7.8	8.2	8.6
Golf		4.3	4.5	5.8	5.0	5.3	5.5
Gymnastics		3.3	3.5	3.7	3.9	4.1	4.3
Horse racing: Walking		2.1	2.2	2.3	2.4	2.5	2.7
Galloping		6.9	7.3	7.7	8.1	8.5	8.9
Judo		9.8	10.3	10.9	11.5	12.1	12.7
Running: Cross-country		8.2	8.6	9.1	9.6	10.1	10.6
Horizontal, 9 min/mi		9.7	10.2	10.8	11.4	12.0	12.5
6 min/mi		13.9	14.4	15.0	15.6	16.2	16.7
Skiing, hard snow: Level, walking		7.2	7.6	8.0	8.4	8.9	9.3
Uphill, maximum speed		13.7	14.5	15.3	16.2	17.0	17.8
Squash		10.6	11.2	11.9	12.5	13.1	13.8
Swimming: Backstroke		8.5	9.0	9.5	10.0	10.5	11.0
Breaststroke		8.1	8.6	9.1	9.6	10.0	10.5
Crawl, fast		7.8	8.3	8.7	9.2	9.7	10.1
Tennis		5.5	5.8	6.1	6.4	6.8	7.1
Volleyball		2.5	2.7	2.8	3.0	3.1	3.3

(in kcal/min)

68 150	71 157	74 163	77 170	80 176	83 183	86 190	89 196	92 203	95 209	98 216
4.4	4.6	4.8	5.0	5.2	5.4	5.6	5.8	6.0	6.2	6.4
6.6	6.9	7.0	7.5	7.8	8.1	8.3	8.6	8.9	9.2	9.5
9.4	9.8	10.2	10.6	11.0	11.5	11.9	12.3	12.7	13.1	13.5
7.0	7.3	7.6	7.9	8.2	8.5	8.9	9.2	9.5	9.8	10.1
8.2	8.6	9.0	9.3	9.7	10.0	10.4	10.8	11.1	11.5	11.9
10.0	10.4	10.9	11.3	11.8	12.2	12.6	13.1	13.5	14.0	14.4
4.4	4.6	4.8	5.0	5.1	5.3	5.5	5.7	5.9	6.1	6.3
11.5	12.0	12.5	13.0	13.5	14.0	14.5	15.0	15.5	16.1	16.6
11.4	11.9	12.4	12.9	13.4	13.9	14.4	15.0	15.5	16.0	16.5
9.1	9.5	9.9	10.3	10.7	11.1	11.5	11.9	12.3	12.7	13.1
9.0	9.4	9.8	10.2	10.6	11.0	11.4	11.7	12.1	12.5	12.9
5.8	6.0	6.3	6.5	6.8	7.1	7.3	7.6	7.8	8.1	8.3
4.5	4.7	4.9	5.1	5.3	5.5	5.7	5.9	6.1	6.3	6.5
2.8	2.9	3.0	3.2	3.3	3.4	3.5	3.6	3.8	3.9	4.0
9.3	9.7	10.1	10.6	11.0	11.4	11.8	12.2	12.6	13.0	13.4
13.3	13.8	14.4	15.0	15.6	16.2	16.8	17.4	17.9	18.5	19.1
11.1	11.6	12.1	12.6	13.0	13.5	14.0	14.5	15.0	15.5	16.0
13.1	13.7	14.3	14.9	15.4	16.0	16.6	17.2	17.8	18.3	18.9
17.3	17.9	18.5	19.1	19.6	20.2	20.8	21.4	22.0	22.5	23.1
9.7	10.2	10.6	11.0	11.4	11.9	12.3	12.7	13.2	13.6	14.0
18.6	19.5	20.3	21.1	21.9	22.7	23.6	24.4	25.2	26.0	26.9
14.4	15.1	15.7	16.3	17.0	17.6	18.2	18.9	19.5	20.1	20.8
11.5	12.0	12.5	13.0	13.5	14.0	14.5	15.0	15.5	16.1	16.6
11.0	11.5	12.0	12.5	13.0	13.4	13.9	14.4	14.9	15.4	15.9
10.6	11.1	11.5	12.0	12.5	12.9	13.4	13.9	14.4	14.8	15.3
7.4	7.7	8.1	8.4	8.7	9.0	9.4	9.7	10.0	10.4	10.7
3.4	3.6	3.7	3.9	4.0	4.2	4.3	4.5	4.6	4.8	4.9

biceps are undergoing concentric contraction, whereas if you return your arm to the straight position slowly, your biceps are undergoing eccentric contraction.

Each muscle consists of a number of motor units. A motor unit is several muscle fibers linked to a motor nerve, which in turn is part of the central nervous system. When the motor nerve is stimulated, the fibers attached to the nerve contract. Several motor units are stimulated at various times so that movement of the limb or limbs occurs. When an athlete wants to flex her arm, the motor units in her biceps muscle are stimulated so that the muscle fibers contract and produce the arm flexion. Since a motor unit fatigues after several stimulations, other motor units are recruited so that the movement can take place smoothly. Thus, the motor units fire asynchronously to produce the desired movement.

Energy expenditure

Daily rates: The number of calories required for daily activities varies according to the amount of activity plus the athlete's age and weight. In determining the athlete's desirable body weight, allow 100 pounds for the first five feet of height and five pounds for every inch thereafter. If the athlete has a large build, add 10 per cent of the total number of pounds; if she has a small build, subtract 10 per cent of the total number of pounds.

Here is a simple method of determining caloric needs:
1. Basal calories = desirable body weight (lbs) × 10
2. Add activity calories:
   sedentary = desirable body weight (lbs) × 3
   moderate = desirable body weight (lbs) × 5
   strenuous = desirable body weight (lbs) × 10
3. Add calories for desirable weight gain, growth (pregnant women), or lactation
4. Subtract calories for desirable weight loss.

Activity rates: Chapter 8 has additional information on the kinds of foods athletes should eat for various activities. Table 5-1 shows the energy expenditure of different sports activities. In order to determine the kcal cost of the activity, multiply the kcal cost for the athlete's weight times the number of minutes she spends in her activity. For example, if the athlete plays basketball for 90 minutes and weighs 110 lbs, her kcal cost of the activity is 621 (6.9 kcal × 90 min).

Response to temperature changes

There have been several studies on women's response to heat stress. A recent study investigated the effects of exercise at different temperatures.[2] The results indicated that the women had little change in body temperature while performing work in either a hot or a normal environment. An additional study on fit men and women showed that men sweated more than women but that the women could cool down better than the men after exercising in the heat.[3] These data suggest that a woman "adjusts her sweat rate better to the required heat loss," that possibly "a greater cardiovascular component of thermoregulation exists in the women," and that women may be "more efficient regulators of their body temperatures." It appears that, as their fitness increases, so does the ability of women to withstand heat stress.

References

1. Hermanson L: Anaerobic energy release. *Med Sci Sports* 1:32, 1969

2. Wells C: Sexual differences in heat stress response. *Phys Sportsmed* 5(9):78, 1977

3. Wyndham CH, Morrison JF, and Williams CG: Heat reactions of male and female Caucasians. *J App Physiol* 20:357, 1965

Further reading

Astrand P and Rodahl K: *Textbook of Work Physiology*. New York: McGraw-Hill, 1970

DeVries HA: *Physiology of Exercise*. Dubuque, Iowa: WC Brown, 1974

Katch FI and McArdle WD: *Nutrition, Weight Control, and Exercise*. Boston: Houghton Mifflin Company, 1977

Lamb DR: *Physiology of Exercise, Responses and Adaptions*. New York: Macmillan, 1978

Mirkin G and Hoffman M: *The Sportsmedicine Book*. Boston: Little, Brown, 1978

CONDITIONING THE ATHLETE

Gail Shierman, Ph.D.

CHAPTER

6

Women have learned that good physical conditioning is vital for participation in all sports and activities. When Title IX of the 1972 Education Amendments Act came into effect and the movement for women's sports gained impetus, the injury rate also increased. This is largely attributed to the lack of proper conditioning. Fortunately, coaches now realize that conditioning not only reduces the injury rate but also improves the quality of the athlete's performance.

Conditioning is the equivalent of physical fitness: The athlete is physically capable of performing her sport with premium efficiency. She can meet the demands placed upon her body both physiologically and biomechanically, not only for the output necessary for her sport but also for critical situations. The athlete is striving for optimum performance throughout.

Components of a conditioning program

A good conditioning program has three major components: muscular strength and endurance, flexibility, and cardiorespiratory endurance. These three should be included in every conditioning program regardless of the sport.

Muscular strength and endurance: Muscular strength is defined as one all-out effort against resistance, whereas muscular endurance is the ability to repeat a movement against resistance several times. For most sports, it is muscular endurance that is important—few activities demand just one all-out effort. Muscular strength and endurance are acquired through strength-training, either on weight-training machines or through exercises. The most common form of strength-training is done on the Universal Gym and the Nautilus machines (see Figures 6-1 and 6-2). These machines allow users to adjust the resistance to individual needs; hence, their popularity is obvious.

Muscular strength and endurance are achieved through repetition and overload. If an athlete repeats an exercise or movement, she increases her endurance. She also must "overload" the muscle group; that is, she must increase the resistance placed on the muscle or muscle group so that it will have to work harder.

There are three different ways to gain strength: isometrically, isotonically, and isokinetically. Isometrics are exercises that are done against a resistance so that body movement does not take place. For example, standing in a doorway and pushing the door frame with the hands is an isometric exercise. Isotonics are any exercises in which movement takes place—weight machines, free weights, or exercises such as sit-ups and push-ups. Isokinetics is movement against a resistance that adapts to the angle of the joint and at a constant velocity. The Cybex II equipment, including the Orthotron seen in many training rooms, is considered isokinetic (see Figure 6-3). This equipment is used mainly for rehabilitation from injuries up to the point of normal strength; the athlete is then changed over to workouts on other weight-training equipment.

Muscular strength and endurance are specific to a muscle or muscle group, so if the athlete's activity requires total body strength and endurance, she must train all parts of her body. Even if she uses only one part of her body for her sport, she should train the entire body. All parts of the body work in a synchronous fashion to produce a movement, so all parts should be strong. Strength-training is also specific to that angle at which the training takes place. Therefore, it is important that the athlete train throughout the range of motion of the joints involved in the movement, so that she will be strong at every angle. If a girl or woman wants to be a good athlete, she must be strong. It is a firm belief of many coaches that strength is the primary component for good athletic performance.

FIGURE 6-1

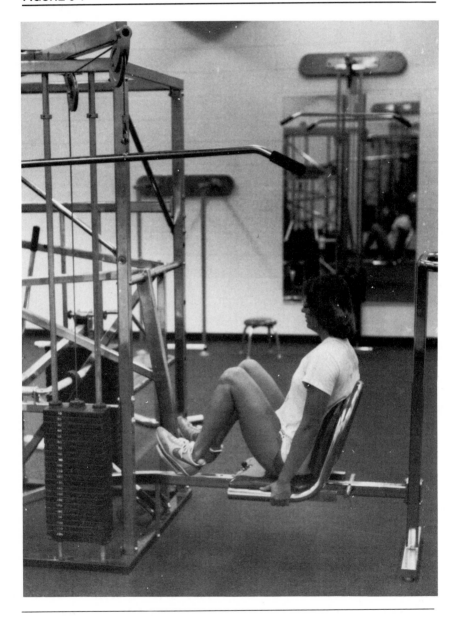

Universal Gym

Flexibility: Flexibility is the range of motion of a joint or how far the joint can flex (bend) and extend (straighten). Some sports require more flexibility than others, but all athletes should have at least moderate flexibility of all body parts. Flexibility is specific to that joint, which means that an athlete can be flexible in one place and not in another. Many athletes, such as those in gymnastics and

FIGURE 6-2

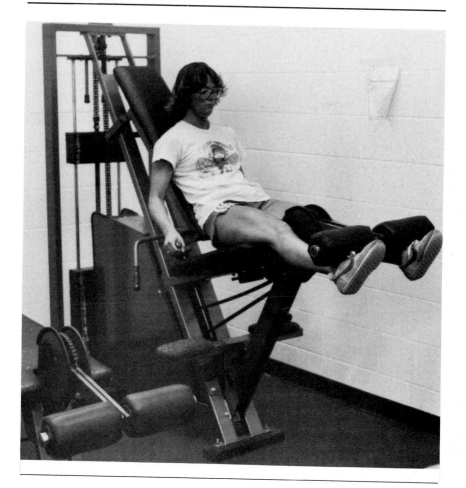

Nautilus

FIGURE 6-3

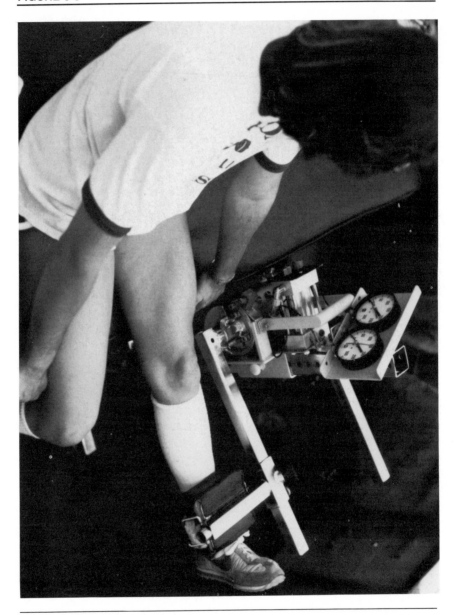

Orthotron

dance, spend a great deal of time stretching all their muscles. If the athlete is naturally flexible all over, she does not need to spend much time stretching or limbering up; she need only maintain what she has. Strength-work would be a better choice, so that her muscles will be strong enough to hold her "loose" joints together and prevent injuries. All flexibility exercises should be performed like yoga exercises, slowly and without any bouncing.

Cardiorespiratory endurance: Regardless of the sport they're involved in, cardiorespiratory endurance should be developed by all athletes. This is the ability of the heart and lungs to function efficiently while participating at any level of the sport without getting tired easily or out of breath. Aerobics is a term commonly defined as including all kinds of activities that require rapid breathing. Some aerobic activities to build cardiorespiratory endurance are running, swimming, bicycling, and aerobic dance. These should be done for at least 30 minutes at a speed fast enough to raise the heart rate and maintain it at 70 per cent of the individual's maximum.

Warming up

The warm-up consists of stretching or flexibility exercises for all parts of the body. The rest of the warm-up is designed for the athlete's sport. Most athletes actually perform their sport-activity during the warm-up, but only to a moderate degree. There is no set length of time for a warm-up, but the athlete should reach the point of sweating slightly. A beginning athlete has to determine by trial and error what feels best for her. It is important that she does not overdo the warm-up period and tire herself out—yet, she should exercise long enough to get the "feel" she needs for her performance. Little is known about the physiological value of the warm-up; there is conflicting evidence about its benefits. However, it appears to be extremely important psychologically.

Rules for optimal conditioning programs

For a beginning athlete, progression is important. If the athlete was active in a sport but laid off for a while, she must begin at a level at which she will not injure herself. Many girls and women get carried away by enthusiasm when they begin their conditioning routines, and injure themselves. This just postpones their participation during the regular season. An athlete should begin the conditioning program at the point at which it feels comfortable, but still requires moderate effort. The athlete should not have any pain during the workouts, but she should feel some stress. If an athlete is not sure how much stress she should feel, she should ask her coach or an older, more experienced athlete in her sport.

As mentioned previously, she should work hard enough during cardiorespiratory-endurance training to get the heart rate up to 70 per cent of maximum. To determine the athlete's maximum heart rate, subtract her age from 220. Take 70 per cent of that number. That is where her heart rate should be to obtain minimum cardiorespiratory endurance or a "training effect." She should try to maintain that heart rate for 30 minutes. If she cannot do it initially, she should do as much as she can and work up to 30 minutes. (Distance runners, of course, require much longer than this.) If the athlete is working at the "training-effect" level, her heart and lungs will become more efficient and her performance will be more efficient. In weight-training, this is known as *overload.* An athlete adds weights (increases resistance) as she progresses in her training program, so that she is getting stronger and can endure muscular effort better.

Conditioning programs should be well balanced and regular. An athlete should do flexibility, strength, and cardiorespiratory-endurance activities daily, but they can vary in intensity—an athlete would not want an intense workout the day before competition. The intensity of the workouts depends upon how often the athlete competes, but generally, alternating days of extreme intensity and moderate intensity is advised.

The woman must acclimatize to the environment: If an athlete changes altitudes, she should try to get there several days in advance, especially if she is going from a low altitude to a high altitude. In this case, the workouts should be lighter and of shorter duration—except for anaerobic activities. Humidity changes and extreme heat or cold will affect the athlete's performance, so it is wise to get to the place of competition a couple of days early. In general, the better-trained athlete acclimatizes better to a different environment.

Exercises for strength

Push-ups: Regular push-ups for women, as for men, are good for building arm and shoulder-girdle strength. Modified push-ups may be used if the athlete is weak, but she should change to regular push-ups as soon as she can.

Sit-ups: Sit-ups should be performed with the hands behind the head, knees bent as much as possible, and the head curling up as the athlete sits up.

Back arches: Lying on the stomach, hands behind head, with a partner holding her legs down, the athlete lifts the upper part of her body as far as she can. She should perform slowly, hold for 10 seconds, and breathe throughout the exercise.

Half knee bends: With hands on hips, the athlete rises up on her toes, then bends the knees halfway to a squat; she returns to the "on toes" position, and then returns to the resting position (feet flat on the floor). This exercise is good for strengthening the legs.

Heel rise: With the toes on a board about two inches high and with heels on the ground, the athlete rises on her toes, keeping the body straight. This exercise is good for leg development.

Exercises for flexibility

Leg stretches: Sitting on the floor, with legs straight out in front, the athlete reaches for her ankles, grasping as low as possible on the leg and pulling the body down as far as it will go and holding that pulled position for a count of 10. Toes should not be pointed. Variations of this exercise include straddle-leg stretches and hurdle-sit stretches.

Side bends: Standing with the feet shoulder-width apart, the athlete bends to the right side with the right arm sliding down the leg and the left arm up over the left ear. She slides down as far as possible, holds, and returns to the starting position. She does the same for the other side. This exercise is good for stretching the sides of the body.

Arm circles: Standing comfortably, the athlete circles the arms, singly, forward and backward, in large circles several times. This exercise keeps the arms and shoulder girdle flexible.

One-half backward somersault: From a sitting position, legs straight in front, the athlete rolls over backward and tries to touch her toes on the floor behind her head, keeping her legs straight. This exercise stretches the backs of the legs and back.

Back clasp reach: From a standing position, the athlete grasps her hands behind her back, leans over forward, and raises her hands up toward the sky as far as possible with arms straight. This exercise is good for flexibility of the arms and shoulder girdle.

Exercises for cardiorespiratory endurance

Running: This is probably the best exercise for improving the cardiorespiratory condition of the athlete. Make sure she runs correctly and tries to increase the time and distance weekly.

Swimming: If the athlete has foot or knee problems, this activity is good for developing cardiorespiratory endurance.

Bicycling: This is a good activity for someone who may have foot or knee problems. It can be done for time over a certain distance, with the distance increased weekly.

Jump rope: This can be done in a small area, for any length of time, and is useful on bad-weather days.

Running in place: This is good if space or weather are problems. Make sure that this exercise is done on floors that "give," rather than on cement floors.

In addition to exercises, there are three types of training programs that have been useful for athletes—interval-training, weight-training, and circuit-training.

Interval-training is just what it says—training done at intervals. It is based on the overload principle. Rather than all at once, the workout is interspersed with rest periods. This type of training program decreases early fatigue and increases aerobic capacity (cardiorespiratory endurance). The athlete can tolerate a greater intensity of work during the workout period. The overload principle is applied by increasing the workload, decreasing rest periods, increasing the number of work-bouts, or increasing the length of the work-bouts. (A bout is one series of an exercise or program of exercises.)

Weight-training is important for developing muscular strength and endurance. Fortunately, women athletes today are learning that weight-training does not cause bulging muscles. This program is done with free weights, on the Universal Gym, or on the Nautilus equipment. Generally, three sets of 10 to 15 repetitions of the exercise done at each station is considered a good workout. Weight-training does not develop flexibility or cardiorespiratory endurance, so an athlete should supplement her weight-training program with other activities or exercises for these areas.

Circuit-training, a series of "exercises" done either with or without equipment, is designed to produce strength, cardiorespiratory endurance, speed, flexibility, or all of these. It is a flexible training program in that it can be adapted to the athlete's sport and to the available equipment. For example, a sprinter could do a circuit-training workout that would include flexibility exercises, short and fast sprints, and some weight-training. Several stations (any number) are set up; the athlete moves from one to another with a short rest interval between each station. Each athlete can work at her own pace and can tell exactly what her physical condition is. Either time or repetition is used as the basis for gauging each station, so the overload principle is applied. The circuit-training program can be used in weight-training programs or entirely without equipment.

Off-season training

Off-season training is necessary for the athlete to maintain a certain degree of conditioning. She must not fall below such a specific point, or when the season begins, she will be totally out of condition and unable to keep up with normal workouts and practices. Although an athlete in top condition does not deteriorate quickly, she should do moderate workouts two to three times a week during the off-season.

Further reading

Jensen CR and Fisher AG: *Scientific Basis of Athletic Conditioning*. Philadelphia: Lea & Febiger, 1975

Klafs CE and Lyon MJ: *The Female Athlete*. St. Louis: Mosby, 1978

PROPER CLOTHING AND EQUIPMENT

Marlene J. Adrian, D.P.E.

CHAPTER

7

T he neuromuscular abilities of the athlete are most important in determining the success and control of her performance, but proper clothing and equipment do influence the final outcome.

The functions of proper clothing and equipment are to enhance performance and to protect the performer. If the performer feels safe, she will be more apt to move with the speed and force necessary to accomplish the movement goal. If the performer feels no binding or restriction from her clothing or equipment—or even believes that they allow her to perform her bodily movements more effectively—she will indeed execute her movements in a more efficient and effective manner.

Clothing and equipment worn by the female athlete fall into two categories, basic clothing and protective equipment (see Figure 7-1). Protective equipment consists of such adjunct apparel as shoulder pads, eye guards, field hockey goalkeeper toe boots, and other items designed specifically to protect the performer from injury by extrinsic forces. Basic clothing consists of brassieres and underpants; shirts, sweaters, and jackets; shorts, knickers, and pants; skirts, tunics, leotards, dresses, and kilts; socks and tights; gloves; and footwear of all types. Although designed primarily for functional purposes, basic clothing does, in fact, help protect the performer from injury due to intrinsic forces, and provides some protection against extrinsic forces.

Basic clothing

Unfortunately, proper basic clothing for female athletes is not always easy to obtain. One reason may be the dress worn by women and girls as recently as the 19th century. Women participated in sport and dance wearing long skirts or dresses that maintained the femininity of the performers but limited their performance. Rather than having the sport or dance determine the clothing, the clothing determined how the sport or dance could be performed. During those days, a woman used an "ankle screen" to prevent exposing her ankles when mounting a bicycle. In the 1890s, bloomers revolutionized the dress of those engaging in gymnastics, other outdoor sports, and in physical education classes. Bloomers provided some freedom for the legs, but the upper body was not always equally free from encumbrances.

It's no wonder, then, that athletic clothing for women has been less than satisfactory. A commom problem has been excessive restriction, possibly because female athletes move more rapidly and through greater ranges of movement than designers expected. In many cases, clothing failed to meet the unique movement requirements of a specific activity. In addition, female athletes increased in muscularity, becoming more mesomorphic, so that traditional patterns of the female garment industry no longer fit. The cut of the pattern was particularly restrictive across the shoulders and under the arms. There was excess material across the hips and breast and not enough length in shirts and pants. Some female athletes have been successful in obtaining perfect fits with apparel based upon a male pattern. However, for the majority of female athletes, the male pattern isn't satisfactory, either. The garment industries of the 1970s have risen to the challenge of providing proper clothing for female athletes, and we should have fewer problems in the 1980s. Because the sporting goods manufacturers have shown the greatest concern for proper clothing, sporting goods and dance stores probably are the best places to obtain appropriate attire.

Basic clothing should allow nonrestricted movement, be nonabrasive and nonirritating, provide an appropriate heat loss/heat retention balance, be lightweight, and provide the initial level of protection to the performer.

Nonrestricted movement: The only valid way to be sure that clothing will not restrict is to use it in all the possible movements of the sport or dance before purchasing. To simulate all the possible movements one will encounter:

• Vigorously swing the arms forward and overhead; swing to the outside and to the inside as high as possible; and swing the arms horizontally at shoulder level forward and backward. If you are testing long-sleeved garments, bring the arms across the chest with the elbows flexed.

• When testing gloves or mittens, extend the fingers and flex the fingers as quickly as possible to note any resistance to movement. Stand on the balls of the feet and extend the body and arms to touch the ceiling.

• Trunk-twisting movements should be done right and left as vigorously as possible, followed by slower forward flexion and backward extension movements.

• Next swing one leg forward and backward as far as possible and then to the side and across the body. Do the same with the other leg. Assume a lunging position with one leg fully extended and the

FIGURE 7-1

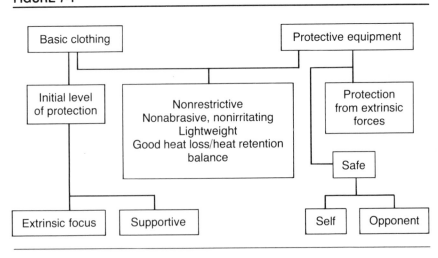

Criteria for selection of basic clothing and protective equipment.

other in a 90-degree flexed position. Repeat movement for the other direction.

- Assume a semisquat or full squat position, depending on the activity for which the apparel is intended.
- When evaluating shoes, prance about—that is, vigorously walk in place, rising on big toes at each push off. Jog about, execute some quick turns, and then sit and rotate the feet in every possible direction. And finally, jump into the air and abduct both legs; that is, raise them to the side as far as possible.

Some specific trouble spots with respect to restrictive clothing: The "one size fits all" clothing—specifically, leotards, tights, and socks—may be too binding for safe wear. Look for signs of numbness or change in skin color. One might need to wear the clothing for at least five minutes to note these detrimental effects on the circulatory system. Spandex and other stretch materials need to be tested before purchase to prevent similar circulatory or restrictive problems. Stretch materials are often used in clothes intended for speed skating, skiing, gymnastics, fencing, and bicycling. These materials are strong, provide some support to the body, and are lightweight. Therefore, how clothes made from these materials fit is important.

Inadequate space for arms is a common problem. Sometimes, sleeves bind because of underestimating the girth at the biceps and triceps muscles. Too often, sleeveless shirts cut under the arms. All shirts should be checked for adequate breadth across the chest and shoulders.

In purchasing clothing that is considered the uniform for the sport, one usually will have only sizing problems. When the right size is selected, the clothing should be nonrestrictive, because it's been designed for the sport. If there is no specific uniform for a sport, one may select proper apparel from that designed for a similar sport. In choosing underclothing, the cut of the underpants must be such that the person can move vigorously without the pants creeping upward.

The fitting of athletic shoes was a serious problem for girls and women prior to 1976, when the female athletic footwear market became big business. Manufacturers had been producing athletic shoes on a men's last—naturally, they didn't fit women; in particular, many found the heels too large. A woman's last is now being used by the leading sport-shoe manufacturers. However, because of the increased number of styles and companies, selection of a proper shoe and shoe size is difficult. This is especially true for jogging shoes; extensive advertising of them is confusing to prospective buyers.

The first and most important factor is that footwear fit properly. An American Society for Testing Materials (ASTM) standard, "Fitting of Athletic Footwear, Recommended Practice," has been published and is available from ASTM headquarters.* Sporting goods retailers should have a copy of the standard to assist them in securing a perfect fit for each customer. (ASTM also has "Recommended Practices in Ski Boot and Ski Equipment.")

Don't believe the myth that shoes always hurt at first, but that they are "broken in" after a few wearings. Shoes that hurt during the try-on will more than likely hurt after weeks of wear—if one can tolerate them that long. Man-made materials usually are stiffer and less formable than leather. But even leather and other fabrics that stretch should not be painful, though they may feel a bit stiff at first.

Nonabrasive and nonirritating characteristics: Although natural-fiber textiles are known for their softness, two man-made fibers, rayon and the acrylics, are also soft. In addition, the blends of man-made fibers and natural fibers give cloth a soft, nonabrasive quality. Therefore, most female athletes will find it easier to obtain nonabrasive clothing than nonrestrictive clothing. Sometimes, however, materials used to produce water repellency, odor prevention, or nonwrinkly characteristics have made the fabrics abrasive. Heavy seams or hems may also cause chafing of the skin, particularly around the neck, arms, and waist. Poorly sewn seams sometimes appear in cheap, or not so cheap, athletic footwear. One should carefully inspect merchandise for these features before purchasing it.

Chemically induced skin irritation from clothing is not common, but athletes might be allergic to wool, or might find the electrostatic charge of some man-made fibers irritating.

---

*ASTM is a national voluntary standards-setting organization. Manufacturers, consumers, and researchers collaborate in the writing of practices, testing procedures, and products to insure safety for the consumer. Their address is 5 Race Street, Philadelphia, Pa. 19106.

Heat loss/heat retention balance: In 1940, the textile industry used 90 per cent natural fibers and 10 per cent man-made fibers. By 1976, this had changed to 30 per cent natural fibers (29 per cent of this was cotton) and 70 per cent man-made fibers (predominantly polyester and nylon). What does this mean to the sporting world and the female athlete? These synthetic materials usually have a tighter weave than do the natural materials—cotton, linen, silk, and wool. Therefore, they don't allow for air passage—they don't "breathe." This causes alterations in the athlete's perspiration/evaporation process and inhibits heat loss. In addition, shoes and uniforms treated for odor control add a film of nonabsorbency to the material. Waterproofing and noniron finishes are also detrimental to heat balance, as these make the material less permeable to air and moisture.

If the athlete feels discomfort—flushed face, hot body, clammy skin—she should determine whether the clothing is as much at fault as the strenuousness of the activity and the temperature and humidity factors. Is there a decided difference between scrimmage and competition under the same environmental conditions except for the replacement of a nonbreathing uniform for the cotton scrimmage clothing?

While it is true that many uniforms do not cover more than the torso and that most individuals adjust quite well (like acclimatizing) to man-made fibers, some individuals have a difficult time maintaining adequate heat balance when wearing these materials. This is especially true for the less physically fit, older persons, and those engaging in the more vigorous sports and dance activities. Because such activities as fencing, softball, baseball, football, and modern dance require clothing that covers the majority of the body, and because much of the clothing is synthetic, primarily of stretch materials, the physician and athlete need to be aware of the first signs of a heat-balance problem.

Fourteen generic man-made fibers are produced in the United States, with nine of them used in sport clothing. Nylon is the most versatile of the materials, the strongest, and most durable. It is used not only in manufacturing indoor-sports uniforms and shoes, but in winter-sports clothing, and in weight loss clothing. The latter type may be dangerous and should not be used without care; I recommend that a physician's guidance be obtained. If a person exercises at a high energy output level and cannot evaporate the sweat through her clothing, the body becomes so hot that excessive sweating with loss of body fluids is the result. It's like being in a pup tent with the sun and outer air radiating a 100-degree temperature.

A relatively new addition to the sports world is olefin. Like other synthetics, it is abrasion resistant, strong, with low water absorbency. It does, however, have the lowest specific gravity of all fibers—less than 1.00—and has a wicking characteristic. This is the ability to draw body moisture from the skin and up through fabric interstices to the outer surface. Therefore, it remains dry to the skin, but removes perspiration moisture from the skin. Olefin socks and underclothing, then, would facilitate evaporation of perspiration if olefin were the only clothing layer. Even when combined with wool or some other natural fiber, the moisture is transmitted to that other fiber while olefin keeps the skin dry and warm. Cotton also has a wicking characteristic, but it absorbs and retains moisture. Some nylons are now being advertised as having a wicking action. The permeability of the material should be an important consideration when purchasing clothing.

Man-made fibers used in the uppers of footwear have not, in most cases, allowed for adequate air passage. Not only do the feet get hot and begin to perspire excessively, but the environment makes an ideal breeding place for bacteria and fungi. The shoe industry is therefore making more leather uppers again, and is coating other natural materials with polyurethanes that are permeable to water vapor.

As more and more improvements are made in man-made fibers and more blends and finishes are being made, basic clothing for sports and dance will show an improvement in the moisture-and-heat-loss characteristics. Adequate heat-retention materials are already being manufactured. In strenuous activity in the cold, one must, however, wear lightweight, moisture-absorbent or wicking materials next to the skin, then a material for heat retention, and possibly an additional lightweight material to prevent the passage of air and moisture.

Light weight: In all sports and dance, basic clothing should be as lightweight as possible and still provide necessary warming or cooling. The less weight, the less restriction there is apt to be, and the less muscle effort required for the activity. The performer will fatigue less readily and psychologically will feel better in lightweight sportswear. This has been especially evident in swimming, speed skating, skiing, and soccer. In most activities, lightweight shoes are an asset. Female athletes without lightweight clothing are probably putting out 10 per cent more effort than they would otherwise need. How lightweight the clothing can be without being unsafe depends upon the activity requirements, as described in the next section.

Initial level of protection: Basic clothing must provide an initial level of protection against extrinsic forces and provide support against intrinsic forces. This initial level of protection exists merely because basic clothing covers the skin. Shearing forces (abrasions) to the skin from skidding, colliding with another person, or falling can be reduced by means of durable, abrasion-resistant, man-made fibers. The smoother surface of these materials may also lessen friction and allow sliding to occur, which can reduce impact on bones. Nylon-blended materials have been designed for such a purpose for persons playing on artificial turf. If natural fibers such as cotton were used, the material would have to be bulkier and of greater weight to offer the same protection as the nylon blends. The athlete must remember, however, to weigh the disadvantages of inadequate heat loss against the small amount of protection that the basic clothing provides.

Materials used in the manufacturing of footwear for sports and dance need to possess three features: adequate traction (coefficient of friction between shoe and locomotion surface), adequate shock-attenuation characteristics, and adequate support.

A shoe to be used on a wooden gymnasium floor is not the same one selected for use on a wet, muddy, grass field. If you cannot check the shoe surface interface at the store, discuss it with the salesperson—manufacturers have such research data to aid in the selection of shoes. Try the shoe on the proper surface and determine whether or not there is optimal friction. If not, return the shoe—don't make it do. And remember that too great a frictional force is as unsafe as too little.

Footwear-testing for shock-attenuation characteristics are being studied by ASTM, which has found vertical forces acting on the foot during jogging and running to be something like two to four times body weight. Joggers on asphalt and concrete streets and sidewalks need greater shock attenuation than those running on grass or specially designed tracks. Therefore, it is probably safest to ask manufacturers for shock-attenuation values for each shoe model, and then to select a shoe that is lightweight, nonrestricting, nonabrasive, that breathes, gives adequate traction, and has the highest value for shock attenuation. Also, of course, consider the support it offers. Strong uppers, especially the counter, should provide support or lateral stability to the foot and ankle. Klein has suggested that because quality control may be lacking in mass-produced sporting shoes, the female athlete should set the shoes on a table and note whether both uppers are 90 degrees to the tabletop.[1] Shoes that roll inward (pronate) are considered unacceptable.

Support is offered to other parts of the human body by man-made fibers high in elasticity. Nylon and Spandex are the more commonly used materials in "stretch uniforms," swimsuits, support hose, and foundation garments. As little as 20 per cent Spandex blended with other materials can provide adequate elastic properties, especially for support-type brassieres.

The lack of an adequate supportive brassiere can cause discomfort as well as trauma to the breast. Haycock, Shierman, and Gillette filmed women walking and jogging on a treadmill while wearing their own bras, special bras, and no bras.[2] That data suggest that persons with inadequate support of the breasts, especially large or pendulous breasts, will experience trauma to the breast and supporting ligaments. As a result of this work and of complaints by female athletes and joggers, there now are several manufacturers of "athletic bras."

Depending upon the size of the breast and the muscle and ligament structures surrounding and supporting the breast, a special athletic bra, a regular bra, or no bra might be safe for athletic participants. The no-bra situation will probably occur in dance, in which case leotards can provide support if the breasts are small, and in swimming when both the stretch material of the suit and the water support the breasts.

To test a bra for adequate support, select one that covers the breasts; perform or simulate the activity you'll be doing and note whether there is any slapping down or lateral movement of the breasts; after five minutes of activity, stop and feel the breast and surrounding structure for signs of discomfort or ache or pain; check again for discomfort, ache, or pain after the usual activity period. If any signs of discomfort are felt, consider acquiring a garment that provides greater support. Remember also to check for excessive restriction of the breast, abrasiveness, or allergenic effects. Here, also, the bra's seams and metal parts can present problems.

Protective equipment

Some of the same criteria exist for protective equipment as for basic clothing. However, two criteria replace the initial level of protection of basic clothing. These are protection from extrinsic forces and safety to person and opponent. Because of the many sports women engage in, protective equipment is available from head to toe (see Figure 7-2).

Sports and dance often involve high forces that can cause trauma to the body. Although proper training can strengthen the muscles, ligaments, and bones, thus preventing some injuries, some impact forces are too great to withstand without the aid of protective equipment acting as a shock attenuator.

Athletes most apt to need protective equipment are those who traumatize the body repeatedly within a short period of time—such as during an hour of running or jogging—and those who are subject to a single high-level trauma—such as is encountered in football tackling or in falling.

How does one determine whether the risk is too great without protective equipment? Use the procedure of establishing and comparing benefit-and-risk scores. Arbitrarily select a scale of 0 to 10 and list all the benefits of wearing a particular protective device, awarding a numerical value to each benefit. Do the same for risks. The numerical value is a subjective estimate based upon the probability and severity of trauma to the area that would be protected by the device. The more frequent the occurrence and the more severe the impact, the greater will be the awarded score. Applying this procedure to the sport of volleyball, one can determine whether or not metal breast protectors should be worn or have much value for a female athlete.

RISK FACTORS	APPRAISAL OF RELATIVE DANGER	AWARDED RISK SCORE
possible trauma from:		
ball in flight from pass	velocity of ball is low; ball deforms easily	0
spiked or served ball	high ball velocity; ball deforms, breasts deform; contact area is relatively large	3
fall onto floor	breasts rarely encounter the initial impact force; breasts deform; contact area is large	1
collision with teammate	breasts are rarely struck; only if bony body part is struck might the impact area be small; breasts deform	1
	Total risk	5

BENEFIT FACTOR	APPRAISAL OF BENEFITS	AWARDED BENEFIT SCORE
breast protector	prevents contusions	5
	prevents temporary pain	2
	Total benefit	7

Therefore, it is not likely that any protective device beyond the supportive basic clothing is beneficial to volleyball participants. Contrast this with boxing and the decision to wear or not to wear a mouth guard.

RISK FACTORS	APPRAISAL OF RELATIVE DANGER	AWARDED RISK SCORE
possible trauma from:		
opponent striking		10
jaw	frequent occurrence; high velocity at impact; moderate to high mass	
mouth	broken teeth; cut mouth	

BENEFIT FACTOR	APPRAISAL OF BENEFITS	AWARDED BENEFIT SCORE
mouth protector	no orthodontist fees; no permanent disfigurement; no early loss of natural teeth	10

Certainly, doctors and athletic personnel have an obligation to be sure athletes wear mouth protectors while boxing.

Each sport and dance activity can be evaluated using this procedure. By this means, a rational decision can be made about protective equipment in a given activity. If such equipment is deemed necessary or desirable, the problem becomes one of selecting the best equipment available. The following are general guidelines for the selection of appropriate equipment for face and eyes, chest and torso, arms and hands, legs, and feet.

Face and eye protection: These protective devices should be lightweight, act as a unit with the head (move with, not independently of, the head), and protect vital areas—nose, eyes, cheekbone, chin, or other parts of the face or head or neck. The major criterion is that penetration is not allowed. For example, the two face masks in Figure 7-3 are sold commercially for use in softball. Note how one looks more effective and safer than the other. In addition, the equipment must be strong enough not to crack or break. For example, football helmets are designed to withstand multiple impacts, whereas a motorcycle helmet that suffers a single impact should be replaced.

Face and eye protective equipment must be made of nonirritants, have no sharp or metal parts that might injure the wearer or another athlete, and provide complete vision. The best way to check the visual field is through peripheral vision: Fix on a point level with the eyes and directly ahead. Place both arms in front at shoulder level and then move them apart until the hands cannot be seen. Note this position. Perform this test with and without the selected eye protectors. Not only does loss of peripheral vision due to poorly designed eye protectors decrease one's ability to perform, it also increases the danger to the performer.

FIGURE 7-2

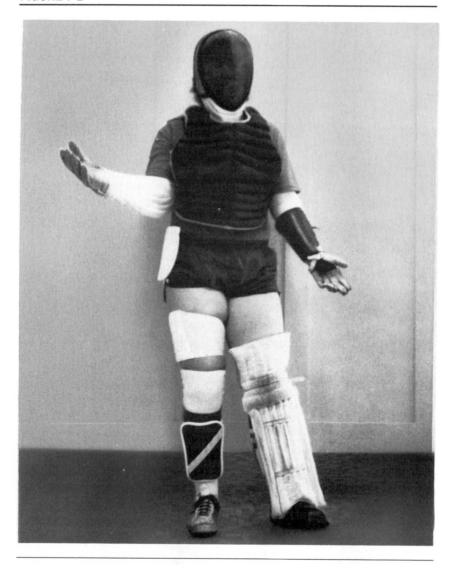

Protective equipment covering all parts of the human body:
fencing mask, softball chest protector, archery forearm guard and
finger glove, epeé arm and hand practice sleeve, hip pad, thigh
pad, knee pad, shin guard, field hockey goalkeeper's leg pad and
toe boot.

Motorcycle helmets obliterate sound and obscure vision. Both factors decrease the safety of the wearer. Motorcycle riders, when aware of such factors, will learn new modes of performing until new designs, possibly including "external ears," will become available for use.

Chest and torso protection: Protection here is more inadequate than with any of the other areas. The problem is that variety of body size results in difficulty of fit, and inadequate fit and the bulk required for protection reduces movement capabilities. The protector should cover the neck and clavicle area if another piece of clothing does not, and should also provide enough material to protect the sides of the torso. The material should absorb most of the impact and yet allow the person to move and not be injured by the hardness of the protector material.

Arms and hands protection: Elbow guards are recommended during skate-boarding, fencing with sabres, roller derby, and on

FIGURE 7-3

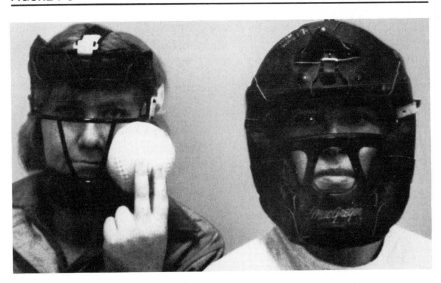

Face protectors: Inadequate safety design allows ball to strike cheek bone. Safe design provides additional head protection.

persons with prior elbow injuries that need protecting. Wrist and forearm wraps and other devices are primarily recommended during the long hours of practice, when trauma might occur because of the frequency as well as the severity of impacts. For example, volleyball coaches recommend long-sleeved shirts for practice and competition, and goalkeepers in field hockey, lacrosse, and ice hockey have bulky forearm and hand protection. Except for these protective applications, the arms are relatively free of protective equipment to allow quick movement.

The hands need to be protected whenever practice or long-term competition could cause blisters or excessive trauma. Golf gloves, gymnastics gloves, softball and baseball mitts and gloves, ski gloves (especially for rope-tow use), fencing gloves, and handball gloves available at sporting goods departments or stores usually meet the desired safety characteristics.

Leg protection: Leg protection consists of pads for the thighs and knees and guards for the shins and ankles. Protectors should be light in weight, nonslip, and not uncomfortable; they should not collect perspiration or rub and cause blisters or other irritation and should provide ample protection without restricting movement. Thigh pads do not always meet these demands, especially the comfort and stability criteria. These pads are most beneficial in uneven parallel bar practice, softball and baseball sliding, football, and fencing.

Most knee pads appear to be well designed. They have been shown to be nonrestrictive, to stay in place, and not cause irritation. Two types are available, to be selected according to playing surface. On artificial floors and for volleyball a slick, friction-free design is advocated so that impact forces may be tempered with sliding components. However, more research is needed to determine exactly how much force can be dissipated without adding restrictive bulk to the protective device.

Shin guards for sports such as field hockey, soccer, and rugby come in a multitude of designs. Select those that feel comfortable, cover the area, and have sufficient shock-attenuation quality to protect against strong impact. Beginners might want greater coverage about the ankles.

Foot protection: Protection for the feet comes in three categories: heel cups, orthoses, and reinforced shoes.

Heel cups and extra soles or other padding are used to absorb impact from repeated trauma such as in jumping and running. They are essential in overuse conditions and for young girls—young gymnasts, for example, might wear shoes when doing vaulting exercises.

Orthotic devices may be required for those with foot deformations or weaknesses and when excessive trauma is expected. However, if playing surfaces are resilient and the athlete/dancer has developed strong feet, orthoses should be unnecessary. Be wary of manufacturers attempting to sell expensive orthoses to everyone. It is true, however, that extra-shock-attenuation shoes usually are required for jogging along concrete or asphalt streets. Reinforced shoes are necessary for the field hockey player who is acting as goalkeeper.

In general, in choosing basic clothing and protective equipment look over the rules of the sport; they frequently list protective-equipment requirements. You might also check what the college and university athletes are wearing and what professional athletes wear. There is some danger, however, in using the latter as a guide because these highly skilled performers may accept higher risk scores without using protective equipment. Their bodies may be stronger and better able to tolerate trauma.

Specific, detailed information can be obtained from sports magazines, *Athletic Purchasing and Facilities* magazine, and the sports safety series from the American Alliance for Health, Physical Education, and Recreation, especially the monograph *Safety in Team Sports*.[3] Read the advertisements; determine whether the devices have been adequately tested in the sport or dance situations; demand evidence that the product meets the safety qualifications of the activity. If possible, select an ASTM-approved product.

Physicians, athletes, and recreational sports and dance participants need to bring to the attention of manufacturers any inadequacies of clothing and protective equipment. The president of the company or other high-level administrator, such as marketing manager or research and development director, should be contacted and told what is unacceptable. In addition, if lack of safety is part of the complaint, the Female Athlete Subcommittee of the ASTM's Sports Equipment and Facilities Committee should be contacted.

References

1. Klein KK: Beware of unbalanced shoes. *Phys Sportsmed* 6(11):155, 1978

2. Haycock C, Shierman G, and Gillette J: The female athlete: Does her anatomy pose problems? In *Proceedings of the 19th Conference on the Medical Aspects of Sports,* pp 1-8. Chicago: AMA, 1978

3. Borozne J, Morehouse CA, and Pechar SF: *Safety in Team Sports,* Monograph #3 Sports Safety Series. Washington: American Association for Health, Physical Education, and Recreation, 1977

NUTRITION

Elizabeth D. Munves, Ph.D.

CHAPTER

8

F or many centuries, individuals have believed that specific foods could influence athletic performance. And it is only recently that the science of nutrition has been able to make recommendations based on research. Food is the source of all nutrients; they are the building blocks of growth and development and provide the fuel for the rigors of athletic training and competition. Studies have demonstrated the relationships among nutrients, and from this has developed the concept of a balanced diet in which all nutrients are important to health and physical performance. It is essential that recommendations and regimens for dietary intake be based upon scientific fact instead of anecdotal opinion. Use of the latter can result in lopsided nutrition that will adversely affect the athlete. A balanced diet cannot be left to chance—it has to be planned. However, there is no "best" diet, and it is possible to adapt individual preferences to the plan for the optimum diet. Maintenance of a desirable nutritional intake is a year-round affair, even when a designated sport is out of season.

A proper diet

The athlete's nutritional needs are the same as that of all adults, with additional calories required according to the intensity of training and competition. Simply stated, there must be an adequate supply of calories, protein, fats, carbohydrates, minerals, vitamins, and water in suitable proportions and at appropriate times. The major nutrients, their functions, and their sources are listed in Table 8-1.

Calories: The energy need is determined by the sum of the requirements of the body plus the demands of the sport. This can vary considerably among individuals and also in the same individual according to variations in activity. Thus, each woman needs to become aware of her activity pattern. Keeping an activity diary for a week or two provides an accurate basis for calculating energy expenditure. An estimate of the athlete's basal calorie needs— those calories required just to maintain the body's process—can be made by using either a nomogram or a simple formula. The non-athlete and the athlete who is not training should add approximately 20 to 30 per cent more calories for light activity or work each day. The number of additional calories needed when the athlete is in training or competition can be estimated by multiplying the minutes engaged in a specific sport times the calorie cost of that activity per minute. The level of training can also influence calorie needs—the better-trained athlete is more efficient in the use of her muscles. However, she is also apt to move those muscles at greater speed, thereby increasing the energy expended. At best, one can only derive an estimate to be used as a guideline in preventing the accumulation of excess calories. Again, depending on the individual and her sport, the total calorie requirement can range from 2,200 to 5,000 calories. Individual energy requirements and the calorie cost of various sports are described in Chapter 5.

Calories are supplied by protein, fat, and carbohydrates. Each gram of protein and carbohydrate supplies four calories, whereas each gram of fat provides nine calories. A desirable distribution of calories would be 15 to 20 per cent from protein, 30 to 35 per cent from fat, and 50 to 55 per cent from carbohydrate. Thus, carbohydrates and fats are the major sources of calories. How these are distributed for maximum effectiveness during training and competition is treated below.

Carbohydrates: These fuel-rich substances are composed of carbon, oxygen, and hydrogen. The simplest forms of carbohydrates are sugar molecules, known as monosaccharides. There are three: glucose, fructose, and galactose. When two of these simple sugars are combined, the carbohydrate is called a disaccharide; in chains

TABLE 8-1

Major Nutrients: Their Sources and Functions

Nutrient	Major sources	Primary functions
PROTEIN		
Complete	Fish, poultry, meat, milk, cheese, eggs	Growth and repair of tissue; precursors of hormones, enzymes, and antibodies
Incomplete	Legumes, cereals, vegetables, nuts	Milk production during lactation; energy source (insignificant, inefficient, and expensive)
FATS		
Saturated fatty acids	Meats, dairy products, butter, most nuts, chocolate, non-dairy creamers, coconut oil, palm oil	Energy source; energy stored as adipose tissue
Polyunsaturated fatty acids	Oils (corn, safflower), soft margarine, walnuts	Carriers of fat-soluble vitamins A, D, E, and K
Monounsaturated	Olive oil, peanuts, peanut butter, mayonnaise	Enhance flavor and satiety value
CARBOHYDRATES		
*Polysaccharides	Breads, cereals, cereal products, legumes, tubers, baked goods, nuts	Enhance flavor; source of fiber; carriers of B-vitamins
Disaccharides (sucrose, lactose, maltose)	Cane and beet sugars, molasses, maple syrup, milk and milk products, malt products, fruits, vegetables	
Monosaccharides (glucose, fructose, galactose)	Breakdown of fruits, vegetables, and milk	

*Also includes indigestible fiber, such as cellulose, hemicelluloses, and pectins.

82

VITAMINS

Vitamin	Sources	Functions
Fat-soluble:		
A	Provitamin A in green leafy vegetables; butterfat, cheese, fortified margarine	Essential for integrity of epithelial cells; aids in resistance to infection; constituent of visual pigment
D	Cod-liver oil, eggs, fortified milk and margarine, sunlight	Promotes growth and mineralization of bones; increases absorption of calcium and phosphorus
E (tocopherol)	Seeds, vegetable oils, green leafy vegetables, margarines	Acts as an antioxidant to protect some vitamins and unsaturated fatty acids
K	Green leafy vegetables, grains, some meats and fruits	Essential in blood clotting
Water-soluble:		
B_1 (thiamine)	Pork, whole-grain cereals, legumes, enriched breads, cereals, rice	Coenzyme in reactions related to removal of carbon dioxide, thereby energy metabolism
B_2 (riboflavin)	Milk, cheese, whole-grain cereals, eggs, meat, enriched breads, cereals, rice	Constituent of two coenzymes for energy metabolism; involved in protein metabolism
Niacin	Liver, whole grains, legumes, meats, enriched breads, cereals, rice (can be formed from tryptophan)	Constituent of two coenzymes involved in oxidation of alcohol, many sugars, and many other aspects of energy metabolism
B_6 (pyridoxine)	Meats, vegetables (green), poultry, fish, potatoes, corn, whole grains	Constituent of coenzymes involved in amino-acid metabolism
Folacin	Green leafy vegetables, whole-grain cereals, liver, yeast	Coenzyme involved in nucleic-acid and amino-acid metabolism
B_{12}	Organ meats, muscle meats, fish, milk (not present in plant foods)	Normal development of red blood cells; coenzyme involved in nucleic-acid metabolism
Pantothenic acid	Distributed widely in plant and animal foods	Constituent of coenzyme A, which is necessary for energy metabolism; needed for normal skin growth and normal development of central nervous system
Biotin	Meats, vegetables, nuts, legumes, whole-grain cereals	Part of coenzymes required for fat synthesis, amino-acid metabolism, and glycogen formation
C (ascorbic acid)	Citrus fruits, fruits, tomatoes, salad greens	Necessary for intracellular matrix of cartilage, bone, and dentin; important in collagen synthesis

TABLE 8-1 cont.

Major Nutrients: Their Sources and Functions

Nutrient	Major sources	Primary functions
MINERALS		
Calcium	Milk, cheese, dark green vegetables, legumes	Bone and tooth formation; nerve transmission; blood clotting
Phosphorus	Meat, poultry, grains, milk, cheese	Bone and tooth formation
Magnesium	Whole grains, vegetables, beans, nuts	Participates in protein synthesis; influences nerve and muscle reactions; essential for bone formation
Iron	Liver, lean meats, legumes, green leafy vegetables, whole-grain and enriched cereals	Constituent of hemoglobin; necessary for energy metabolism
Zinc	Meats, eggs, milk, whole grains	Essential component of at least eight enzyme systems that affect metabolism of nutrients
Sodium	Salt and other seasonings; many additives; milk	Influences body-water balance; affects function of nerves; acid-base balance
Potassium	Fruits, meats, milk	Acid-base balance; affects functions of nerves; influences body-water balance
Fluorine	Drinking water from certain areas; tea; seafood	Formation of dentin; may be important in maintenance of bone structure
Iodine	Marine fish and shellfish; vegetables grown on iodine-rich soil; iodized salt	Constituent of thyroid hormones

Additional minerals known to be required:
Sulfur, chlorine, copper, silicon, vanadium, tin, nickel, selenium, manganese, molybdenum, chromium, cobalt.

of three or more they're called polysaccharides. The carbohydrate in food is reduced to the monosaccharide state in the gastrointestinal tract and then passes from the intestine to the bloodstream and then to the liver, where it is converted from fructose and galactose to glucose. Glucose is the only available form of carbohydrate that circulates for energy. Up to a certain point, excess glucose may be converted to glycogen and stored either in the liver or in the muscles. A surplus can be shunted into the "metabolic pool," where it becomes part of fatty acids and is stored as adipose tissue, or less frequently, contributes elements to the synthesis of amino acids. The importance of these reactions will be appreciated when the diet for specific sports is presented.

Fats: Fats, too, are composed of carbon, hydrogen, and oxygen, but in combinations different from carbohydrates. They exist as fatty acids, and depending on their structure, they are solid (saturated fat) or liquid (unsaturated fat). An essential nutrient (one that must be supplied in the diet) is linoleic acid, an unsaturated fatty acid. Fats also serve as carriers of the fat-soluble vitamins, A, D, E, and K. Fat is a concentrated source of energy, and its storage and mobilization provide a unique energy substrate for the endurance athlete. Fat in women is stored around the reproductive and other organs; some fat is beneath the skin to act as a thermal regulator; in the trained athlete, fat is also stored in muscle. The body composition of the average American female is approximately 25 per cent fat, whereas the male is 15 per cent fat. With training, fat is reduced—some highly trained female athletes have less than 5 per cent body fat.

It is thought that the American diet is too high in fats, especially saturated fats. Approximately 40 per cent of our diet consists of fats; this level of intake is believed by many researchers to be a significant factor in coronary heart disease.

Protein: Protein is needed for the maintenance and repair of body cells and tissues and as a component of enzymes and hormones that regulate body functions. Protein provides four calories per gram and is not regarded as a major source of energy. Protein is composed of 23 amino acids, 14 of which are synthesized in the body; the rest must be supplied by the diet. During digestion, protein is broken down into its component amino acids, which are absorbed through the intestinal wall and then circulated by the bloodstream. The life of amino acids is relatively short—probably only a few hours—and protein cannot be stored. To a varying degree, there is continual exchange of amino acids within cells and tissues; this reaction is referred to as dynamic equilibrium. Thus, the diet must provide adequate amounts of essential and nonessential amino acids.

Foods are classified as complete proteins—those that contain all the essential amino acids—and incomplete proteins—those lacking one or more. Complete proteins come from animal sources; plant foods generally provide incomplete proteins.

A strict vegetarian diet that is carefully planned can provide all the essential amino acids. The lacto-ovo-vegetarian—one who eats eggs and milk products—obtains all the essential amino acids from these foods, which enhance the quality of vegetable proteins.

Contrary to popular belief, exercise does not increase the protein requirement—the exercising muscle needs only energy, which is provided primarily by carbohydrates and fats. Many studies have shown that protein is not lost during exercise. A small increase in protein in the diet might be needed during strength-training when muscle mass is increasing. The protein content of the average American diet is almost twice that of the recommended allowances, so there is no need to plan an increase above the athlete's usual intake.

Excessive protein ingestion increases the fluid required for digestion and urinary elimination of nitrogen byproducts. This can have undesirable effects, as will be discussed later regarding the pregame meal.

Vitamins: Vitamins combine with enzymes to regulate the metabolism of nutrients within the body. If the diet includes a variety of foods within the suggested plan discussed later, it will contain adequate amounts of vitamins. There is no scientific evidence that the vitamin requirement increases significantly with exercise. Massive doses of vitamin-combinations or even of specific vitamins, have not been shown to improve performance and endurance, nor do they prevent injury or infection. Beliefs and practices among athletes fluctuate, and today the trend seems to be for overdoses of vitamins C, E, and B_{12}—vitamins found in good supply in our foods. The claims for increased athletic efficiency with megadoses have not been supported by research. Megadoses of vitamins are considered drugs, not foods, and may have deleterious effects. Toxic effects of fat-soluble vitamins have been documented, and some side effects related to renal function have been reported in individuals taking megadoses of vitamin C. It is true that a vegetarian who consumes only plants and cereals may have a diet deficient in B_{12}; however, most vegetarians eat milk, cheese, or eggs, which are sources of B_{12}.

Minerals: Minerals are essential for many body reactions—muscle contractions, control of heart beat, conduction of nerve impulses, and regulation of body fluids. The mineral content of the body is in delicate balance; some excess minerals are excreted in the urine and sweat, while some are stored, so that they are available in times of stress and/or inadequate intake. While the need for many minerals has long been recognized, how they function, how much we need each day, and the foods that contain them are currently being studied. Minerals required by the body are divided into two categories: those needed in large amounts and those referred to as trace minerals. The ones needed in large amounts are sodium, potassium, magnesium, and calcium. These are all present and easily available in our foods. The trace minerals are equally important and believed to be readily available from foods. One trace mineral, iron, is especially important to the female athlete, as it is to all women, and efforts must be made to ensure adequate intake.

Sodium is found in body fluids and serves as a regulator of body water. If an individual is low in sodium she will become dehydrated and experience muscle cramps that interfere with training. However, sodium-deficiency is unlikely—our problem is that we take in too much sodium, as much as 60 times the minimum requirement. The practice of taking salt tablets during training and competition to prevent sodium loss is unnecessary, and in fact, may have serious consequences.

Potassium plays an important role in the function of muscle cells, and deficiency can result in muscular weakness and fatigue. It has been suggested that extra potassium is required for exercise, but this does not mean large doses—the amount present in potassium-rich foods is sufficient.

Magnesium assists in the control of muscle contraction and is part of the mechanism that converts carbohydrates to energy.

TABLE 8-2

Selected Sources of Iron
(RDA for Women—18 mg)

FOOD			AMOUNT	IRON MG
Meats	Liver	Calves	3 oz	11.25
		Beef	3 oz	7.5
		Pork	3 oz	18.97
		Chicken	3 oz	9.0
		Lamb	3 oz	13.37
	Turkey, roasted		3 oz	1.5
	Pork chop		3 oz	2.7
	Hamburger		3 oz	3.0
	Beef, roast		3 oz	2.2
	Chicken		3 oz	1.3
	Bologna		3 oz	3.5
	Fish, haddock		3 oz	1.0
Eggs			1	.9
Vegetables	Kidney beans		½ cup	2.4
	Baked beans		½ cup	2.4
	Lima beans		½ cup	1.4
	Spinach		½ cup	2.0
	Mustard greens		½ cup	1.2
	Peas, green		½ cup	1.6
	Peas, split		½ cup	1.7
	Broccoli		1 stalk (med)	1.4
	Potato, baked		1 med	1.1
Fruits	Apricots, dried		3 whole	1.2
	Raisins		1 packet (½ oz)	.5
	Prunes, stewed		½ cup	1.9
	Apple		1 med	.4
Grains/ cereals	Bread, enriched		1 slice	.6
	Bread, whole wheat		1 slice	.8
	Rice, enriched		1 cup	1.4
	Cornflakes, enriched		1 cup	.6
Other	Milk		8 oz	.1
	Cheese, cheddar		1 oz	.2
	Nuts, peanuts		½ cup	1.5
	Honey		1 tablespoon	.1
	Molasses, blackstrap		1 tablespoon	3.2

The iron in foods of animal sources is absorbed more efficiently than iron in foods of plant origin. Portions indicated are those most commonly used.

Heavy exercise has been shown to lower magnesium via sweat loss, but these losses can easily be replaced by proper diet.

Calcium, in addition to being an essential component of the bones and teeth, also helps to control muscle contraction and acts as a regulator in numerous metabolic reactions. Many teenage girls have diets low in calcium as they switch from milk to peer-acceptable carbonated drinks. The National Research Council has recommended a daily level of calcium intake and the specific foods needed. Calcium requirements are not increased by exercise.

As previously indicated, iron is important to the female athlete; the recommended intake for women is 18 mg a day. Iron deficiency is the most common nutritional deficiency seen in the United States in recent years. We have apparently increased our needs while our intake of iron-rich foods has decreased. Deficiency has been seen in women from moderate- and high-income families as well as in those from low-income families. A small amount of iron, totaling less than 1 mg/day, is lost regularly from the body through exfoliated cells, hair, and in bile, but the female may lose another 5 to 45 mg during her menstrual period. Iron is needed to carry oxygen to the cells, and the athlete must prevent deficiency in order to ensure endurance and optimum physical performance. There are few iron-rich foods; iron is found in small amounts in a number of foods. Meat, supplying iron in the form of heme, is one of the better sources. A vegetarian, then, needs to plan her diet carefully. Milk products, while they will help the vegetarian's amino-acid pattern, are poor sources of iron. It would be wise to medically monitor the iron levels of the female athlete and provide iron supplements, if they are necessary. Table 8-2 summarizes food sources of iron.

Nutritional requirements for healthy women

As nutrients essential for health have been identified, recommendations have been made for their use. The first Recommended Dietary Allowances (RDA) were issued in 1941 under the auspices of the National Research Council. Levels of intake, by age and sex, were identified as "recommended amounts," and to allow for variations in individual needs, were set well above what were believed to be the minimum levels. Thus, although nutrition programs use

TABLE 8-3 A

Food and Nutrition Board, National Academy of Sciences-National Research Council

Recommended Daily Dietary Allowances,ᵃ Revised 1979

Designed for the maintenance of good nutrition of practically all healthy people in the U.S.A.

PROTEIN · FAT-SOLUBLE VITAMINS

	Age (years)	Weight (kg)	Weight (lbs)	Height (cm)	Height (in)	Protein (g)	Vitamin A (μg R.E.)ᵇ	Vitamin D (μg)ᶜ	Vitamin E (mg α T.E.)ᵈ
Females	11-14	46	101	157	62	46	800	10	8
	15-18	55	120	163	64	46	800	10	8
	19-22	55	120	163	64	44	800	7.5	8
	23-50	55	120	163	64	44	800	5	8
	51+	55	120	163	64	44	800	5	8
Pregnant						+30	+200	+5	+2
Lactating						+20	+400	+5	+3

WATER-SOLUBLE VITAMINS

	Age (years)	Weight (kg)	Weight (lbs)	Height (cm)	Height (in)	Vitamin C (mg)	Thiamin (mg)	Riboflavin (mg)	Niacin (mg N.E.)ᵉ	Vitamin B₆ (mg)	Folacinᶠ (μg)	Vitamin B₁₂ (μg)
Females	11-14	46	101	157	62	50	1.1	1.3	15	1.8	400	3.0
	15-18	55	120	163	64	60	1.1	1.3	14	2.0	400	3.0
	19-22	55	120	163	64	60	1.1	1.3	14	2.0	400	3.0
	23-50	55	120	163	64	60	1.0	1.2	13	2.0	400	3.0
	51+	55	120	163	64	60	1.0	1.2	13	2.0	400	3.0

Pregnant				+20	+0.4	+0.3	+2	+0.6	+400	+1.0
Lactating				+40	+0.5	+0.5	+5	+0.5	+100	+1.0

MINERALS

	Age (years)	Weight (kg)	(lbs)	Height (cm)	(in)	Calcium (mg)	Phosphorus (mg)	Magnesium (mg)	Iron (mg)	Zinc (mg)	Iodine (μg)
Females	11-14	46	101	157	62	1200	1200	300	18	15	150
	15-18	55	120	163	64	1200	1200	300	18	15	150
	19-22	55	120	163	64	800	800	300	18	15	150
	23-50	55	120	163	64	800	800	300	18	15	150
	51+	55	120	163	64	800	800	300	10	15	150
Pregnant						+400	+400	+150	g	+ 5	+ 25
Lactating						+400	+400	+150	g	+10	+ 50

a The allowances are intended to provide for individual variations among most normal persons as they live in the United States under usual environmental stresses. Diets should be based on a variety of common foods in order to provide other nutrients for which human requirements have been less well defined. See Table 8-3 B for suggested average energy intakes. See Table 8-3 C for estimated safe intakes of some vitamins and minerals.

b Retinol equivalents. 1 retinol equivalent = 1 μg retinol or 6 μg carotene.

c As cholecalciferol. 10 μg cholecalciferol = 400 I.U. vitamin D.

d α tocopherol equivalents. 1 μg d-α-tocopherol = 1 α T.E.

e 1 N.E. (niacin equivalent) = 1 mg of niacin or 60 mg of dietary tryptophan.

f The folacin allowances refer to dietary sources as determined by Lactobacillus casei assay after treatment with enzymes ("conjugases") to make polyglutamyl forms of the vitamin available to the test organism.

g The increased requirement during pregnancy cannot be met by the iron content of habitual American diets nor by the existing iron stores of many women; therefore, the use of 30 to 60 mg of supplemental iron is recommended. Iron needs during lactation are not substantially different from those of nonpregnant women, but continued supplementation of the mother for two to three months after parturition is advisable in order to replenish stores depleted by pregnancy.

the RDA as a guideline, intake of a specific nutrient below these levels does not necessarily mean that a diet is deficient. The allowances are revised every five years, and as our knowledge about nutrition has increased, the number of nutrients in the table has expanded. The RDA does not contain all the nutrients that are known to be needed; it includes only those for which there are significant data for making recommendations. Table 8-3 (A, B, and C) cites the current RDA.

TABLE 8-3 B

Mean Heights and Weights and Recommended Energy Intake

Category	Age (years)	Weight (kg)	(lb)	Height (cm)	(in)	Energy needs (with range) (kcal)	(MJ)
Females	11-14	46	101	157	62	2200 (1500-3000)	9.2
	15-18	55	120	163	64	2100 (1200-3000)	8.8
	19-22	55	120	163	64	2100 (1700-2500)	8.8
	23-50	55	120	163	64	2000 (1600-2400)	8.4
	51-75	55	120	163	64	1800 (1400-2200)	7.6
	76+	55	120	163	64	1600 (1200-2000)	6.7
Pregnancy						+300	
Lactation						+500	

The energy allowances for the young adults are for women doing light work. The allowances for the two older age groups represent mean energy needs over these age spans, allowing for a 2 per cent decrease in basal (resting) metabolic rate per decade and a reduction in activity of 200 kcal/day for women between 51 and 75 years and 400 kcal for women over 75. The customary range of daily energy output is shown for adults in parentheses, and is based on a variation in energy needs of ±400 kcal at any one age, emphasizing the wide range of energy intakes appropriate for any group of people.

Energy allowances for children through age 18 are based on median energy intakes of children of these ages followed in longitudinal growth studies. The values in parentheses are 10th and 90th percentiles of energy intake to indicate the range of energy consumption among children of these ages.

From Recommended Daily Dietary Allowances, revised 1979. Food and Nutrition Board, National Academy of Sciences-National Research Council, Washington, D.C.

Nutritionists soon realized the RDA was not a teaching tool, and a food plan was developed that would include groups of foods containing nutrients in RDA-recommended amounts. It is important to have a variety of foods within each group; for example, not all meats contain the same vitamins and trace minerals. Still, following such a plan permits considerable flexibility and allows for individual likes and dislikes. The food groups are:

Fruits and vegetables: Fruits and vegetables are all excellent sources of vitamins and minerals and small amounts of carbohydrate. They also provide cellulose, an indigestible carbohydrate that contributes to elimination. Within this group, emphasis is placed on one serving of a fruit, such as citrus, melon, tomatoes, or berries to provide vitamin C, and one serving of a dark green leafy vegetable, such as spinach or raw salad greens, to supply vitamin A, folic acid, and minerals. Four daily servings of foods in this group are suggested.

Cereals and grains: This group includes cooked and cold cereal, grains such as rice and barley, grain products including pasta (spaghetti, macaroni, noodles), and breads, flour, and baked goods. These foods provide an inexpensive carbohydrate source of energy, as well as some protein, minerals including trace minerals, and some of the B-vitamins. Whole-grain cereal also provides fiber. Whole-grain products are emphasized, but if refined products are selected, they should be enriched (thiamine, riboflavin, niacin, and iron are added). If calories are needed, foods from this group are excellent choices because of their nutrient density. Four or more servings are recommended.

The protein group: This group includes fish, poultry, meat, eggs, and vegetarian sources of protein such as legumes and nuts. Legumes consist of beans (navy, kidney, lima, and soya), lentils, peanuts, and dried peas (yellow, split pea, black-eyed). If plant proteins are used, they need to be eaten in combinations that will provide all essential amino acids. Other nutrients supplied are B-vitamins and iron. Meats and eggs are high in saturated fats, so a prudent approach would be to limit these foods to one or two a week and emphasize fish, poultry, and vegetable proteins. Two or more daily servings (3 to 4 oz/serving) are recommended.

Milk and milk products: This group consists of milk in its various forms—whole, skim, 1 per cent fat, 2 per cent fat, yogurt, and cheese. These foods are rich sources of calcium (the best), riboflavin, and protein. Milk products made from milk-fat—butter and cream cheese—are not usually considered in this category as they do not provide the nutrients mentioned above. The fats that are in milk and cheese are saturated fats, and may need to be limited. Skim milk and skim-milk cheeses are excellent choices for the athlete. The adult woman should include two servings from this group in her diet each day.

Table 8-4 suggests how the Four Food Plan can be adapted for a woman who needs fewer than 2,000 calories. Keep in mind that this meal plan provides a balanced diet: one that contains all the

TABLE 8-3 C

Estimated Safe and Adequate Daily Dietary Intakes

Vitamins

	Age (years)	Vitamin K (μg)	Biotin (μg)	Pantothenic Acid (mg)
Adolescents	11+	50-100	100-200	4-7
Adults		70-140	100-200	4-7

Electrolytes

	Age (years)	Sodium (mg)	Potassium (mg)	Chloride (mg)
Adolescents	11+	900-2700	1525-4575	1400-4200
Adults		1100-3300	1875-5625	1700-5100

From Recommended Daily Dietary Allowances, revised 1979. Food and Nutrition Board, National Academy of Sciences-National Research Council, Washington, D.C.

nutrients the competing athlete needs. No single category of food contains all nutrients, so it is essential that the suggested number of portions be taken from each group.

The athlete in training and competition needs to modify this plan in two ways: to increase calories and/or plan for days of competition. The pre- and postgame diet is discussed below. However, the athlete may need a caloric intake higher than what the diet illustrated in Table 8-4 provides. The best way to do this is to increase the number of portions from the cereal group and to increase the size of portions of the other three. This will increase calories as well as vitamins and minerals.

of Additional Selected Vitamins and Minerals[a]

Trace elements[b]

	Age (years)	Copper (mg)	Manganese (mg)	Fluoride (mg)
Adolescents	11+	2.0-3.0	2.5-5.0	1.5-2.5
Adults		2.0-3.0	2.5-5.0	1.5-4.0

Trace elements[b]

	Age (years)	Chromium (mg)	Selenium (mg)	Molybdenum (mg)
Adolescents	11+	0.05-0.2	0.05-0.2	0.15-0.5
Adults		0.05-0.2	0.05-0.2	0.15-0.5

a Because there is less information on which to base allowances, these figures are not given in the main table of the RDA and are provided here in the form of ranges of recommended intakes.

b Since the toxic levels for many trace elements may be only several times usual intakes, the upper levels for the trace elements given in this table should not be habitually exceeded.

Other food items

Fats: These include butter, margarines, oils, and meat fats such as lard and bacon. These foods are high in calories yet add flavor and zest to meals. Dairy and meat fats are primarily saturated. In addition to calories, vegetable oils and some margarines supply essential fatty acids, and dairy fats are a source of vitamin A. For those watching calories, intake should be limited.

Sugars: Sugar is available as granulated, brown sugar, and molasses; in candy, honey, jam, soft drinks, and in desserts and sugar-coated cereals. Our per capita consumption of sugar is rising each year. This is considered unwise, as forms of sugar provide only calories; the minuscule amounts of other nutrients in brown sugar and molasses are too small to be of value. Sugar is absorbed quickly into the circulating blood, and stimulates the secretion of insulin. This hormone removes excess blood sugar, causing a rapid drop, and within a few hours the individual is hungry. This phenomenon is known as reactive hypoglycemia. The role of sugar in the diet of the athlete is discussed below.

Alcohol: While alcohol contains calories—seven per gram—it should not be considered a food. Research has indicated that alcohol has a direct toxic effect on the liver and can result in the accumulation of fat. It acts on the central nervous system, and even small amounts have been shown to affect judgment and coordination, resulting in impairment of performance.

Caffeine: Caffeine is found in coffee, tea, cola drinks, and chocolate. Even though caffeine acts as a central nervous system stimulant, there is no evidence that it improves the performance of athletes. In fact, its undesirable effects, increasing the work of the heart and inducing strong diuresis, means it should be used only in moderation by the athlete.

Special foods

Can any foods improve the status of the woman athlete? There is no scientific evidence that specialty items, such as concentrated protein powder, kelp, brewer's yeast, bee pollen, bone meal, desiccated liver, and megadoses of vitamins, to name a few that are popular, do anything to enhance performance and endurance and improve health. The athlete who depends on a single (or several) specialty items to provide her with all she needs and who neglects to eat regular foods forfeits essential nutrients.

Questions also arise concerning the benefits of foods described as organic or natural. Organic foods are those grown without chemical fertilizers. From a nutritional standpoint, there is no advantage to this. Both kinds of foods undergo the same digestive process, and the muscle cell is unable to differentiate between them. Natural foods are usually defined as those that have not been processed, but are consumed as produced. From a nutritional and health standpoint, there are advantages and disadvantages. Grains and cereals that have not been refined (a process that removes the layers rich in B-vitamins and some of the trace minerals) may be superior. However, raw milk, which is unpasteurized, may carry harmful bacteria. (Indeed, before pasteurizing of milk was required, brucellosis was quite common.) Even though the small amount of vitamin C in milk is markedly reduced by pasteurization, the health benefits far outweigh the small nutritional loss. The additional nutritional value of other natural food items—raw sugar, specific kinds of honey—is insignificant. It is important not to confuse flavor and taste with nutrient intake. With respect to "natural foods," only a few items are nutritionally worth the higher cost.

Weight control

The goal of the athlete is to maintain her best competitive weight; scientifically, this refers to the percentage of body fat. As I said before, the norm is around 25 per cent for women. At the present time, there is no known desirable percentage of body fat for women athletes, but above 25 per cent is considered excessive. The lowest percentage of fat, about 2 per cent, has been reported for gymnasts. This may be effective for competition, but the long-range implications for health are unknown.

When compared against women of so-called desirable weight, the athlete may appear to be overweight, as she generally has a greater muscle mass, which weighs more than an equal amount of fat. A more precise way of clinically estimating body fat is by measuring the skinfold at designated sites with calipers specially

Four Food Plan Menu—1,760 Calories

TABLE 8-4

	Group 1 Fruits and Vegetables	Group 2 Cereals and Grains	Group 3 Protein Group	Group 4 Milk and Milk Products	Fats	Other: Desserts Sugars
Breakfast	Orange juice, 4 oz—60 calories	Cereal, dry or cooked, ¾ cup—90 calories; Toast, 1 slice—36 calories		Milk, ½ cup—85 calories	Margarine, 1 tsp—35 calories	Sugar, 1 tsp—23 calories; Tea, 1 cup (clear)—0 calories
Lunch	Apple—80 calories Lettuce, 1 leaf—0 calories	Bread, 2 slices (sandwich)—72 calories	Tunafish salad, 2 oz (sandwich)—110 calories	Milk, skim, 8 oz—85 calories	Mayonnaise, 1 tsp—35 calories	
Dinner	Baked potato—145 calories; Green salad—5 calories; Green peas, ½ cup—55 calories	Roll—85 calories	Roast chicken, 4 oz—200 calories	Milk, skim, 8 oz—85 calories	Margarine, 2 tsp—105 calories; Salad dressing, 3 tsp—85 calories	
Snacks	Banana—100 calories	Crackers, 3—36 calories		Cheese, ½ oz—50 calories		Ice cream, 3 fl oz—100 calories
Number of Servings	6	6	6 oz	3	7 tsp	2

designed for this purpose. Using conversion tables that are ordinarily supplied with the calipers, the true percentage of body fat can be determined.

Weight loss: A weight-loss program should be carefully planned lest muscle mass be lost as well as adipose tissue. The overweight woman athlete must understand that a proper program takes time. This can best be accomplished by reducing calorie intake and increasing calorie expenditure. The woman in training may have only a little additional time to devote to physical activity each day. She does not want to jeopardize the effect of training or impair her health, so she cannot create a large daily calorie deficit. To lose one pound of adipose tissue requires a deficit of 3,500 calories. Thus, a 500-calorie daily deficit will cause a one-pound loss per week.

An individual, realistic program should be developed for each woman, determined by her age, nutritional needs, and physical activity. The best way is to keep a food and activity record for one week. The total calorie expenditure is determined, and the schedule is examined for time that may be available for extra physical activity. A revised energy-expenditure and energy-intake plan that will bring about a desired rate of fat loss yet maintain the individual in optimum health and condition is then drawn up.

A weight-loss diet containing fewer than 2,000 calories is probably not necessary for the athlete in training or competition. Off-season, it may be possible to decrease intake somewhat more (to 1,600 to 1,800 calories; see Table 8-4) and increase the usual energy expenditure. The caloric intake should be determined by the amount of activity possible. While the calorie expenditure of physical activity may seem too low to be effective, an extra hour each day can add considerably to a weekly or monthly loss.

Most popular weight-loss diets are undesirable as they are usually nutritionally inadequate. If they are high in protein or high in fat, they affect the overall metabolic process, thereby resulting in the production of excessive ketones and the depletion of glycogen stores. Such regimens adversely influence performance.

Very low-calorie diets—those containing 1,200 calories or fewer—or even a starvation program, have no place in the life of a woman athlete.

An effective weight-loss program must include continuous energy intake and expenditure records. Only in this way can the individual become aware of her problems, plan changes, and evaluate the success of the plans. Eventually the regimen will be the basis for life-long weight maintenance.

Weight gain: Some athletes find it more difficult to gain weight than to lose weight. To gain a pound of muscle mass requires an excess of 2,500 calories plus physical activity. Again, one needs to begin by analyzing a carefully kept food and activity record. The activity program should be assessed for its calorie expenditure and the diet should be assessed for nutritional adequacy and calorie content. It also must be examined for the possibility of adding calorie-dense foods without affecting overall nutritive intake. Foods that could fit into this pattern are low-bulk carbohydrates and vegetable oils. However, it is possible for these foods to create a feeling of satiety and thereby reduce the total intake. For some, a calorie-dense—sandwich and beverage—bedtime snack can be added; this increases intake without affecting the daily pattern. It is not necessary to emphasize protein; as more calories are consumed, adequate amino acids are provided in extra amounts of food. No more than 500 to 1,000 calories above the number of calories expended per day should be added. In fact, a small daily increment over a long period is probably the most effective.

Because the woman athlete wants to gain lean body mass, not fat, her weight-gain efforts should occur during a vigorous training program. The weight gain can be monitored by regularly measuring skinfolds to ensure that fat content remains the same and that the increased exercise is sufficient to form muscle mass.

Both weight loss and weight gain for the athlete should be medically supervised.

Diets in relation to sports events

There are as many customs of eating in relation to sports events as there are athletes. Some of the practices are personal adaptations of physiological principles, and others are dictated by myths. It is important that nutrition not interfere with competitive performance, yet provide needed energy. On the day of competition, the influence of physical and psychological stress, with its attendant nervous tension, needs to be recognized. Ritualizing eating is the athlete's means of coping with this stress. However, one must be sure that such patterns are not in conflict with scientific fact.

The following principles should be followed in planning pregame nutrition:

● There should be enough energy to maintain an adequate blood-sugar level and to avoid any feelings of hunger and weakness during the period of competition.

● The food and fluid intake should ensure an optimal state of hydration.

● The stomach and lower bowel should be empty by the time of competition.

● Any food that might result in gastrointestinal upset should be avoided.

● Foods that are acceptable to the athlete—those she thinks will help her win—should be included.

Carbohydrate-loading: Fuel for competition is provided by carbohydrates and fats. It has been shown that carbohydrate reserves can be a limiting factor during high-level performance when activity is sustained for more than one hour, as in cross-country skiing, long-distance running, or bicycle-racing. However, it has recently been shown that dietary manipulation prior to competition can increase the glycogen level in muscles. A week-long regimen to accomplish this has come to be known as "carbohydrate-packing." Carbohydrate is restricted for the first few days, and the diet consists of mainly protein and fat. Concurrently, the athlete maintains a vigorous training schedule. She exercises those muscles used for her specific sport, thereby depleting their glycogen stores. By midweek, she will probably tire easily, and her performance will not be her best. At this point, she changes to a high-carbohydrate diet, one that is adequate in protein and fat, but stresses unlimited carbohydrates. This diet, including the regimen described in the following paragraphs, is maintained until the day of competition. The research on carbohydrate-packing has shown that glycogen levels can be almost tripled through dietary manipulation. While this technique is believed to be effective, most suggest that the routine be used sparingly—one or two times a year for the most important events. If used too often, it is possible that the metabolic processes may become conditioned to prefer carbohydrate fuel instead of free fatty acids. Also, the method has not been effective with all athletes.

The precompetition diet: The plan should begin at least 48 hours before competition; some have even recommended it begin at 72 hours. Foods high in sodium should be limited; this includes processed meats—luncheon meats, hot dogs, and the like—most seasonings and condiments, and obviously, highly salted items. Salt increases the fluid content of the body, and, while it is essential that the athlete be well hydrated, excess fluids are undesirable. Water intake should be generous: eight glasses per day.

At least 48 hours prior to competition the meals should stress carbohydrate, yet be balanced. This allows for maximum glycogen storage to provide a ready source of energy. Conditioning and training are usually reduced a day or so prior to competition. Thus, muscles can fully recover and store glycogen. The recommendation is to limit high-fiber foods—raw vegetables and fruits, whole-grain cereals and seeds—during this period. This minimizes the need for bowel elimination during an event. Also, flatulence-causing foods should be avoided. Flatus, a mixture of gases in the gastrointestinal tract, can be distracting and can adversely affect performance. Foods that contribute to this include beans, legumes, and members of the cabbage family—broccoli, brussels sprouts, cabbage, sauerkraut.

The pregame meal: This meal, consisting of regular foods, should be eaten up to three to four hours prior to the event. This permits foods to be digested and absorbed. The athlete is probably under significant nervous tension, a state that can influence the digestive process. There can be a decrease in blood flow to the stomach and small intestine and decreased motility, as well. On the other hand, tension can increase the motility of the lower intestinal tract, causing diarrhea. Gastrointestinal reactions to stress are highly individual and vary among individuals at different times. Food likes and dislikes and concerns about food are apt to be exaggerated at this time.

The pregame meal should be high in carbohydrate yet low in sugar; it must be low in protein and fat. This principle is in direct contrast to the practice of a pregame steak dinner. Desirable carbohydrate foods are breads, cereals (either dry or cooked), pasta (spaghetti, macaroni), potatoes, rice, fruit, and fruit juices. Even though sugar is a carbohydrate and a quick source of energy, it is a poor pregame food, as it causes rebound hypoglycemia. Fructose, the sugar found in fruits, has to be converted to glucose by the liver and thereby is available more slowly; thus, it does not contribute to this problem. A meal high in protein is usually high in fat as well and is undesirable. Protein foods require the elimination of fixed acids by the kidneys and thereby withdraw water from the body. Fatty foods slow the emptying time of the stomach and should be avoided at pregame time.

By taking bouillon or broth at least three hours before the event, an adequate salt intake is provided. Two to three cups of water should be taken also. The athlete should enter an event well hydrated; as during exercise, fluid is lost in sweating and exhaled breath. However, too much fluid can create the need to urinate.

Some athletes have tried liquid pregame meals that are easily digested and nutritionally adequate. There are several on the market that were initially developed for hospital patients and contain carbohydrates, fats, and proteins. They have been successfully used up to 2½ hours before game time.

During competition: Athletes may need to eat during events to maintain energy and prevent dehydration. Glucose, dextrose pills, cubes of sugar, honey, and hard candy are not the best diet, as these draw fluids to the intestinal tract and are apt to add to the problem of dehydration. Thus, the athlete should drink a limited amount of sweetened uncarbonated liquid, such as fruit juices, in small amounts at frequent intervals. A suggested pattern is to sip hourly half a cup of fruit juice.

A number of sports, such as tennis and swimming, may extend over one day or two days with several hours between events. If it is possible to do, eating regularly scheduled meals as close to normal as possible is the best regimen. This schedule should be modified by the guidelines enumerated for the pregame meal. Supplementing the program with sweetened beverages during the contest helps maintain optimum blood sugar and muscle glycogen as well as hydration.

Postgame meal: This meal is often neglected in the overall planning. The athlete can be either keyed up or depressed, and she may not be ready to eat. Often there are travel deadlines to meet and, for the traveling team, it may not be easy to obtain desired food. However, whenever possible, a dinner-type meal should be offered, one that is high in calories, offering protein, carbohydrates, vitamins, and minerals, in a comfortable place with friends, when the athlete is relaxed enough to eat. This may be from one to several hours after the contest. Beverages containing stimulants should be avoided as the athlete may still be tense.

A few questions about nutrition may remain. The following are the ones most frequently raised.

Is a training table necessary? Strictly speaking, the athlete should be able to select an appropriate diet from available foods. Additional calories could come from extra portions. However, a training table, if under the supervision of a dietitian, can become a teaching experience, can ensure that the athlete does not consume a lopsided diet because of mistaken notions, and provides regular meals. The psychological benefit of creating an esprit de corps among the team cannot be minimized.

How many meals a day is best for the athlete? Present evidence indicates that an athlete's performance is better when she eats at least three meals a day; perhaps more frequent but smaller meals might be beneficial. However, skipping a meal, breakfast for example, has been shown to adversely affect performance.

Does the athlete need special foods? The nutrients needed by the athlete can be provided in a balanced diet as described in the Four Food Plan. Items containing concentrated nutrients, such as protein and sugar, are not recommended, as they may adversely affect normal hydration. Taking these items can also distort the total food intake so that the athlete may not eat a complete balanced diet.

Does the woman athlete have any special nutritive needs? The only special concern for the woman athlete is her need for iron. Because of loss during menstruation, she has to include an adequate intake of iron each day. Her iron status should be monitored, and it may be necessary to prescribe a supplement. She should continue to emphasize an iron-rich diet, even though she may take a supplement.

Will taking vitamins improve performance? Vitamins are needed by the athlete and the nonathlete, but these can be provided by a balanced diet. Large doses of all vitamins, or of specific ones, have not been shown to affect athletic performance. In fact, megadoses of fat-soluble vitamins are known to have toxic effects.

Further reading

Nutrition in general

Adams C: *Nutritive Values of American Foods in Common Units,* Agriculture Handbook No. 456, Agriculture Research Services, USDA. Washington: Government Printing Office, 1976

Church CF and Church HM: *Food Values of Portions Commonly Used,* 12th ed. Philadelphia: Lippincott, 1975

Deutsch RM: *Realities of Nutrition.* Palo Alto: Bull Publishing, 1976

Mayer J: *A Diet for Living.* New York: David McKay, 1975

Nutrition Reviews Present Knowledge in Nutrition, 4th ed. New York and Washington: The Nutrition Foundation, 1976

Stare FJ and McWilliams M: *Living Nutrition,* 2nd ed. New York: Wiley, 1977

Stuart RB and Davis B: *Slim Chance in a Fat World—Behavioral Control of Obesity.* Champaign, Ill: Research Press, 1972

White, PL: *Let's Talk About Food.* Chicago: AMA, 1974

Nutrition for the athlete

Buskirk ER: Nutrition for the athlete. In *Sports Medicine,* Ryan A and Allman FL, eds, p 141. New York: Academic Press, 1974

Huse DM and Nelson RA: Basic, balanced diet meets requirements of athletes. *Phys Sportsmed* 5:52, 1977

Mayer J and Bullen B: Nutrition and athletics. In *Proceedings of the 6th International Congress of Nutrition,* Edinburgh, Aug 9-15, 1963. London: E & S Livingstone, 1964

Mirkin G and Hoffman M: *The Sportsmedicine Book.* Boston: Little, Brown, 1978

Nutrition for Athletics: A Handbook for Coaches. Washington: American Association for Health, Physical Education, and Recreation, 1971

Roundtable: Nutrition practices in athletics abroad. *Phys Sportsmed,* 5:33, 1977

Slovic, P: What helps the long distance runner run. *Nutrition Today* 10:18, 1975

Smith NJ: *Food for Sport.* Palo Alto: Bull Publishing, 1966

Wagner R: Nutrition for athletics. *Coach and Athlete,* p 28, March 1976

MEDICAL ILLNESS

Allan M. Levy, M.D.

CHAPTER

9

Although the female athlete is subject to all the illnesses that affect the general public, I am limiting this discussion to conditions that cause serious problems in the sports world.

Upper respiratory infections

The No. 1 cause of loss of training or performance time is the upper respiratory infection or common cold. There are many misconceptions about its transmission, including the notion that becoming chilled or wet can cause a cold. Yet, volunteers exposed to a cold environment and to rhinovirus organisms had no increased incidence of colds.[1, 2] Similarily, submerging volunteers in ice baths failed to increase incidence. So there need be no fear of catching a cold because of strenuous activity followed by a hot shower and a trip outside in frigid weather.

The most important predisposing factor is fatigue. The incidence of respiratory infection usually rises as the season goes on and the athlete becomes more fatigued by training and the demands of performance. The individual who is overtrained can expect a much higher incidence of infections because the body does not have the ability to mobilize resistance factors when it is severely and chronically fatigued.

As there is little we can do to shorten the duration of a respiratory infection, our efforts should be concentrated on prevention through maintenance of good body condition, adequate rest, proper diet, and sensible training. Avoidance of contact is the best prevention, especially prior to a major event. This should also be practiced when going to an area where respiratory infections are epidemic. We now know that skin transmission of infection occurs, and it is therefore important to wash the hands frequently.

Many Americans believe that high doses of vitamin C help prevent colds and clear symptoms more rapidly. However, there is no evidence that vitamin C has either effect. There is also no evidence that vitamin E or megavitamin therapy can lower the incidence or change the course of colds.

Once the respiratory infection has started, treatment should be completely symptomatic. Aspirin is useful for fever, headache, and malaise and is probably the most important drug available. Decongestants and cough preparations may be used as necessary. It should be remembered that many of the cold preparations contain antihistamines and that these act as depressants in many people. While these agents may be helpful in maintaining unbroken sleep at night, they should not be used by the athlete during training or events, as they can interfere with performance and may actually depress reflexes to the point at which injury occurs. During play, nasal sprays or cold-preparations made with ephedrine-like drugs should be used.

Should an athlete with a URI practice? One must balance the effect of rest on the course of the illness against the psychological and physical effects of loss of training time.[3] There is interesting evidence that nonsmokers have no loss of respiratory function during a URI but that there's a definite decrease in those who are smokers.[4] This would be a factor to consider. Fever is another factor—it is wise to restrict activity if the athlete has a temperature above 100 degrees F.

Among the significant complications of upper respiratory infections are sinusitis, tracheobronchitis, and pneumonia. Sinusitis may be viral in origin, secondary to the viral URI itself; here, treatment is symptomatic. However, there may be a true bacterial sinusitis—an acute severe illness with fever, pain, and toxicity. The usual organisms are pneumococcus or streptococcus. This must be vigorously treated with antibiotics because the complications can be grave.

Patients with tracheobronchitis should have a throat culture to determine the cause and should be treated accordingly. Particularly important are the use of cough suppressants before practice and at bedtime—the cough is due to tracheal irritation and would be aggravated by rapid breathing.

Pneumonia is the most severe of the complications. Bacterial pneumonias can be treated with antibiotics, and mycoplasma pneumonia responds well to erythromycin or tetracycline, while treatment of viral pneumonia is symptomatic. Viral etiology is less common in the adolescent. Pneumonia has a long recovery period, and complications may occur if the athlete is rushed back to activity and pushed beyond her capacities.

Many people call the common URI "flu." However, influenza is a definite illness characterized by fever, malaise, and cough. Should athletes be immunized against flu? Effectiveness of the vaccine can vary from 0 to 80 per cent, depending on the specificity of the vaccine for the infecting strain. While it might be of value to immunize a team that is going into an epidemic area, one must remember that the incidence of side effects can run as high as 20 per cent. In general, I don't feel that mass immunization of the athletic population is of any value.

Another common problem of athletes is allergy, including allergic rhinitis, or hay fever, and asthma. Either of these may seriously interfere with performance. There is marked interference with respiratory capacity and oxygen exchange, usually accompanied by marked fatigue. Whether this is due to increased histamine release or to a poor sleep pattern secondary to respiratory problems is unclear. What is certain is that both performance and training levels drop precipitously if there is marked interference with oxygenation of the body.

Allergic conditions may be accompanied by urticaria or eczematous rashes, especially when the allergen is ingested. Any food or medication is capable of producing an allergic response, but protein molecules seem to be the prime offenders.

Again, use of antihistamines in the athlete must be carefully weighed. The side effects of drowsiness and reflex slowing cannot be tolerated during activity. If none of the several chemically different antihistamines are free of side effects in a particular patient, then try the ephedrine-like drugs.

In asthma, treatment with cromolyn sodium seems to present the best approach, although aminophylline is still widely used with success. It may become necessary to use short courses of steroids to break the attacks and allow rapid resumption of full activity. The same medication regimen should be used for both practice and performance so that the athlete may standardize the effect.

Closely related to these conditions is something called exercise-induced bronchospasm (EIB). Clinically, this appears to be an attack of asthma brought on by exercise. It is characterized by wheezing and shortness of breath similar to that of a true asthma attack. While its mechanism of action is not allergic, EIB occurs in about 40 per cent of patients with nasal allergies and 90 per cent of true asthmatics at full stress.[5] This is probably because the bronchial lining of an allergic person is more sensitive to changes than that of the nonallergic. The mechanism in EIB is inability of the respiratory system to adequately warm and moisten the large amounts of air inspired during heavy activity. The drying and lowering of temperature in the respiratory tract trigger the spasm, with the resultant asthma-like symptoms.[6] This is borne out by the fact that EIB is extremely rare in swimmers, and victims of it may swim strenuously without problems.

One of the illnesses that has received much publicity and is the subject of much misinformation is infectious mononucleosis. One of the first cries we hear after persistently poor athletic performance is: "She must have mono." The disease is caused by the Epstein-Barr virus. Diagnosis is made by the heterophile antibody test, which, however, is not conclusive. We now know that many cases are heterophile-negative. (When clinical manifestations are unusual and the heterophile is negative, certain Epstein-Barr-specific blood tests can nail down the diagnosis.) The disease primarily attacks adolescents and young adults, and is common in college and military personnel, probably because of their proximity in confined areas. Contrary to popular opinion, the disease is only mildly contagious and occurs in only 3 per cent of the college population each year. In addition, the recurrence rate is extremely low.[7]

The disease can vary from an unrecognized period of fatigue and "feeling lousy" to a severe siege of high fever, painfully sore throat, and marked debilitation. The first symptoms generally are headache, generalized aching, fatigue, and the sore throat that is present in 85 per cent of patients. There is usually some fever. Physical signs include reddening and swelling of the throat and swollen red tonsils with heavy white patches. Enlargement of the cervical lymph nodes, especially those of the posterior chain, is always present. There is often swelling of the eyelids and a puffiness about the eyes. Enlargement of the spleen is almost always present, and liver function is always abnormal, although jaundice occurs in only about 10 per cent of cases. A red rash that can last up to 14 days may be seen in 10 per cent of the patients. In rare cases there can be central nervous system involvement mirroring encephalitis.

Once the acute phase is over, the greatest problem to the athlete is the increase in spleen size, its marked softening, and its tendency to rupture with minimal trauma. In severe cases, rupture may be spontaneous—its incidence is highest in the 10th to 21st days of the illness. The size of the spleen can be followed by flat-plate X-rays of the abdomen or, if it is available, by diagnostic ultrasound. The spleen usually returns to normal size in about four weeks. This is the limiting factor in an athlete's resumption of full activity, even of a noncontact sport.

Treatment of the disease is basically symptomatic, with rest, fluids, and aspirin paramount. In some cases, cortisone has been used—but there is no agreement on its routine use in athletes. Cortisone can shorten the course of the illness, and this is some doctors' argument for its use in the athlete who has an important contest coming up. And cortisone's use in severe throat obstruction, persistent high fever, and marked enlargement of the spleen is very worthwhile. However, I don't feel that it should be routine in an athlete just to get her back to training faster.

Gastrointestinal problems

GI ailments are next in importance. These can range from mild upsets that cause only loss of concentration and disruption of training schedules to severe conditions that may send the athlete to bed or to the hospital. GI ailments are divided into two groups, infectious and functional. Although the functional group probably accounts for more cases and more lost time, the infectious problems are more violent and I deal with them first.

The most common form of infectious gastroenteritis is viral in origin. It is usually characterized by nausea, vomiting, abdominal cramps, and diarrhea. It rarely lasts more than 24 to 48 hours and treatment is totally symptomatic. Food intake should be stopped until the nausea is gone, and then kept light and aimed primarily at replacing fluids. Antinauseant, antispasmodic, and antidiarrheal medications are available if symptoms are severe. A day or two off from training may be necessary if symptoms and subsequent weakness are severe. The most debilitating side effect has to do with the loss of electrolytes, particularly potassium, during the diarrheal phase. This may be severe enough to markedly interfere with muscle function in subsequent training.

Of a much more serious nature is true bacterial diarrhea, which is usually more severe and almost always much more prolonged than viral forms. We usually begin to think in terms of bacterial etiology when the symptoms continue past the 48-hour mark, and when fever becomes prominent. The diagnosis is made by isolating the organism in stool culture. Treatment is an appropriate antibiotic. Debilitation is very severe with this type of illness, and consequently the recuperative period will be much longer than with viral diarrhea. Resumption of activity depends on the return of strength. And not only are dehydration and electrolyte loss factors, but the lack of carbohydrate intake during illness delays return to activity.

On the functional side, GI ailments can result from emotional factors and changes in habits. Emotional factors seem to center around the pressure and tension of competition. Symptoms can vary from loss of appetite to nausea and diarrhea. Diarrhea must be controlled so that it won't interfere with competition. Loss of appetite and nausea interfere with precompetition food ingestion. Under normal conditions the emptying time of the stomach is close to four hours, and we tend to schedule precompetition meals on this basis. However, nervous tension can prolong emptying time, and the meal may not be absorbed on schedule. It is important that a light, quickly absorbed carbohydrate meal be taken early enough to avoid nausea.

In GI ills brought about by change in habits, travel is the precipitating factor. Time-zone change affects both body functions and eating patterns, and geographic change brings varying mineral and bacterial content of drinking water. Local variations in water-purification techniques can also trigger changes in bowel function. There are also changes in diet—regional cooking styles and restaurant food may be very different from the training diet at home. Lastly, change in the time of an event can be a major upheaval, thus aggravating any of the problems mentioned.

I should briefly mention a syndrome called exercise-induced diarrhea, most commonly seen in runners. It has many causes, one of which is milk intolerance. A high milk intake is common in athletes and may lead to cramping and diarrhea if the person lacks the enzymes that break down the disaccharides of milk. There are many other causes of the syndrome, but all of them are magnified by the fact that in exercise the blood flow to the bowel is drastically reduced, magnifying any mild bowel dysfunction.

Diabetes

One of the most controversial subjects has been whether a diabetic should fully participate in athletic programs. Although there have been many successful diabetic athletes, there has been great reluctance on the part of most family physicians to allow diabetics to compete. In recent years, it has been firmly established that continuous training and exercise are not only not harmful but actually of great value in the stabilization of diabetics. This includes even the so-called "brittle" diabetics, who seem to respond very well to regimented programs of activity.

The noninsulin-dependent maturity-onset diabetic has the same blood-sugar response to exercise as nondiabetics: Blood-sugar levels rise during short-duration, high-intensity exercise. On the other hand, in long-duration, moderate-intensity activity, there is a gradual decline in glucose levels.

This type of diabetes is felt to be due to insulin resistance brought about by weight gain and lack of physical activity. Exercise causes a marked decrease in insulin resistance, and combined with weight loss resulting from the exercise, can often lower blood sugar to levels that no longer require medication.

In insulin-dependent diabetics, hypoglycemia is a much more common occurrence. Apparently there is more rapid mobilization of depot insulin from a muscle that is being exercised. This causes a rise in the circulating insulin level, which reduces blood sugar by causing more rapid uptake by the muscles and inhibiting release of replacement glucose by the liver. The other major source of energy to the muscle is metabolism of free fatty acids. The mobilization of free fatty acids in the body is inhibited by the antilipolytic action of insulin. The combination of these factors serves to sharply reduce the circulating glucose level and can precipitate symptoms if the rate or degree of drop is severe enough. The rate of fall of glucose is much more rapid in insulin-dependent than in orally medicated diabetics.

It is clear, then, that the ideal pre-exercise state for the diabetic is to have a low level of insulin activity and a hyperglycemic blood condition. The insulin activity should be from a prolonged depot source and not from a short-acting dose that would peak during activity. If a combination dose is given, the short-acting component should be timed so that it does not hit during the activity period. The increased mobilization of the depot insulin should be adequate; in order to limit this increased mobilization, the insulin should not be injected in a limb that will be exercised. (The abdominal wall would seem the ideal site.) On the other hand, if the athlete is severely insulin-deficient and is ketotic prior to exercise, then ketosis and hyperglycemia will both increase during the exercise phase. A careful balance between the two conditions is necessary to control the patient. If an athlete has noticeable urine sugar and acetone on the morning of an event, she should probably be checked and adjusted before competing. However, a 1+ urine sugar level is probably safer for the athlete than a clear urine, in that it indicates a level of hyperglycemia that will protect against the increased insulin release.

A diabetic athlete starting a training program will probably find her insulin requirement reduced by as much as 40 per cent during training. Often, athletes taking 15 units or less can completely discontinue insulin. (Likewise, orally medicated diabetics can often stop their medication.) Once this level is reached, however, it is usually easier to achieve control by a change in carbohydrate intake than to change insulin dosage from day to day.

Lastly, there is the question of pregame meals and interval feedings. In recent years, high-carbohydrate pregame meals have been the rule. These are safe even for the diabetic athlete and help to

115

establish her hyperglycemia. However, food ingestion causes an insulin peak at about 35 to 40 minutes, with a short but sharp drop in blood sugar. If activity starts at this time, there will be rapid hypoglycemia. Sugar absorption will peak at 1½ to two hours, and this should probably be the timing of the meal. If the activity is intense and prolonged, there should be interval feedings at 30- to 60-minute intervals. Dilute solutions of glucose are the most rapidly absorbed and maintain blood-sugar levels. The athlete should be aware of early signs of hypoglycemia, such as fatigue, hunger, headache, or dizziness, and of difficulty in concentrating. If she develops symptoms, she should stop competition at once in order to avoid a severe reaction.

If these concepts are individualized to the needs of each athlete, there is absolutely no reason to withhold the benefits of exercise and training, or the rewards of competition, from anyone on the basis of diabetes.

References

1. Jackson GG: Understanding of viral respiratory illnesses provided by experiments in volunteers. *Bact Rev* 28:403, 1964

2. Douglas RG, Lindgren KM, and Couch RB: Exposure to cold environment and rhinovirus common cold. *N Engl J Med* 279:742, 1968

3. Roundtable: Upper respiratory infection in sports. *Phys Sportsmed* 3(10):28, 1975

4. Fridy WW: Airway function during mild viral respiratory illnesses. *Ann Intern Med* 80:150, 1974

5. Roundtable: Respiratory allergy in athletes. *Phys Sportsmed* 6(5):56, 1978

6. Saunders N and McFadden ER Jr: Asthma, an update. *Disease a Month* 24:11, 1978

7. Roundtable: Infectious mononucleosis in athletes. *Phys Sportsmed* 6(2):41, 1978

CARDIOVASCULAR CONSIDERATIONS

Arthur S. Leon, M.D.

Statistics have shown that there are more than 4 million people in the United States with various degrees of disability due to coronary heart disease (CHD). These figures include 2.5 million persons under the age of 65. About 700,000 persons die from this disease every year.

Autopsy studies of teenage and under-25-year-old soldiers killed during the Korean and Vietnam wars showed that atherosclerosis begins much earlier in life than was once thought. Many of these youngsters—all presumably in excellent health—showed thickening and narrowing of arterial walls. A number of factors in our modern life-style are believed to be contributing factors—a diet high in animal fat, heavy cigarette smoking, lack of exercise, and stressful living conditions.

Whether exercise or participation in athletics has any dramatic effect on coronary mortality remains to be seen—a number of studies are aimed at finding out. Some of the things that happen to the heart and the body during exercise make us think that it can.

Acute response to exercise

There are two basic types of exercise. The first is static or isometric exercise, in which muscular contraction increases muscular tension but results in little or no change in muscular length or joint movement; examples are lifting, pushing, or carrying heavy objects. The second type of exercise is dynamic or isotonic, in which rhythmic muscular contractions result in changes in muscle length and joint movement; examples are walking, running, swimming, and bicycling. The acute and chronic cardiovascular effects of these types of exercise differ greatly.

Isotonic exercise: Isotonic exercise increases the metabolic activity of the contracting muscle, necessitating an increased rate of blood delivery in order to supply oxygen and other nutrients for energy and to remove carbon dioxide and other metabolic breakdown products and dissipate heat. The circulatory adjustments to meet these demands impose a great strain on the cardiovascular system. For example, cardiac output has been demonstrated to increase fourfold over resting levels in young female athletes during maximal exertion. This is mediated by an increase in heart rate and stroke volume. Increased cardiac output may be maintained at 85 per cent of maximum for several hours by a trained athlete during endurance events such as marathon running.

Reflex adjustments cause an increased proportion of the cardiac output to be distributed to the working skeletal muscles. This is accomplished by a marked dilatation of arterioles (vasodilation) in the exercising muscle beds and a concomitant constriction of arterioles in areas less affected by the exercise (inactive muscles, the gastrointestinal tract, and kidneys), leading to a net reduction in peripheral vascular resistance and a shunting of blood to the active muscles. This redistribution of blood flow, coupled with increased extraction of oxygen by the exercising muscles, causes a widening of the total body arteriovenous oxygen difference; that is, an increase in the amount of oxygen extracted from the arterial blood. These changes are accompanied by an increase in systolic blood pressure, while diastolic blood pressure remains unchanged or decreases during heavy dynamic exercise.

Maximal oxygen uptake (VO_2 max), or aerobic capacity of the body, represents the maximal transport of oxygen from the lungs to the tissues during dynamic exercise and can be calculated from the product of maximal cardiac output and maximal arteriovenous oxygen difference. VO_2 max represents the best physiological measurement of functional capacity of the cardiorespiratory system. Factors affecting the aerobic capacity include heredity, age, sex, and exercise training.

VO_2 max increases with age up to 20 years. Beyond this age, there is a gradual decline; at 60 years of age, an individual's VO_2 max is usually about 70 per cent of the level at age 20. However, this decrement can be retarded by regular isotonic exercise. Before the age of 12, there is no significant difference in VO_2 max between males and females; following this, aerobic capacity of the average female is about 85 per cent of that of the average male. Contributing factors to the lower levels in females are probably lower hemoglobin levels, less lean body mass, and less physically active life-style. Because of greater stroke volume, endurance athletes have a VO_2 max that is about twice as high as that of the average sedentary person. Cardiac patients have reduced VO_2 max, generally because of reduced stroke volume.

Coronary blood flow reflects increased metabolic demands by the heart muscle, and it increases proportionately with the cardiac output, heart rate, and with the heart rate-systolic blood pressure product; it may be four- to fivefold higher than resting levels during maximal dynamic exercise.

Isometric exercise: The cardiovascular response to isometric exercise differs significantly from the response to isotonic exercise. With onset of static muscular contractions, there is a marked increase in both systolic and diastolic blood pressure; this is associated with marked arteriolar constriction (increased peripheral vascular resistance). Cardiac output shows only a small increase as compared to the increase with dynamic exercise, and it is due solely to an increase in heart rate, with stroke volume remaining essentially unchanged. Such physiological changes are generally poorly tolerated by patients with cardiac disease and limited reserve.

Adaptive effects of chronic exercise training

When the body is subjected to regular habitual physical exercise, biochemical and physiological adaptations occur that result in a more efficient acute response to exercise and in an enhanced maximal capacity; these differ for isotonic and isometric exercise. Dynamic exercise training may also result in beneficial alterations in carbohydrate and lipid metabolism and in psychological benefits not seen with static exercise.

Isotonic exercise training: Sufficient amounts of regular endurance exercise result in significant increases in the capacity of the body to utilize oxygen (VO_2 max) in both healthy people of all ages and cardiac patients. An average increase in VO_2 max of 10 to 20 per cent is usually obtained in training programs for healthy sedentary people. The higher the initial level, the more difficult it is to set a training increment. This increase in VO_2 max along with a reduced oxygen requirement for a given submaximal level of activity results in greater vigor and endurance and less inclination to fatigue.

Both an enhanced maximal cardiac output and maximal arteriovenous oxygen difference contribute to the increases in VO_2 max induced by training. An increase in maximal stroke volume due to improved cardiac function accounts for the increased cardiac output; the other contributor to cardiac output, the heart rate, is actually reduced by training.

Training adaptations in the active skeletal muscles and red blood cells contribute to the increased maximal arteriovenous oxygen difference. In the skeletal muscle, there is an increase in the size and the number of mitochondria and the concentration of contained aerobic enzymes. Muscle myoglobin is also increased, which adds to the efficiency of delivery of oxygen from the cell membrane to the mitochondria. The biochemical adaptations in skeletal muscle also decrease the rate of glycogen utilization and lactic-acid formation, which contribute to a greater tolerance of exercise. Training may also increase the blood volume and its oxygen-carrying capacity, as well as enhance the red blood cells' ability to release oxygen.

A reduction in heart rate at rest and during exercise is important in decreasing cardiac work and myocardial oxygen and coronary blood flow measurements and thereby improves the efficiency of the cardiovascular system. For a patient with coronary heart disease, the net effect is an ability to perform a higher level of work before reaching the limits imposed by impaired coronary flow.

A short-term drop in blood pressure immediately after exercise results from vasodilation. However, a significant sustained reduction in resting blood pressure can be expected only when there is an associated weight loss.

Exercise studies in animals have demonstrated an increase in extent and size of coronary arteries and more capillaries to myocardial muscle fiber. There are few studies on the effects of exercise training on the human coronary artery tree, although autopsy studies have demonstrated larger coronary arteries in physically active as compared to sedentary men. Coronary arteriography before and after training in coronary patients has generally failed to demonstrate that exercise improves coronary circulation in the presence of advanced coronary artery disease; however, as I've already indicated, improved cardiovascular efficiency reduces coronary blood flow requirements.

The role of regular dynamic exercise in maintenance of proper body weight, reduction of body fat, and appropriate adjustment of appetite is now widely appreciated. Dynamic exercise increases caloric expenditure and, through associated hormonal action on the fat cell, increases the breakdown and mobilization of the fat stores for use as fuel (antiobesity effect). Changes in body composition with dynamic exercise training consist of a decrease in total body fat with no change or a slight increase in lean body tissue.

Other beneficial metabolic effects of regular isotonic exercise include: enhanced insulin tissue sensitivity and glucose uptake by muscle and fat cells, which improves glucose tolerance and helps prevent and control maturity-onset diabetes (antidiabetic effect); reduction in elevated levels of blood triglycerides, probably by increased utilization as fuel by the exercising muscle and decreased synthesis (antilipemic effect); and increased ratio of cholesterol carried in high-density (HDL) to low-density (LDL) lipoprotein.

This last-mentioned effect is important in view of the inverse relationship of HDL levels and direct relationship of LDL levels to risk of coronary heart disease, with the demonstration in laboratory studies that HDL has the effect of removing cholesterol from artery walls while LDL deposits it there. Thus, a higher ratio of HDL to LDL should help protect against atherosclerosis and coronary heart disease.

Training programs also often stimulate other favorable health habits, such as cessation of smoking and attention to proper diet. Psychological benefits include: a feeling of well-being, self-control, self-confidence, and improved body image; better handling of stress; distraction from day-to-day problems; and promotion of sound sleep.

Isometric training: Isometric exercise training consisting of repetitious muscular contractions against resistance results in an increase in muscle mass and an associated improvement in muscle strength. However, no significant cardiovascular benefits can usually be demonstrated after a conditioning program of static exercise. In fact, aerobic capacity and endurance may actually be diminished, because blood supply is not increased proportionately to the greater muscle mass. Nevertheless, strength development may be beneficial for athletes, for orthopedic patients during rehabilitation, and for individuals requiring muscular strength on the job and for recreational purposes.

Amount of exercise necessary

A number of factors must be taken into consideration in setting up an exercise training program. These include the reasons for exercising, recreational interests, inherited physical endowment, previous training status, age, and health of the individual entering the program. It is generally recommended that any vigorous exercise program be preceded by a thorough cardiovascular evaluation, including exercise electrocardiographic tests for all individuals with known cardiac problems, those habitually inactive individuals older than 35, and younger adults with coronary risk factors (high serum cholesterol, elevated blood pressure, cigarette smoking, or diabetes mellitus). The purpose of the cardiovascular evaluation is to detect any contraindications to vigorous exercise—such as serious cardiac rhythm disturbances—to establish special precautions, and to prepare safe, individualized exercise prescriptions based on the capabilities and limitations of each individual.

Dynamic exercise routines involving large muscle groups (legs, back, and shoulders) should be selected on the basis of the individual's willingness and ability to pursue them on a regular basis for a lifetime; examples are walking, jogging, bicycling, and swimming. The competitive elements of sports and games should be discouraged in high-risk populations. Isometric exercises should also be discouraged in cardiac and hypertensive patients. Cardiac patients requiring strength development should use a low-resistance, high-repetition routine such as lifting of light weights, paying attention to exhaling with each contraction in order to avoid the blood pressure-raising effects of straining (Valsalva maneuver). Cardiac patients should be instructed to stop their workouts immediately if they develop symptoms of chest pain, nausea, dizziness, or excessive shortness of breath. All workouts should be preceded by a warm-up period and followed by a cool-down period to reduce the chance of muscular injury or circulatory problem. Warm-up/cool-downs usually involve five to 10 minutes of limbering-up exercises and walking or other low-intensity activities.

Other important precautions that reduce the chance of orthopedic and cardiovascular complications are: beginning a training program for habitually sedentary adults with low-intensity, short-duration workouts and only gradually progressing to the desired level; avoiding exercise during illness; temporarily cutting back workouts after a layoff and gradually working back to previous levels; dressing appropriately and altering workouts according to weather conditions; and avoiding exercising for at least two hours after a heavy meal.

During the past 20 years, there has been a great deal of research on the kind of isotonic exercise training that increases VO_2 max. This has led to quantification of requirements in terms of required intensity, duration, and frequency. Work is now under way to determine the optimal means of achieving the metabolic benefits of isotonic exercise.

The intensity or relative oxygen requirement of the workout is the most important variable in improving cardiovascular performance or VO_2 max. A threshold for improvement is approximately 50 to 60 per cent of an individual's VO_2 max with very little additional improvement at levels higher than 70 to 80 per cent VO_2 max. Because there is a linear relationship between heart rate and oxygen cost (percentage of VO_2 max), checking pulse rate during or immediately following exercise is commonly used to regulate intensity of a workout. A heart rate that is 70 per cent of an individual's maximal heart rate (determined by exercise testing or estimated by subtracting age from 220) correlates with 60 per cent VO_2 max, and 85 per cent of maximal heart rate with 75 per cent VO_2 max. As a rule, one would expect a training effect in young people at a minimal training heart rate of 140 beats per minute, in middle-aged people with 120 bpm, and in older people with 100 to 110 bpm. Theoretically, different modes of isotonic exercise give a similar training effect at a similar exercise intensity.

The relative risk of musculoskeletal injuries or cardiovascular complications increases with exercise intensity; thus, a prudent program should be designed to provide the greatest benefit with the least risk. An exception is the athlete preparing for competition who is trying to achieve a maximal training effect in the shortest possible time. In general, the small sacrifice of training benefits at a lower intensity can be compensated for by increasing the duration and frequency of exercise.

Duration of exercise is another important variable in eliciting a training effect. The lower the intensity of exercise, the longer the duration necessary, and conversely, with extremely high exercise intensity (greater than 90 per cent VO_2 max), improvement in VO_2 max can be obtained with training sessions lasting only five to 10 minutes daily. The optimal duration of exercise for the usually recommended moderate exercise intensity of 70 to 80 per cent VO_2 max is about 30 minutes a session. This should be sufficient to produce sweating and mild fatigue and breathlessness.

A minimum frequency of three evenly spaced workouts (70 to 80 per cent VO_2 max and 30 minutes' duration) per week is necessary to improve VO_2 max; improvement becomes evident within four weeks. Some additional improvement is observed with five days a week of training, but a sixth or seventh workout has little additional value and substantially increases the risk of musculoskeletal problems. A minimum of two workouts per week is required to maintain an acquired level of VO_2 max.

MEDICAL ASPECTS OF SPORTS FOR THE SCHOOL-AGE ATHLETE

Walter J. Kennedy, M.D.

CHAPTER

11

It is important to understand the anatomical and physiological similarities and differences between girls and boys at the different growth periods—prepubertal, pubertal, and adolescent. An advantage of such understanding is that it helps avoid confusion and misunderstanding concerning girls' participation in co-ed sports programs or in contact sports.

During the growth years prior to puberty, there are no significant structural or functional differences between the sexes that affect their athletic performance, or prevent them from competing against one another in contact sports. Anatomical data, tests of strength, cardiovascular endurance, and motor skills show few differences between girls and boys up to the age of 12 years.[1] Furthermore, fewer injuries are found in preadolescents than among high school or college athletes. Studies also show organized sports for prepubertal youngsters to be safer than those of the so-called sandlot variety.[2]

Because of the earlier maturation of girls, they reach their physiological growth peak before boys and, at between 10 and 14 years of age, have greater height and weight than boys of the same age and often surpass them in athletic ability.[3] However, boys become considerably stronger after puberty, develop larger muscles, greater muscular and cardiovascular endurance, and are more proficient in almost all motor skills, so that they outdo girls in almost all athletic performance ratings.[4,5]

With maturity, the differences between male and female body structure and configuration become more obvious. Greater muscle bulk in the male results in broader shoulders. He also has a greater amount of subcutaneous fat in the abdominal and upper regions of the body, while the female has substantially more fat in the hips and lower regions of the body.[2] At full maturity, the average woman is five inches shorter than her male counterpart, and weighs 30 to 40 pounds less. However, she is 40 to 50 pounds lighter in lean body weight, and has considerably more adipose tissue—22 to 26 per cent body fat versus 12 to 16 per cent in the male.[5] The lungs, heart, liver, and kidneys of females are smaller than those of males, and the erythrocyte and hemoglobin mass are relatively and absolutely less.[3]

The divergent changes in body structure and strength that occur after puberty and that set the sexes apart in apparent athletic ability are no doubt due to increases in androgen secretion in the male and estrogen in the female. Although the physical and functional differences between the postpubertal female and male appear to be programmed genetically and biologically, it is also likely that cultural and environmental factors play a significant role, as young women in the past have for the most part been directed into sedentary habits.

As girls have become more active physically, there has been some concern that increased exercise might result in a large, bulky musculature. These fears are unwarranted. Wilmore found that women are able to achieve much greater muscle strength without very much change in muscle bulk.[6] His studies also show that the mean strength of young nonathletic girls can be improved by as much as 30 per cent during a 10-week training program.

Until puberty and during early adolescence, the cardiovascular endurance of young girls, as measured by VO_2 max, approximates that of the male. (VO_2 max represents the greatest amount of oxygen an individual can deliver to his working muscles during maximal exercise; it is considered to be the most accurate estimate of endurance.) During later adolescence, girls' endurance decreases, whereas boys' endurance increases. This rather abrupt change can be partially explained by the lower hemoglobin levels and the reduced oxygen-carrying capacity in the female at this age. Another reason might be that girls at this age become more sedentary in their habits; it must be more than physiology, as the endurance capacity of postpubertal girls is known to increase considerably with proper exercise, and can, in fact, exceed that of sedentary males.[1]

Medical concerns

Sports-medicine physicians have long been concerned about heat dissipation in the athlete during strenuous exercise, particularly in warm, humid climates. Therefore, the finding that the body temperature of the female rises two to three degrees higher than that of the male before the cooling process of sweating occurs takes on significance, particularly as the female has fewer functional sweat glands than the male.[7] Those responsible for the health of young female athletes need to be aware that girls may have more difficulty with heat stress when participating in strenuous sports in a warm environment.

In the past, young women have frequently been discouraged from participating in sports and exercise during menstruation. There is no justification for this restriction. Nor is there any evidence to indicate that menstrual difficulties are in any way affected by physical activity, except that exercise might improve regulation of the menstrual cycle.[4]

Although contact sports vary greatly in the degree of force of contact, and therefore in their potential for injury, it is a well established fact that there is no physiological reason to restrict girls from participating in such sports.[4] It cannot be determined from the direct evidence now available whether adolescent girls, in fact, sustain fewer injuries than boys of the same age when each participates in contact sports with others of the same sex. Many factors, not the least of which is conditioning, must be considered in making any determination. This situation parallels that of preadolescent boys in contact sports, in which, despite expectations to the contrary, few injuries were noted; injuries were much less frequent than in high school boys, in whose contests contact forces are much greater. Because the muscle mass and the resulting forces generated by preadolescent boys and adolescent girls are comparable, it may be expected that the adolescent female would sustain fewer injuries.[8]

Matching the growing female athlete

As girls continue strength-training and become increasingly aggressive during strenuous contact sports, they may sustain more injuries. Nevertheless, the number of potential injuries can be reduced and the youngsters' safety can be better protected if care-

---

FIGURE 11-1

NAME   Jane Doe

DATE OF BIRTH   July 4, 1965

ONSET OF MENSTRUATION (month & year)   August 1, 1976

EXAMINATION DATE February 5, 1980 CHRONOLOGICAL AGE 14 yrs. 7 mos.

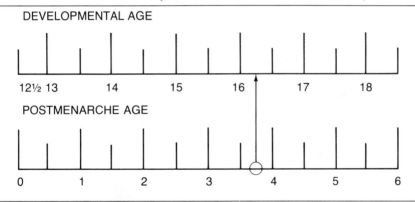

To determine girl's developmental age, physician fills
in form with name, date of birth, month and year menstruation
began, and examination date. Number of elapsed years
and months between onset of menstruation and examination date
is plotted on lower line, and arrow drawn from that point
to top line. This gives girl's developmental age.

Adapted from a form devised by Thomas E. Shaffer, M.D., for use in the selection and classification program of the New York State Public High School Athletic Association. Used with permission.

ful attention is given to proper matching. Grouping of competitors by age alone is not satisfactory. But there is good correlation between a girl's developmental level and her strength, coordination, and nutritional needs.

A quick measure of her development can be made by observing the stage of growth of pubic and axillary hair. A more accurate and more easily obtained method uses menarche as the basis of evaluation. This method assumes all girls to be at the same stage of physical development and to have a developmental age of 12½ at menarche. The stage of development is determined by calculating postmenarchal age and converting it to a developmental age (see Figure 11-1).

Guidelines

In 1975, noting that girls had been denied their proper share of sports activities because of widespread misconceptions, the American Academy of Pediatrics' Committee on the Pediatric Aspects of Physical Fitness, Recreation and Sports, hoping to correct the disparity, issued the following statement regarding participation by girls and young women in sports:

"(1) There is no reason to separate prepubescent children by sex in sports, physical education, and recreational activities.

"(2) Girls can compete against girls in any sports activity if matched for size, weight, skill, and physical maturation so long as the customary safeguards for the protection of their health and safety are carried out.

"(3) Girls can attain high levels of physical fitness through strenuous conditioning activities to improve their physical fitness, agility, strength, appearance, endurance, and sense of psychic wellbeing. These have no unfavorable influence on menstruation, future pregnancy, and childbearing.

"(4) Postpubescent girls should not participate against boys in heavy collision sports because of the grave risk of serious injury due to their lesser muscle mass per unit of body weight.

"(5) The talented female athlete may participate on a team with boys in an appropriate sport provided that the school or community offers opportunities for all girls to participate in comparable activities."[9]

It is difficult to believe that these guidelines could be improved on, and they can be of great assistance to educators and physicians in their decision making concerning participation of girls in sports.

Health and safety rules

All youngsters in interscholastic or other organized sports programs should be assured of optimal protection against injury. Although this concept has been well recognized in the male sports arena for several years, it should be emphasized for those who are newly responsible for the health and safety of young female athletes. The safeguards necessary to protect their health and safety are essentially the same as those first established in 1966 for all growing athletes by the Medical Aspects of Sports Committee of the American Medical Association. These guidelines include proper conditioning, competent coaching and officiating, proper rules and regulations to protect the athlete, good equipment and facilities, and adequate medical supervision.

The primary responsibility for making certain that all girls in sports receive adequate conditioning and are provided proper coaching, officiating, equipment, and facilities rests with community or school administrators and educators. Although the physician's chief concern must be with health supervision and with the prevention and treatment of injuries, she/he must also serve as adviser to community or school personnel on health matters relating to conditioning, coaching, or officiating techniques, or when improper equipment or facilities might provoke injuries.

Those interested in a more detailed discussion of this subject can obtain an informative and comprehensive booklet, "Medical Evaluation of the Athlete—A Guide." This pamphlet, which represents the opinion of sports-medicine experts over the years, can be purchased from the Order Department, OP-209, American Medical Association, 535 North Dearborn Street, Chicago, Illinois 60610.

Common chronic diseases

An exhaustive account of the disorders that confront the physician in sports medicine cannot be given proper consideration here; however, bronchial asthma, diabetes mellitus, and epilepsy deserve individual attention. Bronchial asthma is the most common chronic disease of the growing youngster, and during adolescence affects females and males equally. More than 200,000 youngsters have diabetes mellitus, and slightly more than half are girls. Seven per cent of all children have had a convulsion. In the past, active involvement in sports has frequently been discouraged in children with one of these conditions. Although each of these might require special management during participation in sports, none is cause for disqualification of the child.

TABLE 11-1

Recommendations for Administration of Agents Effective in Prevention or Relief of Exercise-Induced Asthma

Drug	Dosage	Route of administration	Time of administration	Accepted at international competition
Theophylline	5 to 8 mg/kg	orally	1 hour	yes
Dyphylline	15 mg/kg	orally	1 hour	yes
Theophylline-ephedrine combinations	5 to 10 years, ½ tablet; 10+ years, 1 tablet	orally	1 hour	no
Isoproterenol	14 μg/aerosol	aerosol	5 min-30 min	no
Metaproterenol	12+ years, 20 mg/dose	orally/aerosol	1 hour	no
Terbutaline	12+ years, 5 mg/dose	orally	1 hour	no
Cromolyn sodium	20 mg/dose	inhalation	5 min-20 min	yes

Adapted from American Medical Association: *The Asthmatic Athlete.* Chicago: AMA, 1977. Reprinted by permission.

Exercise-induced asthma

Despite the fact that bronchial asthma has been recognized since the second century A.D., the disease continues to cause confusion among both physicians and the general public. Asthma can be triggered by many factors, including exercise. The lack of understanding of exercise-induced asthma often excludes youngsters from sports. Usually, these restrictions are unnecessary. With proper understanding and adequate medication, young people can compete safely.

Duration of exercise can determine its effect on the asthmatic. Short-term exercise of one to two minutes results in bronchodilation, whereas longer-term exercise of four to 12 minutes can result in bronchoconstriction.

Exercise-induced bronchospasm (EIB) is a common complaint in asthmatic children and teenagers, and is unrecognized in others.[10] It can be elicited in an asthmatic by exercise such as running on a sidewalk or treadmill for at least six to eight minutes. A timed vital capacity spirometer or peak flow meter is used to record lung function. Tests are performed before exercise, at one minute after exercise, and at five-minute intervals thereafter. Usually EIB develops 10 to 15 minutes after hard, lengthy exercise. A fall of 15 per cent or greater in lung function after exercise indicates significant EIB.[11]

A simpler but much less accurate method is listening with a stethoscope. However, significant changes in pulmonary function occur before rales can be heard.

With proper medical management most young girls with asthma can participate fully in sports.[12] Total exclusion should be infrequent, and partial exclusion only in severe cases. Occasionally, it may be necessary to limit the extent of exercise to sports in which output of energy is of short duration—softball or baseball, sprints, field events, golf, volleyball, skiing, and especially swimming.

It is important that the asthmatic athlete warm up prior to sports participation to obtain the benefit of bronchodilation, which occurs following exercise of short duration.

With proper medical supervision, exercise-induced asthma can be prevented or reversed. Table 11-1 provides recommendations for various effective agents.

Diabetes mellitus

Because exercise is essential to their good health, it's ironic that girls with diabetes have been discouraged from participating in sports. Exercise, together with dietary regulation and insulin, completes the therapeutic triad so important to management.

Exercise can reduce insulin requirements substantially by increasing the skeletal muscle uptake of glucose from the blood. But the insulin-dependent girl with diabetes should never attempt to control her diabetes through diet and exercise alone, because studies have shown that *insulin is needed* for exercise to be effective.[13, 14]

The importance of maintaining good diabetic control (nearly normal blood-sugar levels) should also be emphasized, because the exercise-induced increase of glucose uptake by the muscle does not occur with marked hyperglycemia. When ketosis is present, exercise can further aggravate the problem and possibly lead to ketoacidosis.[15]

Exercise may also help prevent long-term microvascular complications that might face the diabetic when she becomes older.

The benefits derived from exercise are good reason to encourage sports participation for the youngster with diabetes. But before considering strenuous physical exertion, she should be evaluated by a physician familiar with diabetes. The doctor's appraisal can furnish important data on her health and level of diabetic control and can provide an opportunity to review basic principles of diabetic management. Dietary needs can also be determined, and for this reason, the help of a dietitian would be desirable. By following the guidelines laid out, the youngster (and her family) can assume the responsibility of maintaining the type of control necessary for her to compete in sports.

The methods used by each diabetic athlete and her physician to maintain proper blood-sugar levels and prevent insulin reaction while participating in sports may vary, but the increased uptake of blood sugar by the muscle during exercise should always be considered. The diet should be increased or insulin reduced accordingly.

The youngster with diabetes and one of her teammates, or her coach, should be taught to recognize insulin reaction. The early symptoms are hunger, pallor, sweating, weakness, and lightheadedness; if not treated, they can progress to mental confusion and unconsciousness.

The insulin reaction is treated by giving rapidly absorbed sugar—jelly beans or gumdrops if the youngster is awake; honey, orange juice, or pop if she is stuporous. Proprietary concentrated sugars (Instant Glucose, Gluctose) are marketed in plastic containers. Glucagon, a hormone that raises the blood sugar, is available for injection under the skin and can be used when a diabetic youngster is unconscious from an insulin reaction. When Glucagon is used, be sure to provide easily digested sugar orally when the youngster awakens.

Epilepsy

Children and teenagers with epilepsy are sometimes restricted from physical exertion and sports for fear that the physical activity might increase seizures and cause intellectual damage, or that injury might result from a seizure during strenuous or contact sports. Yet youngsters with epilepsy who are engaging in physical activity have fewer attacks than when they are inactive.

Follow-up of more than 15,000 children with epilepsy over a 36-year period—including patients who participated in vigorous contact sports—has shown no instance of recurrence of seizures related to head injury in any of the athletes.[16]

Aisenson compared the accident rate of 960 residential patients involved in full athletic activities, including strenuous contact sports.[17] Two hundred and ten patients had seizure disorders and 750 were nonconvulsive. His findings indicated no significant differences: The accident rate was 2.8 per cent in the children with seizures and 2.9 per cent in those without.

Although hyperventilation resulting from voluntary overbreathing is known to precipitate petit mal seizures, youngsters with epilepsy do not experience any increase in seizure activity when they exercise. One explanation is that voluntary overbreathing produces alkalosis and that this may be the cause of increased susceptibility to seizures.[16] The breathlessness that occurs in the course of exercise is associated with lactate-pyruvate acidosis, which inhibits seizure activity.

Moreover, exercise has been shown to elevate the seizure threshold and thereby reduce the likelihood of seizure. Electroencephalographic abnormalities found during hyperventilation tend to return to normal during muscular activity. EEG abnormalities found during hyperventilation before exercise are greater and occur earlier than with hyperventilation after exercise.[18]

Youngsters with epilepsy are more likely to have seizures during sleep, and for some this is the only time seizures occur. Also, some children show abnormal EEG readings only when asleep.

The young athlete with seizures has a responsibility to herself to follow proper health and conditioning guidelines to maintain body strength and resistance to fatigue, because fatigue may be a precipitating factor for seizures.

A child or teenager with seizures should be discouraged from participating in sports that entail danger of falling from a high place or diving in deep water. Of the interscholastic sports now available, the young female with seizures should be excluded from two—gymnastics and diving. Swimming should be under adequate supervision.

No credible evidence of increased seizure activity has been found when seizure-prone youngsters of either sex are allowed to participate freely in a well-rounded sports program, and are provided proper conditioning for the activity. Instead, they may gain tremendous physical and emotional benefit as a result of mingling and competing with their normal peers. The great diversity of sports now accessible to the young female with seizures, plus the anticonvulsant medications available today, make it possible for her to participate in all degrees of physical activity. As parents, educators, and physicians, we should encourage such participation in sports.

Sports injuries

With increased participation, more sports injuries have resulted, often requiring examination and treatment. Some of the contusions, hematomas, ligamentous injuries, and fractures are old hat to most physicians, as they are identical to injuries traditionally found in the male. Other conditions—stress fracture, the patellofemoral syndrome, certain types of apophysitis, to name a few—

are being recognized with increasing frequency. This could represent increased astuteness on the part of physicians, but more likely it is due to a swing from football and wrestling to jogging, swimming, gymnastics, track and field, tennis, and similar sports.

Stress fractures: Although stress fractures have been recognized for well over 100 years, they are occurring more frequently, not only in the female but also in the male athlete. The present thinking is that a stress fracture is the result of submaximal cyclic loading on the growing bone, and is due to a series of events rather than one single event. In a recent series, the fibula was involved 25 per cent of the time, the metatarsal 20 per cent, the tibia 20 per cent, and the os calcis 15 per cent.[19] The fibula and the tibia are involved in athletes participating in cross-country, track, and swimming. The femur and the pelvis are involved in jumping sports, and the patella, os calcis, femur, and pelvis in basketball.[20] Typically, the athlete presents a history of pain increasing in crescendo fashion. At first, the pain is relieved by rest, but if the athlete persists in exercise, the pain increases and becomes continuous. Examination reveals tenderness over the painful area, and on occasion, slight swelling. Radiological changes may not be recognized on first examination, but appear later. Usually discontinuing the activity results in healing. The athlete's activity should be restricted long enough to allow healing to be complete.

Anterior-compartment syndrome: Whenever severe pain is present in the lower leg, particularly if there is a history of strenuous running without a proper conditioning period, anterior-compartment syndrome should be considered. It is due to swelling of muscles within a fixed fascial compartment, so that the arterial supply to both muscle and nerve is reduced. The resulting ischemia can lead to necrosis of the involved muscle and to foot drop. The pain in the anterior leg is usually severe and occurs during running exercise. At first, it is relieved by rest, but with continued activity, the pain can become continuous. Whenever localized, compartmental tenderness is associated with pain on stretching, this entity should be considered. If foot drop is not present, relief can be obtained with rest and elevation of the extremity, along with cold compresses. On occasion fasciotomy may be required.

Shin splints: Except for the pain, shin splints are usually of no great significance. They are usually due to stretching of the posterior tibial muscle, with tenderness at the site of its origin on the posterior margin of the tibia, and occur as a result of improper conditioning associated with running on too hard a surface.[21]

The patello-femoral joint: Subluxation of the patella can occur in the adolescent athlete and is more common in girls because of the increased Q angle existing with genu valgum. Frequently, a high riding patella, a flattened lateral femoral condyle, or a poorly developed vastus medialis is a contributing factor in the injury.

The dislocation causes sudden, severe, and disabling pain. Upon examination, the youngster will complain of severe pain if lateral pressure is applied to the patella.

Patellar chondromalacia (patello-femoral pain syndrome) is the most frequent cause of knee pain in girls, and in a recent survey by DeHaven, accounted for nearly one-third of all injuries found in girl athletes.[22] Here, the youngster complains of pain in the patellar area, usually of both knees. Symptoms are aggravated by activity to the knee joint, such as running or climbing stairs. Intermittent buckling of the knees may be described. Physical examination reveals an increased Q angle, high patella, and tenderness on the medial and lateral sides of the patella. Again, severe pain is present when lateral pressure is applied to the patella. Both subluxation of the patella and patellar chondromalacia should be referred to an orthopedist for further care.

Although the patello-femoral joint is frequently involved when an adolescent girl has knee pain, the examiner should also consider internal injuries to the knee (injuries to the semilunar cartilage or cruciate ligaments), as well as epiphyseal injuries—in particular, epiphyseal fracture of the distal femur. One last important point: It should be remembered that occasionally in hip injuries the youngster presents with knee pain referred from the hip.

Apophyseal injuries: Injuries in the area of the pelvis are being recognized more often in females. They are found more frequently in youngsters involved in gymnastics, dancing, or cheerleading. Usually, the injury is an avulsion of the ischial tuberosity at the attachment of the hamstrings. It occurs as a result of forceful flexing of the hip with the knee extended when the youngster attempts to do splits. An X-ray is indicated whenever this injury is suspected in order to determine the extent of the avulsion, as surgery might be necessary with a wide displacement.

The sports injuries discussed here represent only a few of the many conditions that are being recognized more frequently by the physicians who examine young female athletes. It is hoped that their inclusion will remind other physicians to consider them in the diagnostic process.

References

1. Wilmore JH: The female athlete. *J School Health* 47:227, 1977

2. Thornton ML: Should grammar school kids compete in contact sports? *Med Times* 104:112, 1976

3. Shaffer TE: The adolescent athlete. *Pediat Clin N Amer* 20:837, 1973

4. Corbitt RW, Cooper DL, Erickson DJ, et al: Female athletics. *JAMA* 228:1266, 1974

5. Wilmore JH: Strength, endurance, and body composition of the female athlete. In *Proceedings of the 15th Conference on the Medical Aspects of Sports* (Craig TT, ed), pp 34-9. Chicago: AMA, 1974

6. Wilmore JH: Alterations in strength, body composition, and anthropometric measurements consequent to a 10-week weight training program. *Med Sci Sports* 6:133, 1974

7. Harris DV: Women in sports: Some misconceptions. *J Sports Med* 1:15, 1973

8. Thornton ML: Pediatric concerns about competitive preadolescent sports. *JAMA* 227:418, 1974

9. Thornton ML, Eng GD, Kennell JH, et al: Participation in sports by girls. *J Amer Acad Pediat* 55:563, 1975

10. Pediatrics, supplement. *J Amer Acad Pediat* 56, No 5, Part 2, 1975

11. The Committee on the Medical Aspects of Sports: The asthmatic athlete. Chicago: AMA, 1976

12. 19th Conference on the Medical Aspects of Sports. Chicago: AMA, 1978

13. Berger M, Hagg S, and Ruderman NB: Glucose metabolism in perfused skeletal muscle, interaction of insulin and exercise on glucose uptake. *Biochem J* 146:231, 1975

14. Dorchy H, Ego F, Baran D, et al: Effect of exercise on glucose uptake in diabetic adolescents. *Acta Paediatr Belg* 29:83, 1976

15. Wahren J, Hagenfeldt L, and Felig P: Glucose and free fatty acid utilization in exercise. *Israel J Med Sci* 11:551, 1975

16. Livingston S and Berman W: Participation of epileptic patients in sports. *JAMA* 224:236, 1973

17. Aisenson MR: Accidental injuries in epileptic children. *Pediatrics* 2:85, 1948

18. Gotze W, Kubicki S, Munter M, et al: Effect of physical exercise on seizure threshold; investigated by electroencephalographic telemetry. *Dis Nerv Sys* 28:664, 1967

19. McBryde AM: Stress fractures in athletes. *J Sports Med* 3:212, 1975

20. Walter NE and Wolf MD: Stress fractures in young athletes. *Amer J Sports Med* 5:165, 1977

21. Eilert RE: Sports injuries in children. *Surg Rounds* 1:54, 1978

22. DeHaven KE: Athletic injuries in adolescents. *Pediat Ann* 7:96, 1978

GENERAL ORTHOPEDIC PROBLEMS

**Irving Strauchler, M.D., and
Andrew Weiss, M.D.**

CHAPTER

12

The largest percentage of sports injuries involves the musculoskeletal system, and the cost of these injuries in terms of financial loss, disability, time, and suffering is astronomical. The age-old quip "The easiest way to treat an injury is to prevent it" still holds true. The ingredients for safe sports activities are a well-conditioned, healthy athlete; proper, functioning equipment; a safe, appropriate playing area; and proper supervision. When these criteria are not met, injuries are more likely to occur.

The key to treatment is correct diagnosis, and the key to diagnosis is awareness. Above all, the athlete and her physician must be aware of the kinds of injuries that can occur and their diagnosis and treatment. The day is long gone when the coach or trainer was the athlete's primary healer and the athlete was referred to a physician only when all other means failed. (The trainer is, however, the first line of defense and, in the athlete's best interest, must develop a close working relationship with the athlete as well as her physician.)

With few exceptions, the best time to examine and diagnose an injury is the moment after it has occurred. The longer examination and diagnosis are delayed, the more difficult it is to make the diagnosis and the more difficult and prolonged the treatment will be. Swelling, muscle spasm, limitation of motion, and muscle atrophy very rapidly cloud the picture.

The hand

The hand plays a cardinal role in most sports because it is responsible for the final performance of most complicated tasks. It also acts as the first line of defense in protecting the athlete during falls and against impact in contact sports.

The hand is a complex organ capable of the greatest sensory input and mobility: It is able to grasp at one moment and act as a fist the next.

Anatomically, the hand consists of: 14 phalanges (finger bones); five metacarpals (knuckle bones); eight carpals (wrist bones); and multiple long tendons to each finger.

No hand injury in which pain and swelling last for more than a few hours should be considered minor. These injuries should be evaluated by a physician as soon as possible and appropriate studies (such as X-rays) ordered.

The hand examination: The following information should be obtained from the athlete:

• How did the injury occur?
• Was any part of the hand deformed and returned to its normal position?
• Have there been previous hand injuries?
• What points hurt the most?
• What makes the pain better and what makes it worse?
• What deformities are present?
• Is there full range of motion in the hand?
• Are there any areas of numbness?

All hand cuts and abrasions should be cleaned as soon as possible and evaluated for possible injuries to deeper structures, such as nerves and tendons. Relatively small cuts, especially those made by broken glass, can do tremendous internal damage while superficially appearing minor. Superficial abrasions should be carefully cleaned to prevent embedded dirt from producing a tattoo-like scar. The hand should be splinted, wrapped, and kept elevated for several days after treatment.

The female athlete must remember that extensive manicuring, especially cuticle cutting, combined with the trauma of field or contact sports can greatly increase the chance of infections about the nail (paronychia). This, in turn, can lead to more serious infec-

145

tions, such as felons, which are fingertip pulp infections. These can require surgical treatment.

An improperly treated cut can result in a serious hand infection, especially cuts caused by accidental or deliberate contact with teeth. These sometimes minute lacerations about the knuckles can lead to fulminant infections. The athlete's treatment involves leaving these contaminated wounds open, splinting, elevation, and appropriate antibiotics.

Proper protective hand gear—padded hand strapping as for boxers and gymnasts in training—a clean, safe, appropriate playing area, and proper supervision are all necessary to reduce the incidence of hand injury and infection.

Fingertip injuries: The woman athlete must keep her nails trimmed and cleaned. Long nails may be chic but show a lack of consideration for fellow athletes and for herself. Torn or split nails

FIGURE 12-1

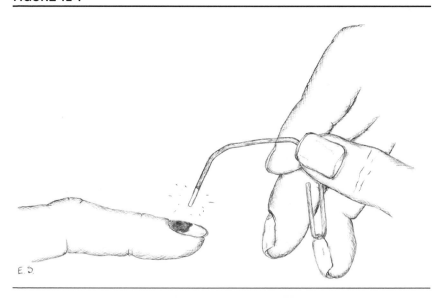

A subungual hematoma can be treated by making a small hole through the nail over the hematoma with a heated tip of an unfolded paper clip.

should be immediately trimmed to prevent sharp edges from cutting or catching.

A crush to the fingertip can cause fracture as well as a large subungual hematoma, which is painful and disabling. It can be treated by carefully making a small hole through the center of the nail or over the center of the hematoma with a small piece of heated metal such as an unfolded paper clip (see Figure 12-1).

The nail root occasionally is pulled out from under the cuticle area; after gentle cleaning, it can be replaced. When the nail injury and fracture occur together, an attempt should be made to keep the nail in place with a splint.

In fingertip amputation, the patient and the separated part should be taken to the hospital immediately for definitive care and, in selected cases, reimplantation.

A mallet finger (jammed finger or baseball finger) is caused by the extended finger being forcibly flexed by a softball or piece of sports gear. The injury is usually to either the extensor tendon or to the bone with which it joins the finger. The injuries are treated surgically if the avulsed bone fragment is large. In most cases, however, the physician treats these injuries conservatively with a small padded splint holding the distal interphalangeal joint in slight hyperextension. This must be *continuously* maintained for six to eight weeks and then at night-only for several more weeks (see Figure 12-2).

Twisting injuries to the finger can cause painful tears in the collateral ligaments supporting the finger joints and inflammation to the joint capsule (capsulitis). Only the involved joints must be immobilized in slight flexion, and gentle range of motion exercises can be begun after approximately 10 to 14 days. The inflammatory process may be prolonged, with residual stiffness the end result. Such injuries should be treated by a physician.

A very useful device is the bent paper clip splint, which is a paper clip formed appropriately for the shape and size of the involved finger joint and padded with cloth tape. This provides easy and convenient immobilization while allowing some sports activity (see Figure 12-3). These splints also allow sports activity when used after finger fractures are partially healed.

A finger caught on a player's jersey in contact sports can lead to avulsion of the finger's deep flexor tendon. There is pain, inability to bend the fingertip, and fullness at the base of the finger. These injuries require early diagnosis and surgical treatment.

A particularly serious type of hand-ligament injury involves the base of the thumb, the metacarpal phalangeal joint, and is known as gamekeeper's thumb. The name is derived from the practice of British gamewardens of killing rabbits by twisting their necks between the thumb and index finger. This occasionally causes stress injuries to the inner thumb ligaments. It results in significant disability because the injured area is stretched each time attempts are made to grasp anything. Most often, in sports, the injury is caused by a fall on the downward directed thumb when the thumb is caught on a piece of clothing or gear and pulled outward, as in a ski-pole injury. A complete tear diagnosed by stress X-rays must be treated with surgical repair.

Simple finger dislocation without complication often can be reduced by the athlete herself, or a teammate, by direct outward pull of the deformed finger. If reduction is accomplished, the finger should be splinted in flexion and seen by a physician as soon as possible. However, if reduction cannot be easily accomplished, the part should be protected and the athlete taken to the emergency room for definitive treatment. The index finger metacarpophalangeal joint is notorious for resistance to closed reduction and often requires surgical treatment.

The treatment of fractures and dislocations of the wrist is beyond the scope of this chapter. Wrist sprains are a common occur-

FIGURE 12-2

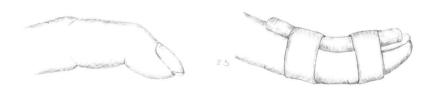

Mallet finger (left) is treated by holding the distal interphalangeal joint in slight hyperextension with a small padded splint.

rence in sports and are usually due to a fall on the wrist rather than a direct blow. If the sprain is severe, X-rays should be taken. If they are negative, the sprain can usually be treated with cast immobilization for several days, followed by gradual resumption of activities when pain and swelling resolve. A small percentage of wrist sprains are due to a more serious underlying injury, such as an occult fracture of the scaphoid bone, which may not be evident on X-rays taken at the time of injury. Another serious cause of traumatic wrist pain is ligamentous injury and carpal collapse. These changes also take time to develop, and if the pain and limitation of motion seen with a sprained wrist persist for more than two weeks, repeat X-ray films should be taken, and the patient seen by a specialist.

FIGURE 12-3

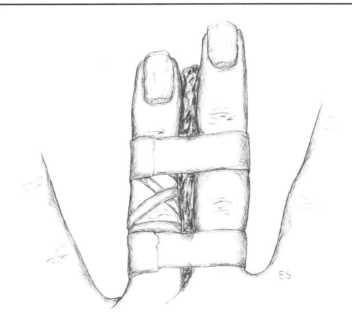

A padded paper clip used as a splint provides immobilization while allowing some sports activity.

Quervain's disease: This is a common occurrence in activities, such as table tennis and racquet sports, that require repetitive wrist and thumb motion. The symptoms are pain in the radial aspect of the wrist aggravated by thumb motion. The tendons that extend the thumb pass through a narrow canal in the radial side of the wrist and, with repeated activity, inflammation begins and a constriction forms in the canal. Treatment is rest and splinting. Unless they bring resolution of symptoms, injections of steroids and local anesthetics into the canal may be necessary. In cases unresponsive to such treatment, surgical release is extremely effective. This condition, unfortunately, is much more common in women than in men.

Carpal tunnel syndrome: This clinical entity is extremely common in middle-aged women and can be caused by a multitude of conditions, including repeated trauma to the wrist. Old fractures in the wrist area can produce this syndrome, as can inflammation of the tendon sheaths passing through the wrist. Symptoms are numbness and tingling in the thumb, index finger, and middle finger, as well as a feeling of clumsiness; at night, the hand feels as if it's falling asleep. Atrophy of the thenar (thumb) muscles is a late manifestation. In early cases, those that occur after injury, initial treatment consists of splinting and analgesics. If this produces no relief, electromyographic studies to confirm the diagnosis should be made, and surgical release of the carpal tunnel should be performed.

The elbow

The elbow consists of three distinct joints: the humeroradial, the humeroulnar, and the radioulnar articulations. Injuries to the ulnar nerve, radial-head fractures, tennis elbow, and olecranon bursitis are the more common problems of the elbow.

The ulnar nerve supplies motor power to the small muscles of the hand and gives sensation to the fourth and fifth digits. It lies in a vulnerable and superficial position along the posteromedial aspect of the elbow. A direct blow to the nerve in the cubital tunnel—or funny bone, as it is more commonly known—usually gives rise to a shocking sensation extending down the arm into the hand. Most such injuries resolve spontaneously within moments. However, severe injury can lead to permanent damage to the ulnar nerve. Prevention consists of using appropriate elbow padding in sports that involve repeated trauma to the elbow.

The elbow transmits the force of falls from the hand to the shoulder and to the upper body. The line of transmission of the force of falls or any other force to which the hand may be subjected is through the radial head and its articulation on the humerus. It is therefore not surprising that the most common fracture in the elbow region is that of the radial head. Most commonly, these injuries are nondisplaced but are extremely painful and require immobilization, analgesics, and, of course, X-ray evaluation in two planes to ascertain that the fracture is not displaced and that no other injury is present.

Tennis elbow is an extremely common condition, not limited to those who are engaged in tennis. It is actually caused by strenuous action of the wrist against resistance, but the involved muscles originate at the elbow, and this is where pain is perceived. Pain also radiates down the outer side of the arm and forearm. Those who engage in any activity requiring repeated and forceful flexion and extension of the wrist—including knitting—are subject to this condition. Most experts believe that tennis elbow is probably a constellation of conditions, all with the common symptom of pain over the lateral aspect of the elbow. These conditions range from a tear in the common tendinous origin of the extensor muscles of the wrist to an inflammation of the lining of the elbow joint (radioulnar synovitis), or to a tear in the muscular insertion of the extensor muscles. Treatment is usually symptomatic, with immobilization of the wrist and elbow in a position of comfort and function, ICE (ice, compression, and elevation), analgesics, and anti-inflammatory drugs. Persistent or recurrent cases can be treated with injections of steroids and anesthetics into the area of maximum tenderness. Long-term rehabilitation involves strengthening of the extensor muscles of the wrist and engaging in sports that limit impact motion to the elbow. Surgery should be considered only for cases that are long-standing, persistent, and unresponsive to conservative treatment.

Olecranon bursitis involves a thin fluid-filled cavity (bursa) over the tip of the elbow (olecranon). This bursa allows mobility of the upper extremity while the elbow is resting on a firm surface. Repeated injury to the olecranon—such as repeatedly landing on one's elbow on a dirt playing field—can lead to abrasions that cause infection in the bursa. This is known as suppurative bursitis. More commonly, it is not an infection that causes the swelling and pain, but merely a sterile inflammatory process secondary to repeated injury to the area. If the fluid accumulation is large and/or painful, it is usually treated with rest, protection, and aspiration. Prevention can be accomplished by appropriate elbow pads when engaged in sports likely to cause this injury.

The shoulder

The shoulder girdle consists of four separate articulations or joints: glenohumeral, the true shoulder joint; acromioclavicular, the collar bone to shoulder joint; sternoclavicular, collar bone to breastbone

FIGURE 12-4

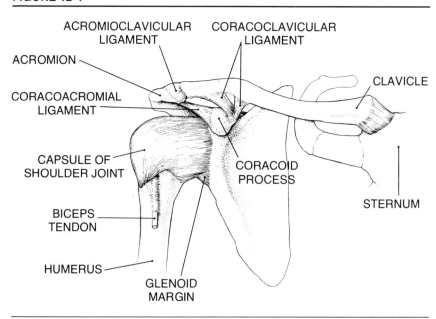

Joints and ligaments of the shoulder.

articulation; and scapulothoracic, shoulder blade to chest articulation (see Figure 12-4). Normal pain-free motion in any one of these joints is dependent on the integrity of the other three.

Contrasting the upper with the lower extremity, one sees that the lower is primarily a weight-bearing apparatus—and therefore strength and stability rule over mobility—while the upper extremity's primary function is getting the hand to where the brain wants it—and therefore mobility rules over stability. This concept is borne out by the structure and function of the respective joints. The shoulder is prone to various subluxations and dislocations. A relative limitation of motion due to scarring in the hip may well be unnoticed, but a relative limitation of motion in the shoulder can be catastrophic to the athlete.

In evaluating injury, it is important to determine exactly what happened: How was the athlete moving? How was she hit? Was a pop felt? Where is the maximum pain? What can't she do?

The shoulder transmits force or energy from the hand, elbow, and arm, up through to the chest and the rest of the body, as in a fall. When the force transmitted overcomes the strength of the soft tissues and bone, something "gives." The direction of the force and the position of the shoulder at the time of impact determine the exact nature of the injury.

The clavicle: Also called the collar bone, the clavicle is the anterior strut connecting the mobile shoulder girdle to the chest. At the medial end, it forms the sternoclavicular joint supported by strong ligaments to the sternum or breastbone. When the shoulder is thrust forward, a fall can cause dislocation at this point. Anterior dislocation produces pain and a bony prominence localizing the pathology to this area; while posterior dislocation is painful, and while there is no obvious deformity, there can be compression of the vital, deep structures of the chest. Therefore, the posterior indication can be more dangerous. Immediate treatment consists of shoulder immobilization and X-ray evaluation. Reduction can usually be accomplished by the physician using direct pressure over the dislocated bone and bringing the shoulder outward and backward.

Clavicular fractures are much more common. Again, the mechanism is a fall on the outstretched hand, especially common in horseback riding, trampolining, and contact sports. There is pain on shoulder motion, and the athlete usually supports the forearm and elbow to prevent shoulder motion. There is visible deformity in the subcutaneous bone, and maximum tenderness is usually present over the area of fracture.

Acute treatment consists of immobilization in a figure-8 soft splint to allow correction of the deformity and give support to the shoulder. This soft dressing should usually remain in place for about two to three weeks. This is usually all the treatment required. There is rarely any long-term disability from clavicular fracture, although often a slightly disfiguring prominence is noted in the area of the healing fracture. This is due to callus (bone scar) formation.

Dislocation at the outer aspect of the clavicular or the acromioclavicular (AC) joint can be disabling and results from the rupture of strong ligaments holding the clavicle to the coracoid, part of the scapula. Landing on the shoulder (head over heels) is the common mechanism of injury, typically seen in contact sports and horseback riding.

The injury is graded 1, 2, or 3. In a grade-1 sprain, there is tearing with no step-off, and the joint remains intact. Local tenderness is the effect of an injury of this grade. In grade-2 dislocations, there is a small step-off but the ligaments are partially intact. A grade-3 dislocation is a complete dislocation of the joint with complete rupture and a significant step-off caused by the weight of the arm pulling the shoulder downward and allowing the clavicle to ride upward.

Grade-1 AC separation can be treated with minimal immobilization, mild analgesics, and limitation of activities for several days until the pain has resolved. In grade-2 AC separation, there is usually more pain and disability, and the shoulder should be immobilized and supported for approximately three weeks to allow healing of the torn tissues to take place. Return to full contact sports should be restricted for another three weeks. In grade-3 separations, surgery is often required to completely reduce the dislocation, although in some cases, the use of devices such as the Kenny-Howard splint for maintenance of the reduction without surgery can be successful. Complete AC separations are significant injuries to the shoulder girdle, and return of 100 per cent shoulder function is often not achieved with either surgical or conservative methods.

Shoulder dislocations and the painful-shoulder syndrome are especially common in women and are discussed in the next chapter.

The knee

The knee has been called the most vulnerable joint of the body from the standpoint of athletic injuries. It is the largest joint in the body, and is not a simple hinge joint, but flexes, extends, rotates, and slides. The femoral condyles sit upon the tibial plateau and are fitted into place by the menisci or knee cartilages, which act like moving washers. The patella or kneecap slides upon the front of the distal femur and increases mechanical efficiency in the quadriceps muscle group. The knee is therefore an anatomically unstable joint in contrast to other joints, such as the hip, which are intrinsically stable. The medial- and lateral-collateral ligaments as well as the anterior and posterior cruciate ligaments are the main ligamentous stabilizers of the knee. Because of tremendous forces acting upon the knee, it and its ligaments must be reinforced by the muscles that span the joint: the quadriceps, the hamstrings, and the gastrocnemius (calf muscle) (see Figure 12-5).

The acutely injured knee: The best time to examine a knee injury is within moments of its occurrence. The longer one waits, the more difficult and painful are the examination and diagnosis. In taking the history, it's important to learn if there have been any previous injuries or knee problems, if the knee was struck or something spontaneously "popped out," and whether there was a popping sensation or tearing sensation within the knee.

One should look for areas of contusion, deformity, or swelling, and the range of motion should be recorded. Medial, lateral, and rotational stability should be ascertained. The maximum area of tenderness is of great importance in making the diagnosis.

Ligamentous injuries of the knee can be divided into three categories: grade 1 or mild injuries, grade 2 or moderate injuries, and grade 3 or severe injuries. Grade-2 ligament sprains involve an effusion, local tenderness, and slight to moderate instability. A grade-3 or complete ligament injury involves marked instability, a lot of pain, and a variable amount of knee effusion—depending on whether the capsule of the knee was also torn with the injury. Athletes with grade-3 injuries should be closely watched and evaluated for vascular damage that may have occurred with a knee dislocation and spontaneous reduction. These injuries, fortunately, are rare. An athlete's ability to walk off the playing field after a knee injury is no indication of the degree of severity. Many athletes with complete ligament ruptures walked off the field under their own power.

Knee injuries should be evaluated by an experienced trainer and physician as soon as they occur, and X-rays are helpful in the diagnosis of possible osteochondral fractures, which can complicate such ligamentous injuries.

FIGURE 12-5

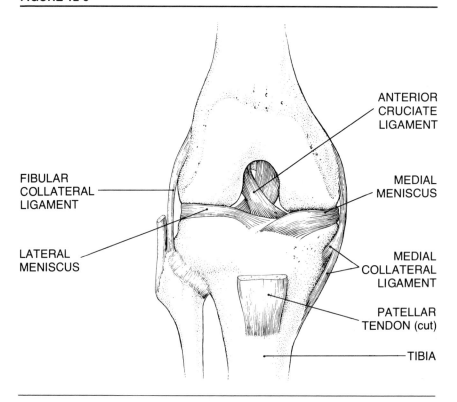

FIBULAR COLLATERAL LIGAMENT

LATERAL MENISCUS

ANTERIOR CRUCIATE LIGAMENT

MEDIAL MENISCUS

MEDIAL COLLATERAL LIGAMENT

PATELLAR TENDON (cut)

TIBIA

Ligaments and menisci of the knee joint.

Other possible injuries are meniscal injuries (torn cartilage), dislocations of the patella, and osteochondral fractures or chip fractures within the knee joints. Athletes with torn cartilage usually have a knee effusion with pain on motion and perhaps a locking sensation.

The details of differential diagnosis are beyond the scope of this chapter, but we should mention that the newer techniques of arthroscopy—looking into the knee joint with a special optical instrument—and arthrography—injecting special radiographic drugs into the knee—have aided tremendously in the diagnosis of these syndromes.

The ankle

Acute ankle sprains are commonly seen sports injuries because the forces generated by running are tremendous. The stresses to which the ankle is subjected allow little tolerance between normal activity and injury.

The ankle is basically a hinge joint with flexion-extension as its primary mode of motion. Most of its rocking motion occurs at the subtalar joint, between the ankle and the heel. The bony architecture of this hinge joint is that of a mortice and tenon: The mortice is made up of the fibula and tibia, with the talus or uppermost part of the foot acting as the tenon. The bony prominence at the inner aspect of the ankle is known as the medial malleolus, a continuation of the tibia or shin bone. The outer prominence of the ankle is known as the lateral malleolus or the distalmost portion of the fibula, the thin bone completing the bony architecture of the leg.

To allow for free flexion-extension motion at the ankle and still control stability of the joint, the joint capsule is thin anteriorly and posteriorly, while numerous ligaments are present on the inside and outside of the joint (see Figure 12-6). There are many ligaments supporting the ankle on all sides. The most important are the three ligaments constituting the lateral-collateral ligament of the ankle and the four ligaments that make up the deltoid or medial-collateral ligament of the ankle. These two complexes are the most frequently injured.

Contusions: A direct blow to the ankle with a baseball bat, tennis racquet, or similar object most often produces a contusion, and is treated in the manner previously mentioned: with compresses, ice, and limitation of activity until pain has resolved. However, X-rays are necessary to rule out a direct fracture, as an incomplete or nondisplaced fracture can, with continued activity, progress to a serious injury. A blow to the outer aspect of the ankle (the lateral malleolus) can produce a dislocation of the peroneal tendons, which normally cause the foot to turn outward. This dislocation causes

FIGURE 12-6

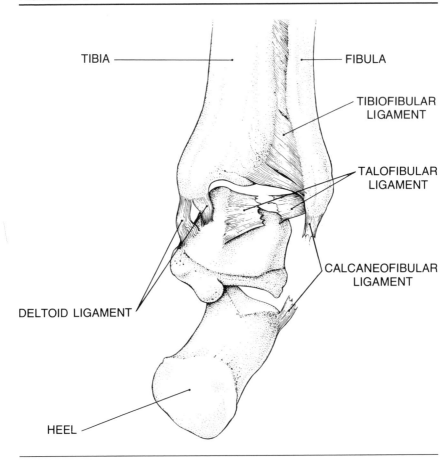

TIBIA

FIBULA

TIBIOFIBULAR LIGAMENT

TALOFIBULAR LIGAMENT

CALCANEOFIBULAR LIGAMENT

DELTOID LIGAMENT

HEEL

Ligaments of the ankle joint.

the tendons to slip out from behind the lateral malleolus and dislocate forward, causing pain and incapacitation. This should be repaired surgically in the acute episode. Direct blows to tendons anywhere in the body and especially to the ankle can lead to inflammation of the tendon sheaths or synovitis, which can be persistent and painful with motion. Treatment consists initially of rest, ice, and strapping, to be followed by steroid injections in one to two weeks if the initial treatment is not successful.

A twisting force of the ankle—inversion, eversion, pronation, supination, or any combination of these four forces—can lead to a spectrum of clinical entities, varying from a mild sprain to a complex fracture-dislocation, according to the magnitude of the force. An inversion (roll-under) injury tears the lateral-collateral ligament of the ankle, while an eversion (rolling outward motion) involves the deltoid or medial-collateral ligament. The most commonly involved ligament is the calcaneofibular, the most anterior part of the lateral-collateral ligament complex (see Figure 12-6). With an acute injury, the ankle is usually swollen and tender to the touch, with an area of maximum tenderness. One can often differentiate between a fracture and a ligament injury. The latter usually causes maximum tenderness just below the bony prominences, while fractures usually cause tenderness centered on the bony prominences of the ankle. As mentioned before, X-rays should always be done to confirm the diagnosis.

A mild ankle sprain (first degree) causes localized tenderness and swelling with minimal disability. The athlete is usually able to walk with some discomfort immediately after the injury. Treatment is icing and strapping, with exercises to strengthen the muscles as soon as the discomfort begins to resolve.

In a moderate or second-degree sprain injury, there is a partial tear of the substance of the ligament, and there is a loss of strength of the ligament. The injured area is extremely susceptible to repeat injury and should be protected. There is usually significant pain and swelling, and the athlete has difficulty walking—usually requiring help to leave the playing field. Physical examination shows marked swelling, limitation of motion, and tenderness maximum at the area just below the bony prominences. The injured ankle should be elevated, splinted, and iced for several hours until definitive diagnosis and evaluation can be done. Often, differentiating between a moderate sprain and a complete ligament injury is difficult, and further examination—stress X-ray or arthrogram under local anesthesia—may be required. Once it has been confirmed that there is no abnormal motion in the ankle and that it is indeed a moderate sprain, icing should be continued for a total of 24 to 48 hours, followed by compressive dressing. The patient should be allowed to ambulate in a plaster posterior splint with crutches. In about three days, when the swelling has been controlled, a short leg-walking cast boot is applied, and the posterior splint removed. The athlete is allowed to place weight to pain tolerance on this cast boot, which should remain in place for approximately two to four weeks, depending on the extent of injury. Conditioning of all uninjured muscles and extremities is a vital part of rehabilitation and should be strenuously pursued.

In severe or third-degree sprains, there is complete rupture of one or more ligaments of the ankle, often associated with a fracture. The athlete is unable to bear any weight on the limb and should not be expected to. The ankle should be immediately splinted to prevent further damage, and the athlete taken to a physician as soon as possible. X-rays should be done; if there is no sign of fracture, an arthrogram may be required to help make the diagnosis. This is often not necessary when gross instability is seen on passive ankle movement. Severe multiple ligament rupture requires surgical repair for best results. With single isolated ligament rupture, the physician may decide on conservative treatment, with cast immobilization for approximately six weeks as an alternative. If X-ray shows a fracture, the minimum period of immobilization is usually six weeks, depending on the extent of the fracture. Accurate reduction must be done, and often there is a period of nonweight-bearing. Again, the athlete should be instructed and coached in an extensive program of conditioning for her uninjured limbs to prevent atrophy. This is a significant injury, and the period of rehabilitation can be considerable.

SPECIAL ORTHOPEDIC PROBLEMS

Irving Strauchler, M.D., and
Andrew Weiss, M.D.

CHAPTER

13

G eneral orthopedic problems are covered in Chapter 12. In this chapter, we review problems that are more prevalent in the female athlete; these are low back pain, scoliosis or curvature of the spine, spondylolysis, spondylolisthesis, shoulder dislocations and related conditions, recurrent dislocation of the patella and patellar tendinitis, shin splints, stress fractures, and compartment syndromes.

Back injury

Back injury/low back pain is a common problem in the athlete and nonathlete alike. It is the greatest single cause of work-related disability and accounts for about 10 to 25 per cent of sports injury.

The spine consists of a series of vertebral bones separated by fibrocartilaginous discs and held together by strong muscles and ligaments. Each vertebral bone consists of an anterior body, a central canal for the spinal cord and the posterior bony arch.

Injury to the attached ligaments and muscles, bones, joints, and nervous tissue, as well as the multitude of referred pain syndromes can cause severe incapacitating back pain. Discovering the origin of this pain in the particular case can be challenging and sometimes impossible.

In evaluating the athlete who has just sustained an injury to the back, one must first obtain a clear picture of what happened. The following questions should be asked: How was the injury sustained? Was the athlete hit? What position was the athlete in at the time of injury? Was there any loss of consciousness? Was there any numbness or feeling of paralysis? Does anything make the pain better? Does anything make the pain worse? What could the athlete do and not do after the injury?

Soft-tissue injury: Direct contusion to the lumbar spine and flank region is frequent in contact sports. The pain is usually localized to the specific area of injury, though occasionally the pain is referred down the leg in a sciatic-type pattern. The athlete can be treated as for other types of contusions, namely with ice, rest, analgesics, and back strapping, if necessary. In severe cases, the athlete should always be observed for signs of internal organ injury such as kidney trauma.

In direct injuries, muscle strain and ligament sprain are also very commonly seen. Often they are not directly due to trauma, and the athlete feels a pop or acute pain as she is twisting or at the extremes of back motion. The pain increases with time, often following a seemingly trivial event. The muscle or ligament involved is the site of maximum tenderness and, if it can be accurately localized, can often be treated with local injections of anesthetic and/or steroids. This cannot be done in the case of diffuse muscle involvement. Treatments also include ice, strapping, and physical therapy, if necessary. Recurrent or chronic muscle strain or ligamentous sprains can be exceedingly difficult to treat. Often, the use of a corset reduces the incidence of recurrence. The athlete with persistent back strain or sprain often must limit her sports activity or change to less strenuous sports.

Fractures: The types of injuries that cause direct contusion, muscle strain, or ligamentous sprain in the extreme can cause fracture either to the lower ribs or to the vertebrae. Any athlete with a significant back injury and significant pain should be X-rayed to rule out the possibility of a fracture. The specific treatment of these fractures is beyond the scope of this book. Any athlete who complains of paresthesias or numbness or weakness in the lower extremity, or of bowel or bladder difficulties after an injury, should not be allowed to stand, should be immobilized in a stretcher with all precaution against any further back injury, and should be immediately seen by a physician in a hospital.

Disc ruptures: In the acute case of maximal muscular effort with flexion of the lumbar spine, there is a tremendous increase in pressure within the fibrocartilaginous disc that separate the vertebral body. The ring that supports the disc can rupture, with resultant compression on the spinal cord or the nerve roots. In this event, the athlete experiences acute severe pain often radiating down the leg and, in rare episodes, causing severe neurological deficits. The athlete should again be placed on a stretcher and taken to a hospital for treatment. The treatment of a ruptured intervertebral disc is beyond the scope of this book. Most such

TABLE 13-1

Causes of Sciatic and/or Back Pain

Trauma
☐ Paraspinal-muscle contusion
☐ Myofascial syndrome (muscle-fascial tears)
☐ Ligament ruptures
☐ Fractures to the spine
☐ Disc ruptures

Referred interthoracic disease
☐ Dissecting aortic aneurysm
☐ Pneumonia with pleurisy
☐ Heart attack
☐ Posterior thoracic tumors

Intra-abdominal referred pain
☐ Stomach and duodenal ulcers
☐ Pancreatitis
☐ Pancreatic tumor
☐ Gallbladder disease
☐ Kidney disease, stones, infections
☐ Abdominal tumors
☐ Retroperitoneal bleeding or abscesses
☐ Diverticulitis/colitis

Pelvic referred pain
☐ Menstrual pain
☐ Endometriosis

cases, especially those with neurological deficit, require surgery.

Arthritis: In the older athlete, degenerative changes in the various joints of the spine can lead to chronic low back pain. Rheumatoid arthritis and the other forms of arthritis can also cause significant back pain. Treatment in most of these cases consists of aspirin or other anti-inflammatory arthritis medication, in addition to a physical-therapy program. Athletics and exercise are an important component of the treatment of arthritis, and an athletic program should be tailored for each patient with arthritis.

Referred pain syndromes: As noted in Table 13-1, there are

☐ Pelvic tumor (uterus, ovary)
☐ Uterine malposition (prolapse, retroversion)
☐ Pelvic infection (PID)

Local tumors
☐ Vascular tumor or malformations
☐ Spinal-cord tumors
☐ Metastases to the vertebral body or other local structures (with or without bony collapse)

Arthritis and miscellaneous
☐ Sacroiliac joint arthritis, vertebral arthritis (spondylolysis)
☐ Osteoporosis
☐ Osteomalacia
☐ Paget's disease
☐ Bony entrapment of the cord or nerve roots
☐ Postsurgical scarring of the spinal cord
☐ Vertebral abscesses

Some causes of sciatic pain without significant back pain include:
☐ Knee pathology (meniscal tear, Baker's cyst)
☐ Hip pathology (arthritis)
☐ Thigh pathology (tumors of the thigh or femur)
☐ Hamstring muscle injury, sciatic nerve contusion, or neuritis
☐ Leg pathology: compartment syndrome, calf-muscle injury, shin splints
☐ Foot pathology such as Morton's neuroma

many causes of chronic low back pain. These can vary from tumors to infections to a variety of internal-organ problems. These causes of low back pain can be differentiated from those previously cited in that they often are not aggravated by back motion and often are not directly related to activity. In a condition such as malposition of the uterus, the pain can be aggravated by prolonged standing and/or running. The differential diagnosis of these syndromes is beyond the scope of this book but they should be kept in mind in treating the female athlete with low back pain.

Back problems specially related to the female athlete

Scoliosis: About 4 per cent of adolescents have some sign of scoliosis, a side-to-side curvature of the spine. Just about half this number—100,000 in the U.S.A.—require some medical observation or treatment.

Although there are many different types of scoliosis, such as those caused by birth defects or neurological disease, the most common, and most important to our discussion, is the hereditary or idiopathic type, which for reasons still unknown is usually more common in the active adolescent girl.

Untreated scoliosis can progress to a severe hunchback deformity with loss of height, late arthritis, and late heart and lung problems due to the deformed chest cavity.

All adolescents should have routine scoliosis screening to pick up the problem early. With early detection, scoliosis can usually be treated and severe deformity prevented. New treatment in progressive cases requires a brace to be worn 23 hours a day and removed only for bathing, swimming, and the like.

For athletes requiring scoliosis-brace treatment, sports, with the exception of competitive contact sports and gymnastics, should be encouraged—although the athlete will find in many instances that the brace limits performance.

Severe curves may progress and require surgery—usually, spinal fusion—and most sports are prohibited for at least one to two years after this operation. The extent of sports limitation varies with the individual. Most youngsters who have had scoliosis surgery have been able to return to sports activity with only certain restrictions.

Physical-education teachers and trainers should be familiar with the method of detecting scoliosis. Girls should be examined so that as much of the back as possible is exposed, usually with shorts and a bra or a two-piece bathing suit. The athlete should be examined from all sides in the standing forward and bending position. Unequal shoulders, a prominent shoulder blade, unequal hips, curve in the spine, or roundback deformities (see Figure 13-1) are all reasons for referral to a specialist for further evaluation.

Roundback deformity or kyphosis is often brushed off as poor posture. This condition, known as Scheuermann's disease, can often progress to an unsightly degree of roundback deformity if not treated properly. The Milwaukee brace has been especially successful in the treatment of this disorder.

Spondylolysis: This is a condition in which part of the posterior protective ring of the vertebral bone separates. In young people, this is most commonly due to trauma (stress fracture). It is generally seen at the junction of the lumbar spine and the sacrum—an area of great stress. The condition is first seen at age five to seven; the incidence increases with age until age 20. It is often seen in gymnasts, bowlers, and weightlifters. The condition may or may not be symptomatic, and its presence in a particular individual may have no correlation with her back pain. The presence of spondylolysis places increased stress on the intervertebral disc at that level, perhaps leading to disc protrusion, and this protrusion more often than the spondylolysis is the cause of neurological difficulties. Treatment of uncomplicated spondylolysis consists of rest, analgesics, occasional back-bracing, and change to a sport less strenuous to the lumbosacral spine.

Spondylolisthesis: With continued stress and stretching of surrounding soft tissue, spondylolysis can progress to a further slipping of one vertebra on the one below; this is known as spondylolisthesis. The condition is graded by the amount of slip present. The slip usually occurs between ages 11 and 15, a period when other changes are taking place in the athlete. Again, as in spondylolysis, it most commonly occurs at the lumbosacral junction (L5-S1) and may be totally asymptomatic; most commonly it presents as low back pain, aggravated by increase with exercise, and with pain radiating into the buttocks. The young athlete may present with back pain and may have only complaints of a tightness or difficulty in fully extending her back and legs, or complain of increased stiffness in her back and legs. In severe cases, she may have tenderness at the lumbosacral junction, and there may be an unusual step-off noted with prominence of the posterior aspect of her pelvis and a decrease in her lumbar lordosis or the normal forward tilt of her abdomen in relation to her pelvis. Severe cases or mild cases showing rapid progression require surgical fusion at this site. Surgical fusion prevents further progress of the disease and prevents neurological complications. With successful fusion, sports activities can often be resumed.

FIGURE 13-1

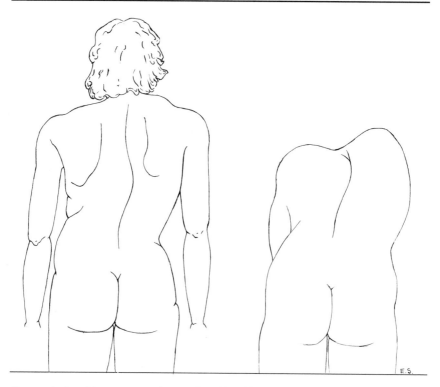

Unequal shoulders, a prominent shoulder blade, unequal hips, curve in the spine, and roundback deformities are signs that scoliosis may be present.

Shoulder dislocations and other conditions

The shoulder joint is unique in that the head of the humerus sits in a shallow, saucer-like hollow, supported mainly by soft tissue. As part of the normal motion, the head of the humerus slides slightly in each direction, to achieve a greater range of motion, supported mainly by the capsule and complex array of muscles and tendons. The deltoid muscle, the large muscle giving the shoulder its normal round appearance, is the outermost layer. Beneath it is a cuff—the rotator cuff—composed of four separate muscles encircling and supporting the head of the humerus. Interspersed between these structures are a number of bursae, which allow for smooth motion between these tissue layers.

Anterior shoulder dislocation accounts for about 90 to 95 per cent of all dislocations of the glenohumeral joint. The mechanism of injury is forced abduction and external rotation as in the overhand throw of the softball or football. There is acute pain and disability, with loss of motion and loss of the normal roundness of the shoulder, with a hollow palpable just beneath the acromion where the head of the humerus usually sits.

Treatment consists of getting the athlete off the playing field immediately, supporting the shoulder in a sling, and getting her to a hospital for X-ray evaluation. This should always be done before reduction to determine the type of dislocation and whether there is an associated fracture. Reduction can usually be accomplished with analgesics and muscle relaxants, although general anesthesia may be required. The reduction must be gentle to prevent further damage. If the athlete feels pain, the reduction will be more difficult and therefore be more traumatic. In first-time dislocations, the shoulder should be immobilized in a "Velpeau-type" dressing, which holds the shoulder and arm supported close against the chest. This should remain in place for four to six weeks to allow the torn capsule and soft tissue to heal. Those with recurrent dislocations require rest and immobilization for shorter periods. Treatment of recurrent dislocation is usually surgical and is beyond the scope of this chapter.

Posterior dislocations fortunately are rare. These are usually produced in a position of forward elevation and internal rotation, and often there is a blow to the shoulder from behind. Traumatic cases are treated with reduction and shoulder immobilization after X-ray diagnosis.

Habitual dislocators, who can dislocate their shoulders on command, are difficult to treat; they usually require the aid of a psychiatrist in addition to an orthopedist.

Rotator-cuff disorders: The incidence of rotator-cuff disorders increases with age and degeneration associated with calcific deposits. Inflammation in the area of degeneration is extremely painful and disabling and is usually referred to as "shoulder bursitis," while in actuality, it's a degenerative tendinitis. Treatment usually begins with anti-inflammatory drugs, analgesics, and rest. If there is no response to this course of treatment, try an injection of local anesthetics and steroids; this often results in long-term relief.

Acute ruptures of the rotator cuff occur with maximal muscular efforts and are more common with those degenerative changes. Range of motion often approaches normal, and diagnosis depends on careful examination. A useful diagnostic test is to ask the athlete to abduct her arm against resistance. This is usually painful, and she will have difficulty holding the stance. Treatment is surgical repair of the ruptured cuff.

Painful-shoulder syndrome: This disorder is extremely common, and its incidence increases with age. It can be due to capsulitis—inflammation of the soft tissue enclosing the shoulder joint; rotator-cuff syndrome—degeneration or rupture; bicipital tendinitis—degeneration and arthritic changes in the long bicipital tendon that runs up the proximal humerus into the shoulder joint; osteoarthritis—arthritic degeneration of any of the four shoulder joints; fracture; and visceral-referred pain. Abdominal or chest pathology that causes diaphragmatic irritation can cause these shoulder pains. Abdominal disorders—gallbladder disease, abdominal bleeding, ectopic pregnancy—and chest disease conditions—pneumonia with pleurisy, heart attack, pericarditis—can cause referred pain. For this reason, shoulder pain not related to shoulder motion or shoulder injury should be treated as a medical emergency.

Frozen-shoulder syndrome: A variation of the painful-shoulder syndrome, this is usually seen in older individuals, although it can affect persons of any age. The syndrome is caused by a vicious cycle—pain that causes a limitation of motion, which in turn causes more pain, and then an increased limitation of motion, until the individual has absolutely no motion at the glenohumeral joint. One can still move the shoulder girdle, however, with limited motion at the other three articulations. Frozen-shoulder syndrome should be treated with intensive, but gentle, physical therapy, analgesics, and anti-inflammatory agents.

Lower extremity problems

Recurrent dislocation of the patella: Conditions that can predispose young women to this condition include genu valgum or knock-knees; overweight; poor muscle development; and increased Q angle, which is the angle of insertion of the patellar tendon into the tibia. This condition is commonly associated with chondromalacia—patellar or cartilage degeneration on the under-surface of the kneecap. Acute treatment consists of documentation of the dislocation either by a physician's examination or X-rays; a careful reduction; aspiration of knee effusion if it is severe; X-rays after reduction if there is a question of an osteochondral fracture; and immobilization of the knee for four to six weeks to allow healing of the torn structures. During the period of immobilization, the athlete should be instructed in quads-setting and strengthening exercises. Many surgical procedures are available for recurrent dislocation of the patella. Each has advantages and disadvantages, the details of which are beyond the scope of this chapter.

Elastic knee-supports, which are commonly available in drugstores, offer some athletes a remarkable degree of support during their sports activities.

Jumper's knee (patellar tendinitis): This syndrome is seen in athletes who do a tremendous amount of jumping, running, and cutting, such as those engaged in basketball, hurdling, and other track sports. There is usually pain over the front of the knee, aggravated by activity and relieved by rest. On physical examination, the characteristic of this entity is point tenderness over the inferior pole of the patella at the junction of the patellar tendon.

Treatment for the acute condition consists of rest, ice, and muscle-strengthening exercises. An elastic kneecap can be applied and often gives the athlete some relief.

Shin splints: This syndrome of pain and discomfort in the leg is produced by running or heavy exercise involving the lower extremities. There is much discussion about the cause of shin splints, and it is probably best to think of it as a wastebasket term referring to different problems all involving leg pain with exercise.

Shin splints are commonly seen in runners, track athletes, ballet dancers, and field-sport players; the condition is more common in women than in men. Shin splints can be due to tears in the attachment of the posterior tibial muscle (aggravated by associated flat feet) and tears in the attachment of deep anterior tibial muscle into the tibial crest.

Conditions that resemble shin splints but are more serious in nature include: stress fractures of the tibia, stress fractures of the fibula, anterior compartment syndromes and/or deep posterior tibial compartments, achilles tendinitis and/or rupture, and plantaris-tendon rupture. In shin splints, acute treatment consists of ice application, rest, and occasional strapping. Analgesics and/or anti-inflammatory drugs are useful in a very painful episode. The athlete's shoe should be checked for proper fit and the foot posture for signs of foot pronation. Thereafter, the athlete should spend more time with warm-ups, especially calf stretching, and running on a softer surface for a decreased distance; she can then gradually work her way up again. In short, shin splints are most often a result of too much, too fast.

Stress fractures

Stress fractures are fatigue fractures produced by multiple minor injuries or stress: The crack in the bone will, with continued force, complete and occasionally displace. Areas most commonly involved are the tibia, fibula, second metatarsal, femur, pelvis, and back. Symptoms consist of pain at the site of stress with activity, and relief with rest. Early on, the X-rays are negative and other diagnoses are entertained.

With time, the bone has an opportunity to remodel and heal the damage. Callus can appear on the X-ray and can be confused with tumor. An aid in the diagnosis of stress fractures is the bone scan, in which minute amounts of radioactive material are injected. The scan picks up a stress fracture long before the X-ray shows any abnormality. A typical stress-fracture patient is the track athlete who has been out of practice during the winter months and decides to get back into shape in a hurry, doing five miles the first day and experiencing only mild aches in her legs. But, after several days, the pain in one leg becomes excruciating. X-rays at first show nothing, but two weeks later, a large amount of callus becomes visible. Had she persisted in pushing herself, a complete fracture might have resulted.

Treatment varies with the area involved and the extent of the stress fracture. Basically, it is treated with rest and analgesics as needed. If X-rays appear menacing, a cast immobilization for a short period of time may be wise.

Compartment syndromes

Muscles are enveloped and supported by tough tissue envelopes called fascial compartments. Their normal useful support can result in severe damage under certain circumstances.

More attention has recently been given to these syndromes. In sports, those most commonly involved are the forearm- and leg-compartment syndromes. Any injury that crushes muscle or interferes with the blood supply causes muscle swelling, which, inhibited by the fascial sheath, leads to extreme pressure and muscle death. This can be seen acutely in fractures and blood-vessel injuries—as when a player with cleat-studded shoes inadvertently steps on another player's forearm.

There is usually swelling, pain, and numbness. This is a surgical emergency, and the only way to prevent disaster is to open the compartment surgically and relieve the compressed muscle.

The most subtle cases are those of the runner whose shin splints persist despite treatment, with pain even during rest. Detailed pressure studies must then be made to confirm the diagnosis of a compartment syndrome.

Popliteus-tendon rupture

This condition can be a great imposter and is confused with a meniscal injury, phlebitis, and achilles tendinitis or rupture. It occurs most often in the middle-aged athlete, especially in tennis and basketball players. The mechanism is a spring for a shot or jumping for rebounds, in which several times body weight is exerted in this area. This muscle is a long, thin calf structure extending down to the ankle. During play, the athlete feels a pop in the calf, with sudden pain and incapacity. Treatment consists of rest, analgesics, ice compression, and elevation. Achilles-tendon rupture also often occurs in the middle-aged athlete.

Tendinitis with healing and repair often precedes an episode of complete rupture. Acute complete ruptures can be treated with prolonged casting or surgical repair.

The ability to push down with one's toes doesn't mean that the achilles tendon is not ruptured. To accurately diagnose the rupture, one must palpate the area of the achilles tendon, perhaps finding a gap or an area of extreme tenderness. In the Thomas test, the athlete allows her leg to be relaxed and the knee flexed at a right angle; the examiner then presses on the calf. If the achilles-tendon muscle-unit is intact, pressure on the calf causes involuntary movement of the foot. Lack of motion is a sign of rupture.

Further reading

Flatt A: *The Care of Minor Hand Injuries*, 3rd ed. St. Louis: Mosby, 1972

Hoppenfeld S: *Physical Examination of the Spine and Extremities.* New York: Appleton-Century-Crofts, 1976

Novich M and Taylor B: *Training and Conditioning of Athletes.* Philadelphia: Lea & Febiger, 1970

O'Donohue D: *Treatment of Injuries to Athletes*, 3rd ed. Philadelphia: Saunders, 1976

Williams JGP and Sperryn PN: *Sports Medicine*, 2nd ed. Baltimore: Williams & Wilkins, 1976

THE FOOT IN SPORTS

Steven I. Subotnick, D.P.M.

CHAPTER

14

S

Sports place increased demands upon the lower extremity, and it is important to have a working knowledge of the basic functional anatomy of the ankle and foot.

Main joints

The ankle: Motion in the ankle joint is mostly on the sagittal plane. The ankle functions as a hinged joint, but there is some motion in inversion and eversion with dorsiflexion and plantarflexion. Thus, a slight arc is described, and the foot at the extremes of plantarflexion and dorsiflexion has a mild amount of inversion along with the major sagittal plane motion. Because the major motion at the ankle joint is in the sagittal plane, multidirectional motions, such as cutting in football or going for a backhand in tennis, place additional stress on the lateral structures of the ankle joint. The ligamentous structures about the ankle joint maintain the integrity of the joint. When movement occurs beyond the normal range of motion, a sprained ligament or fracture may result. The plantarflexed ankle is less stable than the dorsiflexed ankle. The talus is held less securely in plantarflexion. Plantarflexion and inversion, when excessive, lead to sprain or rupture of the talofibular anterior ligament.

Chronic lateral instability of the ankle with repeated ankle sprains may be the sequelae of the first improperly treated ankle sprain. In this case, stress views should be taken; if they show a talar tilt, a lateral stabilization of the ankle would be the treatment of choice. Repeated pain at the anterior aspect of the ankle may be due to anterior impingement exostosis. X-rays would show jamming at the anterior aspect of the ankle. An anterior arthroplasty of the ankle is often helpful for these problems.

The subtalar joint: The joint immediately distal to the ankle joint is the subtalar joint, a very complicated joint with pronatory and supinatory motions. The center of motion changes as the joint position changes. Two forms of motion take place at the subtalar joint: closed kinetic chain motion, and opened kinetic chain motion. When the foot is anchored on the ground, motion of the subtalar joint is in a closed kinetic attitude. Thus, internal rotation of the leg results in pronation of the subtalar joint, causing the calcaneus to evert and the longitudinal arch to be lowered. Subtalar joint pronation also unlocks the midtarsal joint and allows the forefoot to adapt to varying surfaces.

With supination, the leg externally rotates and the calcaneus inverts. The medial longitudinal arch is raised, and the forefoot somewhat adducts upon the rearfoot. The midtarsal joint is locked by subtalar joint supination, and the foot becomes a rigid lever. In the closed kinetic chain attitude, the talus moves with the leg and is locked into the ankle joint mortise.

Most subtalar joint motion takes place with transverse plane rotation of the talus and leg or frontal plane motion of the calcaneus with either eversion or inversion. There is a slight amount of motion of the calcaneus on the sagittal plane. Thus, with pronation, the inclination angle of the calcaneus lowers; with supination, the inclination angle rises.

The subtalar joint, therefore, acts as a universal joint and allows the foot to accept the transverse plane rotations of the leg. Internal rotation of the leg and talus results in calcaneal eversion and foot pronation. External leg rotation results in calcaneal inversion with foot supination.

With an open kinetic chain, the foot is not anchored distally. This occurs during the swing phase of gait. Open kinetic chain pronation at the subtalar joint results in the foot dorsiflexing, everting, and abducting. Open kinetic chain supination is consistent with plantarflexion, inversion, and adduction of the foot.

The midtarsal joint: This joint is immediately distal to the subtalar joint. The midtarsal has two axes, the oblique and the longitudinal. The midtarsal joint is controlled in part by the subtalar joint. A supinated subtalar locks the midtarsal and prevents significant motion from taking place. A pronated subtalar allows for the midtarsal to have more parallel axes, and motion is available. About the longitudinal axis, the main motion is that of inversion or

FIGURE 14-1

Digital Deformities and Joints of the Foot

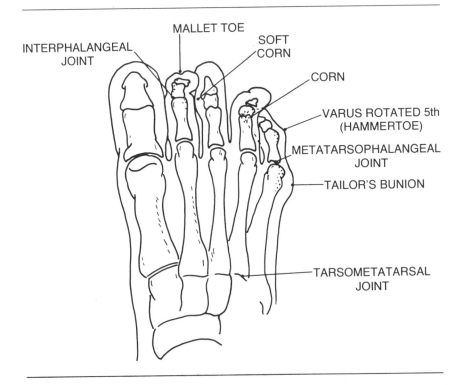

Illustrations in Figures 14-1 to 14-6 by S. G. Newell, D.P.M., from Subotnick SI: *Podiatric Sports Medicine*. Mount Kisco, NY: Futura Publishing Company, 1975. Used with permission.

eversion of the forefoot. At the oblique axis, the main motion is dorsiflexion or plantarflexion. A foot with a tight achilles tendon or an equinus deformity will often pronate to obtain dorsiflexion of the forefoot upon the rearfoot when it is not available at the ankle joint. This motion takes place about the oblique axis of the midtarsal joint.

Neutral position: When the foot is neutral the subtalar joint is neither pronated nor supinated. Likewise, the midtarsal joint is maximally pronated. This means that when standing on the foot, there is a normal medial longitudinal arch and the heel is about perpendicular to the supporting surface. Normally, the subtalar joint allows two-thirds to three-quarters of the motion from the neutral position to be in the direction of inversion and one-third to one-quarter of the motion to be in eversion. A neutral subtalar joint also exists when the bisection of the posterior surface of the calcaneus is in line with the lower one-third of the leg.

In bipedal stance, when the feet are neutral, if one were to remove the outside influence of supporting muscle-tendon units and likewise to cut the ligaments in the foot, the osseous integrity of the alignment of the joints would allow the feet to remain stable; the arches of the foot would likewise be stable. This ideal neutral position is most important on hard, unyielding surfaces and becomes increasingly important as more athletic demands are placed upon the lower extremity. Most people have minor degrees of variation from the ideal and while these variations cause very little problem in everyday activity, in athletics, the variations become more significant.

The tarsometatarsal joint: At the junction of the long bones in the foot—the metatarsals with the midfoot—are the tarsometatarsal joints (see Figure 14-1). These joints allow for some motion on the sagittal plane, but very little motion takes place at these joints.

Metatarsophalangeal joints: At the junction of the toes and the long metatarsal bones of the foot are the metatarsophalangeal joints. Motion in these joints is mostly on the sagittal plane with dorsiflexion and plantarflexion. Some rotation can be expected. An example of this is an unstable first metatarsophalangeal joint with hallux valgus and bunion deformity. Excessive axial rotation of this joint results in permanent deformity and may result in disability for the athlete.

Interphalangeal joints: Within the toes are the interphalangeal joints, and motion is mostly available upon this sagittal plane. Some rotation is available with distraction of the joints.

Muscles controlling the foot

The stirrups: Those long muscles extrinsic to the foot from the leg that help maintain the positions of the major joints in the foot are called the stirrups. On the medial side of the foot and ankle are the flexor group, consisting of the posterior tibial muscle, the flexor digitorum longus, and the flexor digitorum brevis. These muscles pass behind the medial malleolus and enter into the medial longitudinal arch or to the great toe. They help to decrease internal transverse plane rotation of the leg and slow down excessive pronation. In addition, they also help to resupinate the foot. These muscles are often aided by the anterior tibial muscle, which is part of the extensor group.

Peroneal muscles: At the lateral aspect of the ankle and foot are the peroneal muscles—the peroneus longus and brevis. These help to stabilize the lateral side of the foot; they are aided by the gastrocnemius and soleus muscles, which combine to form the achilles tendon. The peroneus longus muscle joins the posterior tibial muscle to form the stirrup of the foot. These two muscles together offer medial and lateral support.

The achilles tendon: The muscles inserting into the achilles—the gastrocnemius, soleus, and plantaris—make up four-fifths of the bulk of the leg. The achilles tendon is an extremely important structure; it tends to stabilize the calcaneus and lateral column of the foot and aids in acceleration and deceleration.

Chronic achilles tenosynovitis with sheath injury that is unresponsive to conservative treatment—heel lifts, elevation, and ice massage—may need surgery to release the sheath of the tendon; this is called a paratenon release. The tendons are usually perfectly normal; it is the sheath that is damaged. If the tendon, however, shows signs of degeneration, incisions are made into it to allow for migration of the fibroblast from the fat to help healing of the tendon itself. Although corticosteroid injections into the achilles tendon may give immediate dramatic relief, cortisone does weaken the tendon, and an injection may lead to partial or total rupture of the achilles tendon. For this reason, I shy away from corticosteroid injections; if an injection must be given, I tell the patient to rest for three to four weeks.

The antigravity muscles: These muscles belong to the extensor group. They function just prior to heel contact to decelerate the foot and prevent a foot slap; they also function during the toe-off and swing phase to clear the forefoot from the ground. The anterior tibial muscle is somewhat medial in its insertion into the first metatarsal, and aids in adduction of the foot. It is counterbalanced by the peroneus brevis, which abducts the foot. The extensors aid in deceleration and extension of the toes.

Taking a long stride or overstriding in sports has a tendency to overstrain the extensor group and may cause extensor shin splint syndrome or tendinitis. Excessive pronation of the foot tends to strain the flexor group, expecially the posterior tibial muscle. Repeated lateral instability of the foot or sprained ankles can injure the peroneal group. Improper flexibility, stretching, or running on the ball of the foot when not physiologically prepared strains the achilles tendon or calf muscles.

Running and jogging result in strengthened gravity muscles, which become tight, while the antigravity muscles become relatively weak. Dynamic imbalance results. It is important to have well-balanced muscles in the lower extremity. These muscle groups must continually be strengthened and stretched.

Intrinsic foot muscles: The short, broad, intrinsic foot muscles are the extensor brevis dorsally and the short flexors and digital stabilizers plantarly. They help decelerate abnormal pronation and stabilize the hallux and lesser toes. Fatigue or malfunction leads to digital contractures.

The plantarfascia: That thick band of tissue immediately beneath the fat on the plantar aspect of the foot is the plantarfascia (see Figure 14-2). It has an origin from the plantar tubercles of the calcaneus and inserts into the plantar aspect of the base of the toes. There are two insertions of the plantarfascia; one, a deep insertion into the capsule, and the other the insertion into the base of the basic phalanges of the toes. The plantarfascia acts as a windlass for the longitudinal arch of the foot.

When the plantarfascia is tight, the longitudinal arch is raised; when the plantarfascia is loose, the longitudinal arch is lowered.

With the toes dorsiflexed, the plantarfascia becomes tighter; with the toes plantarflexed, the plantarfascia becomes looser. Excessive pronation places stress along the medial aspect of the plantarfascia and may result in a partial tear or rupture. Plantarfasciitis may also persist in those patients with high arched feet who, when they run, tend to stretch the plantarfascia beyond its physiological limits.

Functional biomechanics of the foot

Pronation results in the foot acting as a mobile adapter and in the foot dissipating stress into space. One normally contacts on the outside of the heel, then pronates through the contact phase of gait, and resupinates through midstance and toe-off. This pronation is necessary to dissipate stress and to allow the foot to be a mobile adapter for varying surfaces.

Supination takes place after the first 15 per cent of the stance phase of gait, or that period of time when the foot is on the ground. Supination is necessary for the foot to become a rigid lever for a

FIGURE 14-2

Areas of the Foot
Susceptible to Injury

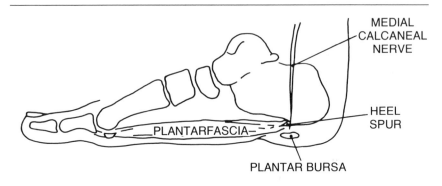

Illustration by S. G. Newell, from Subotnick: *Podiatric Sports Medicine.*

stable toe-off or lift-off. Closed kinetic chain pronation takes place with internal rotation of the leg, and closed kinetic chain supination with external rotation of the leg. Abnormalities of the foot that cause the foot to compensate by excessive pronation or supination change the rotation of the leg and may influence the entire kinetic chain. Thus, an excessively pronating foot causes internal rotation of the leg and may lead to some lateral instability of the patella, or could influence the thigh, hip, or low back. This holds true for excessive supination of the foot. Deformities of the kinetic chain that may occur in the low back, hip, or knee can affect the foot and cause excessive or abnormal motions to take place.

The base of gait: The base of gait is defined as the width between the two feet when one is standing. There is normally a four- to eight-inch distance between the two medial malleoli during normal stance. During walking, this distance may be four inches, but during unidirectional sports, such as running, the base of gait is zero. Thus, when running, one goes from a wide to a narrow base of gait. This causes a functional varus as the support limb angulates toward the center of gravity of the body. This places additional stress on the outside of the heel and accounts for increased pronation during running. In multidirectional sports, in which the center of gravity may be easily upset, a wider base of gait is favored and the feet tend to be externally rotated. The athlete likewise tends to keep the center of gravity lower. There is less functional varus in multidirectional sports.

Angle of gait: This is the angle formed by the feet in comparison with the line of progression. Thus, if one draws a line from the inner aspect of the heel to the first metatarsal head and compares this with the sagittal plane line of progression, the angle of gait is noted. A normal angle of gait is anywhere from 15 to 20 degrees external rotation. Some people tend to have their feet pointed straight ahead, giving a zero angle of gait.

In-toed or pigeon-toed individuals have a negative angle of gait, or adducted angle of gait. Multidirectional sports favor a more external rotated position or abducted angle of gait for increased stability, whereas unidirectional sports, such as long-distance running, normally have an angle of gait of zero. The faster the run, the less time on the feet, the higher the center of gravity, and the narrower angle and base of gait.

Contact stress in running: Because the body is falling through space during running, gravitational forces come into play. During walking, full body weight or half body weight is borne by each lower extremity. During running, three G's pass through the support foot. Running downhill, the gravity force may be as high as four times body weight. Thus, someone accustomed to having full body weight to half body weight during everyday activities places three to four times body weight on the lower extremity during running. This increased stress must gradually be adapted to if one is to avoid overuse injuries.

Man-made surfaces account for many difficulties in sports. They are nonyielding and tend to be static in nature. The foot was meant to function on natural surfaces, such as jungle floors or dirt trails. These surfaces absorb shock, place less stress on the foot, and allow the joints of the foot to open and close with pronation and supination of the foot as it adapts to varying surfaces. Thus, on man-made surfaces with activities such as jogging, almost perfect biomechanical control of the foot is necessary to allow the foot to be a strong functional device. The foot must primarily absorb shock and secondarily adapt to the man-made surface. With prolonged activity on man-made surfaces, the foot tends to fatigue, thus allowing for more pronation and delayed resupination. This causes the support extremity to become unstable and accounts for overuse injuries or fatigue injury.

We have found that people with minor biomechanical variations who have overuse injuries above a certain level, say, 20 miles per week of jogging, benefit from functional foot control with some form of orthosis.

Orthoses: Foot orthoses are devices that support the foot. They are not really crutches, inasmuch as they allow the foot to assume proper positions so that the muscle-tendon units working about the major joints of the foot can move the joints of the foot into proper positioning to allow for maximum efficiency. Various deformities of the foot need various orthotic devices.

Biomechanical deviations or deformities of the leg, subtalar joint, or midtarsal joint can occur. Subtalar-joint problems are those of subtalar joint varum or valgum. This means that the neutral position of the subtalar joint is in an attitude of varus or in an attitude of valgus rather than neutral. The midtarsal joint likewise can have a neutral position of forefoot varus or forefoot valgus. A high-arched foot with a dropped forefoot and plantarflexed first metatarsal is a forefoot valgus foot and needs an orthosis with lateral support. A weak foot or pronated foot is hypermobile, with sagging of the medial longitudinal arch; when the subtalar joint is neutral and the midtarsal joint is maximally pronated or neutral, there is a forefoot varus. The forefoot varus is obvious when one sees the gap underneath the first and perhaps the second metatarsal heads in comparison to the frontal plane. Forefoot varus needs an orthosis that helps build up the medial longitudinal arch; a Morton's extension under the great toe is often very helpful.

Types of orthoses: Orthoses can be soft and compressible, semirigid or semiflexible, or rigid. The softer orthoses are more accommodative and easily tolerated. They are most useful for multidirectional sports and for sports in which there is increased weight upon the ball of the foot or upon the toes. Semiflexible supports are made from a cast of the foot when the foot is held in neutral position. The cast is then balanced, or the support itself is balanced. The semiflexible support is good for jumping, running, or multidirectional sports. A more rigid orthosis is best for standing or walking activities and may be used in unidirectional sports, such as long-distance running at slower speeds. It likewise is made from a neutral cast of the foot.

I prefer giving a soft temporary support to my patients to see how they tolerate it before making any decision as to whether a more permanent and more costly orthosis is necessary.

Fitting the foot—choosing athletic shoes

The right size: Many women have a problem obtaining proper athletic shoes because women's heels are often narrower than men's. Until recently, athletic shoes for female athletes have been men's shoes—only two sizes smaller. Athletic-shoe companies are now manufacturing special lasts for women's shoes with the heel a bit narrower.

This is the way to obtain proper fit when buying shoes: 1) always fit the larger foot; 2) fit for the longest toe; 3) allow for the depth of one thumb or approximately one-third of an inch to extend beyond the longest toe. Remember that one full shoe size repre-

FIGURE 14-3

Modifications in Athletic Shoes to Accommodate Deformities

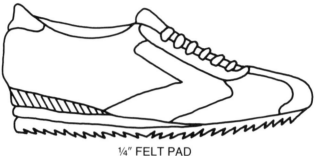

¼" FELT PAD

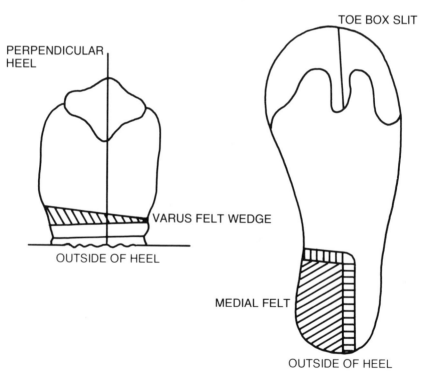

PERPENDICULAR HEEL

TOE BOX SLIT

VARUS FELT WEDGE

OUTSIDE OF HEEL

MEDIAL FELT

OUTSIDE OF HEEL

Illustration by S. G. Newell, from Subotnick: *Podiatric Sports Medicine.*

sents only one-third of an inch, and half a size is one-sixth of an inch. It is best to buy the shoes a bit too large rather than too small. In shoes with a narrow toe box or shoes that place pressure over the toes, you may need to go a full size larger. Allow for the widest part of the foot to be fit. In other words, if you have a narrow heel and a wide forefoot, buy the shoe that has enough width for your forefoot. The heel can be made more secure by placing moleskin or felt padding within the shoe. Likewise, if one foot is larger than the other and you notice that the smaller foot tends to move in the shoe, you may place one-eighth- to one-quarter-inch felt under the tongue of the shoe; this will stop the sliding. Make sure that the shoe has adequate flexibility at the ball of the foot. A stiff shoe may cause problems in the achilles tendon. Increased flexibility can be obtained by drilling one-eighth-inch holes in the soles of the shoes at the balls of the feet. Shoes with a perforated midsole have increased forefoot flexibility.

The shoes: When you are selecting shoes, make sure that they are not deformed. The heel portion of the shoe, when the shoe is on a flat table, should be perpendicular to the ground. An exception to this are the Brooks Vantage shoes, which have a varus wedge on the inner aspect of the heel to account for the functional varus that occurs during running. Thus, with a varus wedge, the medial aspect of the heel is higher than the lateral aspect.

The counter of the shoe, or that portion that grabs the heel, should be firm to prevent excessive rolling of the heel. There should be some padding at the upper aspect of the heel cup to pad the achilles tendon. The shoe should be somewhat stiff from the heel to the ball of the foot. It should be flexible where the toes join the ball of the foot at the metatarsophalangeal joint. There should be adequate thickness of rubber and padding under the heel as well as under the ball of the foot. There should be enough room in the toe box for your toes to have adequate motion.

Modifying shoes for problem feet: Many people have foot deformities that cause problems in athletic shoes. Bunions may require a shoemaker to apply elastic over the protruding aspect of the first metatarsal head. Also, toe boxes may have to be slit for subungual hematomas or hammertoes, and a small piece of elastic placed in the toe box by a shoemaker to alleviate pressure. If your patients have foot abnormalities, they might see a podiatrist who could suggest various forms of shoe modifications for these problems (see Figure 14-3).

Dress shoes: Although they look good, dress shoes for women tend to be nonfunctional and cause a great deal of trouble. High-heeled shoes place a great deal of stress on the ball of the foot and may cause metatarsal pain or may predispose to Morton's neuroma

FIGURE 14-4

Hallux Valgus with Bunion and Other Disorders

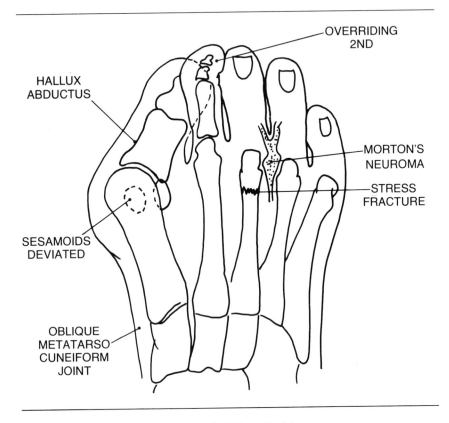

Illustration by S. G. Newell, from Subotnick: *Podiatric Sports Medicine.*

symptoms with compressed or irritated common plantar's nerves (see Figure 14-4). High-heeled shoes may also cause a functional equinus by shortening the calf muscles. This could account for a strained achilles tendon in women who wear high-heeled shoes during the day and low-heeled shoes for jogging or tennis. If high-heeled shoes must be worn, a liberal amount of stretching of the posterior muscles is indicated before and after exercising.

A good everyday shoe is one that is similar to a good running shoe, with approximately one-quarter inch of rubber or outsole material under the ball of the foot and one-half to three-quarters inch under the heel. A tie shoe tends to have a better fit than a loafer-type shoe.

Problem feet

The ankle: There are two common ankle problems in sports. One is that of the inversion ankle sprain in which there is injury or damage to the lateral aspect of the ankle joint over the lateral-collateral ligaments. Often a flared heel on an athletic shoe helps prevent lateral instability and lateral ankle sprains. Sometimes a foot orthosis is necessary to prevent this problem. Ankle sprains are often neglected, resulting in some chronic sequelae; one of the more common problems is that of the sinus tarsi syndrome.

When an inversion sprain occurs, along with damage to the lateral-collateral ligaments, the intraosseous ligament in the sinus tarsi might also be strained. This results in chronic pain at the lateral aspect of the ankle beneath the fibular malleolus. This is often due to the pronated position that the foot is held in following a sprain to prevent a further inversion sprain. Treatment for the sinus tarsi syndrome consists of allowing more neutral foot control. We often use a soft temporary foot support or tape the foot. Along these same lines, acute ankle sprains often need immobilization followed by rehabilitative exercises.

The rearfoot: Common athletic injuries in the rearfoot include achilles tendinitis as well as retrocalcaneal irritation. Achilles strains are best treated with a one-quarter-inch heel lift and stretching to the point of resistance, but not through the point of resistance. If there is excessive pronation causing a torque of the achilles tendon, an orthosis may be helpful. If ambulation is difficult because of the strain of the achilles, then immobilization should be done. Rehabilitation of an achilles tenosynovitis or injury includes stretching and strengthening exercises.

Retrocalcaneal exostosis: Also called runner's bump (see Figure 14-5), this problem is often caused by rolling of the calcaneus in the athletic shoe. There is usually pain at the posterolateral aspect of the achilles insertion into the calcaneus. There may be adventitious bursitis, strain of the achilles at its attachment, or pain from an exostosis on the calcaneus itself. This is initially treated with felt padding and anti-inflammatory medication. Ice massage for six minutes after athletic activity is often quite helpful. One-quarter-inch heel lifts may also be beneficial. If there is excessive motion of

FIGURE 14-5

Retrocalcaneal Exostosis
(runner's bump)

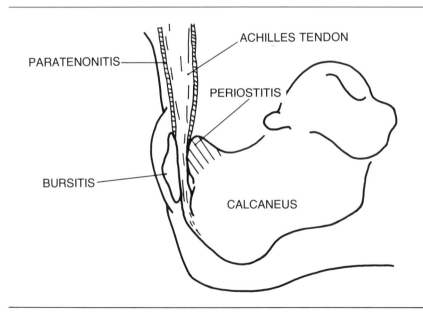

Illustration by S. G. Newell, from Subotnick: *Podiatric Sports Medicine.*

the calcaneus during sports, a temporary orthosis may be used to see if there is correlation between calcaneal movement and the injury. If the results are satisfactory, a permanent orthosis could be used. Sometimes, an adventitious bursitis responds well to a local injection of corticosteroid. If X-rays show excessive retrocalcaneal exostoses and conservative treatment fails, surgery would be indicated.

Heel spurs: Pain on the bottom of the heel is often due to heel-spur syndrome (see Figure 14-2). Heel-spur syndrome includes a myriad of problems, and there may or may not be a heel spur. The most common cause of pain is actually an adventitious bursitis or runner's bruise on the bottom of the heel. The palpable mass on the plantar aspect of the heel responds well to a soft temporary orthosis with a horseshoe pad to alleviate stress. If adventitious bursitis is present and resistant to the padding, a mixed cortisone injection may be helpful to disperse the fibrotic tissue. When X-rays show a heel spur, the initial treatment is the same as for a runner's heel—a soft accommodative orthosis with horseshoe pad. Cortisone injections may be helpful. Standard laboratory tests to rule out collagen disease, gout, and arthritis are necessary.

Plantarfasciitis: Plantar heel pain may also be due to plantarfasciitis. The origin of the plantarfascia is the plantar tubercles of the calcaneus where the heel spur also has its origin. Often, plantarfasciitis is associated with plantarcalcaneal heel spur. Conservative treatment consists of anti-inflammatory medication, resting the foot, and foot orthoses. Taping of the longitudinal arch is very helpful for plantarfasciitis and also for heel-spur problems, as it tends to shorten the distance between the origin and insertion of the plantarfascia (see Figure 14-6). Chronic plantarfasciitis may respond to mixed cortisone injection and physical therapy. Those heel-spur problems and plantarfascial problems that fail to respond to conservative treatment may need surgical intervention. Plantarfascial problems can be prevented or helped by stretching the plantarfascial structures. This is done by raising on the ball of the foot and leaning against the wall or pulling the toe dorsally.

The talus: The most common cause of pain around the talus is an exostosis at the dorsal aspect of the talar neck. This is often the sequela of a sprained ankle or may be due to a pronated foot position with consistent jamming or impingement of the talar neck

FIGURE 14-6

Plantarfascial Tape

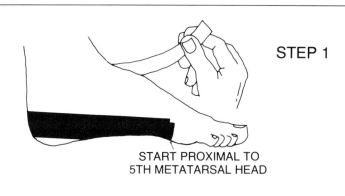

STEP 1

START PROXIMAL TO
5TH METATARSAL HEAD

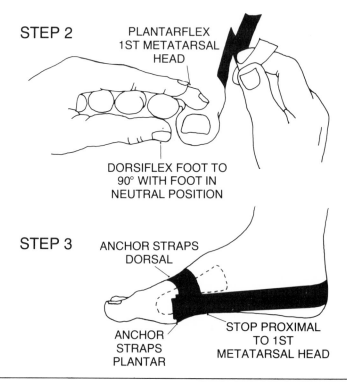

STEP 2

PLANTARFLEX
1ST METATARSAL
HEAD

DORSIFLEX FOOT TO
90° WITH FOOT IN
NEUTRAL POSITION

STEP 3

ANCHOR STRAPS
DORSAL

ANCHOR
STRAPS
PLANTAR

STOP PROXIMAL
TO 1ST
METATARSAL HEAD

Illustration by S. G. Newell, from Subotnick: *Podiatric Sports Medicine.*

upon the tibia. This is more often seen in sports such as football or soccer. X-rays show the exostosis at the talar neck, and physical examination reveals pain with palpation over this area. Various forms of felt padding may be used; an initial injection of corticosteroid into the area may be helpful. If pain persists, excision of the exostosis is indicated.

The posterior aspect of the talus may also be involved with an os trigonum injury, which is principally seen with dancers and gymnasts. If there is pain at the posterior aspect of the subtalar joint, especially with raising on the ball of the foot, the posterior shelf of the talus may be rubbing on the calcaneus or an os trigonum could have been torn loose, especially if there was a traumatic wrenching-type activity. When the os trigonum has been avulsed, there is pain at the posterolateral aspect of the ankle over the posterior aspect of the talus. An injection of lidocaine HCl can be made in the area; if pain disappears, one has made the diagnosis. Often balancing the foot with an orthosis takes care of the problem; if pain persists, surgery may be necessary.

Navicular: The navicular is a large midtarsal bone at the medial longitudinal arch. It may have an enlarged medial protuberance or a second center of ossification called the os navicularis. With twisting injuries, the os navicularis can be partially avulsed from the main body of the navicular, resulting in chronic pain, generally most apparent when the athlete runs on the ball of the foot.

Immobilization and orthoses are indicated for conservative treatment; if healing is incomplete, excision of the os navicularis is indicated. A stress fracture of the navicular may occur—or one of any bone in the foot, and this should be ruled out.

The posterior tibial tendon inserts into the navicular, and posterior tibial tendinitis is often associated with os navicularis.

Arch: Pain in the arch is often due to a pulled plantarfascia, especially the medial band. There may also be pain in the arch secondary to overpronation. Morton's interdigital neuromas, which cause pain in the toes and between metatarsal heads, can radiate pain into the arch. Also, compression of the neurovascular bundle under the medial malleolus, called tarsal-tunnel syndrome, may cause pain radiating into the arch along the medial plantar nerve. A positive Tinnel's sign will be present, with radiating nerve pain initiated by percussion of the neurovascular bundle.

Arch pain is often successfully treated by taping the foot to provide for stability of the arch; then, a temporary orthosis may be followed by a permanent orthosis. X-rays should be taken to rule out stress fracture.

Midfoot: The midfoot and metatarsals are most commonly injured with stress fractures. Stress fractures initially do not show on X-rays, and one usually makes the diagnosis on clinical findings. If there is dorsal swelling on the foot and extensor tendinitis has been ruled out, and if there is pain with motion of the metatarsal, then a stress fracture is probably present (see Figure 14-4).

Treatment consists of immobilizing the foot for the first three weeks with taping and padding and a firm shoe. The patient can run on soft surfaces if there is no pain, but if pain is present, all running activities should be stopped for at least three weeks. Following this, the athlete can usually return to light running on softer surfaces with the foot taped. The foot is taped for six weeks from onset to healing of the stress fracture. A biomechanical examination of the lower extremity should be made to see if there is a long or short leg, or some other biomechanical abnormality predisposing to the stress fracture.

Other midfoot problems include calluses under metatarsal heads that may indicate malpositioning of the metatarsal head. These often respond well to various types of foot orthoses. Occasionally, a very painful callus from a dropped metatarsal head requires a surgical procedure such as an osteotomy of the metatarsal to raise the plantar metatarsal surface to the level of the adjacent metatarsals.

Morton's neuromas are common at the metatarsophalangeal joint. They tend to be caused by excessive rolling of the foot with the plantar nerve impinged upon soft-tissue structures and bone. This causes hypertrophy of the nerve sheath. There may be occasional numbness of the toes or shooting pain into the toes and along the ball of the foot. The most common place for a Morton's interdigital neuroma is in the third interspace or between the third and fourth toes, but it may occur anywhere (see Figure 14-4).

Conservative treatment consists of a long- and slow-acting cortisone injection with a local anesthetic. One, two, or even three injections at seven-day intervals may be necessary. Orthoses are quite helpful. X-rays are taken to rule out stress fracture, and laboratory tests are ordered to rule out systemic problems that may be manifested in the foot.

If conservative treatment fails, local excision of the neuroma is usually successful.

Bunions: Many women bring bunion problems into sports. Or they develop when the woman matures as an athlete. They are due to instability of the first metatarsophalangeal joint. There is pain over the first metatarsal head, and there may be some pain with range of motion of the great toe. If there is pain with motion, a hallux limitus may be present; this could be the precursor of an arthritic joint. Deviation of the great toe is termed hallux valgus (see Figure 14-4).

Mild bunions respond well to balancing of the foot and allowing the intrinsic musculature to stabilize the great toe. Advanced deformity requires surgical revision to prevent further subluxation and joint damage.

There are many bunion procedures, chosen according to the various deformities present. When the proper procedure is chosen and done with due care, the results are quite gratifying. In cases of arthritic joints that must have maximum function, I have used medical-grade silastic implants with good results.

A tailor's bunion is often present on the outside of the foot; this is actually pain over the lateral aspect of the fifth metatarsal head. Stretching the shoe sometimes takes care of this problem, but if there is still pain, surgical reduction is necessary. I usually prefer an osteotomy of the fifth metatarsal neck for this problem.

Toes: Various contractures or instabilities allow corns to form. They can initially be treated by debriding every four to six weeks and having the patient get a shoe with a lot of room in the toe box. If there is significant pain, minor surgical procedures can straighten the toes and remove the corns and calluses.

Foot-related problems

Foot-related problems are those occurring elsewhere in the body that may have their etiology in foot function.

Problems of the leg: The more common problems of the leg that appear to be helped by balancing the foot include shin splints. Shin splints are a combination of various strains or stresses of the mus-

FIGURE 14-7

A Stretch Routine for
Before and After Running

**Total time approximately
20 minutes**

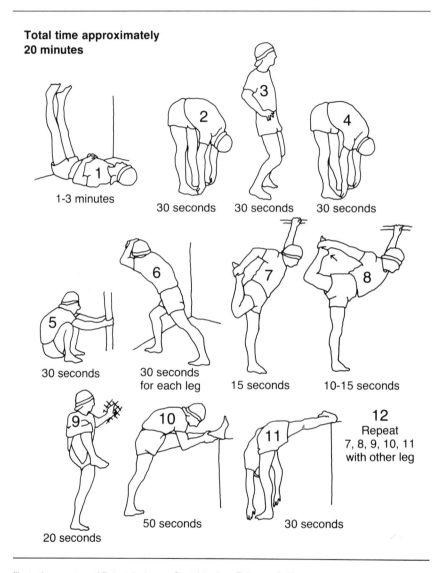

1-3 minutes

30 seconds   30 seconds   30 seconds

30 seconds   30 seconds
for each leg   15 seconds   10-15 seconds

20 seconds   50 seconds   30 seconds

12
Repeat
7, 8, 9, 10, 11
with other leg

Illustration courtesy of Robert Anderson, Stretching Inc., Fullerton, Calif.

cle, tendon, or bone. A more proper term for shin splints is enthesitis. This means an injury to the attachment of the soft tissue to the bones. Medial leg pain is often due to flexor group enthesitis and is helped by supporting the medial longitudinal arch of the foot. Anterior shin-splint pain is due to overstriding or foot imbalance, and orthoses, as well as proper rehabilitative exercises to strengthen the antigravity muscles, are necessary. One must rule out stress fracture. Flexibility exercises before and after sports activities are essential (see Figure 14-7).

Knee problems: Patellar-related running problems often respond dramatically to balancing of the foot. Excessive pronation of the foot allows for internal rotation of the leg and appears to functionally increase the Q angle. Thus, the patella may have increased lateral subluxation. These patellar-related problems respond to exercises to strengthen the vastus medialis. When true pathology is present in the knee joint or at the patello-femoral junction, orthopedic treatment is necessary.

Long-leg/short-leg: Leg-length discrepancies up to one-quarter or even one-half inch may not cause problems in everyday activities. They do cause many problems in the athlete. I have found that a limb-length discrepancy as little as one-eighth inch may throw off a stride and cause an overuse injury. This may result in low back strain or any one of the overuse problems of the lower extremity.

What appears to happen is an overstride on the short-leg side to catch up with the long-leg side. This results in contacting further back on the heel of the short-leg side, with increased stress and contact pronation. Treatment consists of proper heel lifts.

Further reading

Anderson R: *Stretching.* Fullerton, Cal: Anderson, 1975.

Cavanagh PR, Pollack ML, and Landa J: A biomedical comparison of elite and good distance runners. In *Annals of New York Academy of Sciences, The Marathon: Physiological, Medical, Epidemiological, and Psychological Studies* (Milvy P, ed), pp 328-345. New York: New York Academy of Sciences, 1977

James SL and Brubaker CE: Biomechanics of running. *Orthop Am* 4:605, 1973

Nelson RC, Brooks CM, and Pike NL: Biomechanical comparison of male and female distance runners. In *Annals of New York Academy of Sciences, The Marathon: Physiological, Medical, Epidemiological, and Psychological Studies* (Milvy P, ed), pp 793-807. New York: New York Academy of Sciences, 1977

Nicholas JA, Grossman RB, and Hershman EB: The importance of simplified classification of motion in sports in relation to performance. *Orthop Clin N Am* 3:449, 1977

Sgarlato TC: *A Compendium of Podiatric Biomechanics.* San Francisco: California College of Podiatric Medicine, 1971

Subotnick SI: A biomechanical approach to running injuries. In *Annals of New York Academy of Sciences, The Marathon: Physiological, Medical, Epidemiological, and Psychological Studies* (Milvy P, ed), pp 888-899. New York: New York Academy of Sciences, 1977

Subotnick SI: Biomechanics of the subtalar and midtarsal joints. *JAPA* 65:755, 1975

Subotnick SI: *Cures for Common Running Injuries.* Mountain View, Cal: World Publications, 1979

Subotnick SI: Orthotic foot control and the overuse syndrome. *Phys Sportsmed,* 3(1):75, 1975

Subotnick SI: *Podiatric Sports Medicine.* Mount Kisco, NY: Futura Publishing, 1975

Subotnick SI: *The Running Foot Doctor.* Mountain View, Cal: World Publications, 1977

Subotnick SI: The short-leg syndrome. *Phys Sportsmed* 3(11):61, 1975

SOFT-TISSUE INJURIES

Christine E. Haycock, M.D.

CHAPTER

15

A soft-tissue injury is defined as one that is confined to the skin and the underlying soft structures, such as subcutaneous tissue, glandular tissue, and muscle. Such injuries are very common among athletes, but are generally minor in nature. Occasionally, injuries to these areas may be quite severe, especially if damage to vessels, tendons, or nerves is involved. Before discussing treatment, let's define each type of injury.

An *abrasion* is usually confined to the outer layers of the skin. Although it is superficial, it can be quite painful. It may cover a wide area—on, say, the thigh of an athlete who slides into base. If kept free of infection, the abrasion generally heals very quickly. Should the deeper layers of the skin be involved, skin grafting might be required. Ground-in dirt or gravel can cause tattooing of the skin if all of the particles are not removed.

A *contusion* is a bruise, or a blow to the skin and the underlying structures, and although the skin is not broken, discoloration—the classic black-and-blue mark—results, due to breakage of the small capillaries beneath the skin. Contusions generally are not serious and require minimal treatment. They often accompany abrasions.

A note of caution: Although most contusions are minor, they may hide severe damage to underlying structures. Muscles or nerves may be torn, vessels ruptured or thrombosed, subcutaneous fat crushed, and solid organs lacerated. Therefore, regard all contusions as signs of more severe damage until proven otherwise.

A *hematoma* is a collection or pooling of the blood beneath the skin. In athletes, it usually occurs in the subcutaneous tissues. Hematomas, however, may occur in such deeper tissues as breast, vulva, and perineum and may require drainage to release the blood. Provided they don't become infected, hematomas have no serious consequences.

Puncture wounds are small lacerations, but as they are frequently seen in sports in which participants wear spikes, they are worth mentioning separately. A puncture wound is caused by a narrow implement that penetrates the skin possibly damaging underlying structures. Most puncture wounds occurring in sports are superficial, but all require careful exploration to rule out further penetration.

Lacerations (cuts) are serious injuries that may damage vital structures—nerves, tendons, ducts, the eye—and cause permanent damage. Lacerations of organs such as the ears, nose, eyes, and the more specialized areas are covered in other chapters and are not discussed here. The common lacerations of the skin and muscles may produce severe bleeding if a major vessel is cut.

An *avulsion* is a laceration in which the skin is torn away from the area, rather than just cut and left in place. This type of laceration can be difficult to deal with because of the loss of skin, and it may require skin grafting.

The primary consideration in soft-tissue injuries is the cleanliness of the wound. A relatively *clean wound* is one from a sharp edge in a moderately clean arena (usually indoors), so that there is very little contamination of the wound by foreign bodies or dirt.

A *dirty wound* is one occurring on a playing field, such as a softball diamond or hockey field, where dirt probably enters the wound as it occurs.

Treatment

All injuries must be thoroughly cleansed immediately after they happen, on the playing field if necessary. Soap and a lot of water or sterile saline, plus painting with an iodine preparation, will do for most abrasions. Still better would be the immediate use of hexachlorophene or an iodine scrub sponge. (These come in sterile packages, and several can be kept in the emergency kit; only water need be added.) The wound is then covered with dry sterile gauze that is taped in place if the athlete is to continue playing.

If a contusion is also present, the immediate application of cold over the dressing will reduce pain and swelling. If possible, cold packs or ice should be used for at least 15 minutes on a minor bruise, and at least 30 minutes on a large hematoma.

Elevation of an injured limb with the ice in place promotes venous and lymphatic return from the limb, and helps to minimize swelling of the area.

Very small and superficial lacerations can be closed with sterile adhesive strips or "butterflies." Longer or deeper lacerations usually require sutures. All lacerations must be inspected for underlying tendon or nerve damage, with motion and sensation testing as required. In most cases, the athlete must be taken to the emergency room or a doctor's office.

In general, tourniquets are not indicated or required to control bleeding from a laceration; direct pressure over the injured area controls hemorrhage in most cases. Pressure can be maintained by a firmly wrapped or taped dressing. Elevation of the limb and the application of cold also help.

Severe arterial bleeding can often be controlled by applying pressure to the vessel proximal to the injury at designated pressure points, such as over the femoral artery in the medial anterior area of the groin, or over the axillary artery in the upper medial arm. Other such points are the carotid artery in the neck (press against the trachea) to control neck, mouth, or throat bleeding; the temporal arteries slightly above and in front of the ear to control scalp bleeding; the facial artery at the notch in the lower jaw for facial bleeding; and the brachial artery just below the collar bone (press in the hollow and down against the first rib) for shoulder or axillary bleeding. Once hemorrhage is at least reasonably controlled, the athlete should be taken immediately to an emergency department for further care.

Lacerations may also occur in conjunction with more severe injuries such as fractures. Treating the laceration as outlined and splinting the fracture minimize further injury.

The athlete's return to competition depends on the extent of the injury. Obviously, severe lacerations—with or without other injuries—require rest until healing is complete. The location of superficial lacerations determines when the player may compete. A cut elbow or knee requires a minimum of 10 days to heal and at least another week of limited motion (accomplished by a bulk dressing such as an elastic bandage) while participating. Lacerations in non-motion areas require five to seven days to heal and, in contact sports, should be protected by padding for another week.

If a muscle injury accompanies the laceration, the five- to seven-day healing period won't be enough, especially if the injury is in an extremity. Muscle injuries—even if they are just contusions—may sideline the athlete for several weeks. Physical therapy for such injuries is imperative to speed the recovery period. Returning to active sports participation too early is foolish and nonproductive; if the healing laceration is reopened, the athlete will lose even more time while secondary healing takes place.

Exercise of the uninjured areas of the body can be carried out during the healing period under the supervision of a trainer and with the use of such machines as the Universal Gym or Nautilus.

Although most young athletes have been immunized against tetanus prior to injury, it is advisable to administer a tetanus toxoid booster (0.5 ml fluid purified toxoid subcutaneously) if none has been given within a five-year period.

If the athlete has not previously been immunized, the booster is given immediately and followed by repeat doses three weeks and six weeks later to achieve immunization. Tetanus antitoxin (human immune globulin) is seldom required in athletic injuries.

Antibiotics are not indicated for most superficial injuries. Careful observation of the wound for any signs of developing infection is the preferred course. Deep or severe dirty lacerations probably require antibiotic therapy following debridement of the wound, but this is a decision of the treating surgeon. He may also elect not to close the wound with sutures but to pack it open until it is free from infection, and then do a delayed closure. Bites or cuts from teeth, for example, are never immediately closed.

Many team physicians advocate the use of enzymes or anti-inflammatory drugs to speed resolution of edema and inflammation from blunt injuries. Preparations such as chymotrypsin are frequently administered on the playing field immediately after injury. The effectiveness of these agents is not proven, but adverse reactions are minimal, so no harm generally results from their use.

More potent drugs such as steroids, phenylbutazone, or indomethacin should be used only by experts, and then with a good deal of caution, especially in the presence of infection.

Injuries to the abdominal wall require special attention, as they may be accompanied by blunt trauma to intra-abdominal structures. Intra-abdominal injuries require hospitalization for observation and, usually, exploratory surgery for repair.

You should suspect a serious intra-abdominal injury in the presence of persistent pain with weakness, pallor, cold sweat, rapid pulse, arterial hypotension, and other symptoms of impending shock. Vomiting of "coffee ground" material or blood, or rectal or urinary passage of blood, are other ominous signs.

The spleen is the most commonly injured solid structure. A blow of any consequence to the left flank may result in rupture of the organ. The rupture may occur immediately or may be delayed, depending on whether or not the capsule of the spleen has been torn. For this reason, an athlete receiving a blow to the area should be observed carefully and told to abstain from further contact sports for at least one week.

Other solid organs subject to injury are the liver, kidneys, and pancreas, although the latter is only rarely injured during sports play. Rupture of the intestines has been reported, but it is a rare occurrence. Similarly, hemorrhage into the mesentery or retroperitoneal area occurs infrequently.

Women are generally at lower risk of severe abdominal injuries than men, as they typically participate in less violent contact sports. When they do participate, however, their risk may be greater because of their less robust abdominal musculature. The female reproductive structures are fortunately well protected by the bony pelvis and hence seldom injured.

A frequently asked question is whether the female breast is prone to injury and whether injury can lead to future consequences such as cancer. The answer is No. Hematomas requiring drainage and abrasions that become infected are the worst injuries; although painful, they are not serious. No cancer of the breast has ever been proven to have resulted from a blow to the breast.

Occasionally, a contusion of the breast results in fatty necrosis and the formation of a firm nodule of fibrous tissue. This may remain for many years, but is of no consequence. When discovered, such nodules are often removed in the mistaken belief that they may be malignant.

A well-designed bra provides support for painful breasts in fibrocystic disease, and a padded bra can be used to prevent injury in such sports as fencing, field hockey, and football.

Further reading

The American College of Sports Medicine: *Encyclopedia of Sports Sciences and Medicine*. New York: Macmillan, 1971

Ballinger WF, Rutherford RB, and Zvidema GD: *The Management of Trauma*. Philadelphia: Saunders, 1973

Cave EF, Burke JF, and Boyd RJ: *Trauma Management*. Chicago: Year Book Medical Publishers, 1974

McMaster WC: When to use ice for injuries. *Consultant* p 83, April 1977

Novich MM: Management and treatment of athletic injuries. *GP* 30:5, 1964

Novich MM: Tips for treating athletic injuries. *Consultant* p 42, July 1962

REHABILITATION OF THE INJURED ATHLETE

Holly Wilson, M.S., A.T.C.

CHAPTER

16

A

thletic injuries primarily involve the musculoskeletal system, all of whose component parts—bone, muscle
tissue, tendons, ligaments, nerves, and blood vessels—could be
damaged.

Inflammation and healing

Immediately following an injury, the body attempts to protect
itself from additional stress while simultaneously preparing for
repair of the damaged tissue. The first step in the return to normal
is the inflammatory phase, which provides the groundwork for the
second—repair and healing. During the initial phase, some, if not
all, of the signs of inflammation may become evident—skin redness, heat, swelling, pain, and malfunction. They indicate the
physiological processes taking place at the trauma site.

With trauma, tissues are either stretched, torn, or crushed.
Damaged vessels cannot retain fluid—whether it be lymph or
blood—and it seeps into the tissue spaces. In response to the trauma, vessels constrict in an attempt to minimize loss of fluid and
seal themselves. Such constriction is short-lived. Damaged cells in
the area spill their contents—including the important enzymes
that promote the inflammatory process. Histamine causes dilation
of the blood vessels, which in turn causes the skin redness associated with inflammation. Dilation is both helpful and harmful. More

blood is brought into the area, but the larger vessels may not have had adequate time to clot—so blood seeps out. The increased blood flow is beneficial, however, in that it provides oxygen to prevent destruction of healthy tissue through oxygen starvation, as well as nutrients required for repair of tissue. The blood also transports white blood cells to the injury site to help with the cleanup process. Their movement into the area is assisted by one of the enzymes released by the damaged cells. This enzyme increases the permeability of the capillary walls, facilitating the passage of white blood cells through the vessel walls and filtering out the plasma. The white cells assist cleanup by ingesting cellular debris and any micro-organisms that may have contaminated the injury site. A third enzyme destroys the damaged cells.

The swelling that accompanies most injuries is actually serum, lymph fluid, blood, and cellular debris that collects in the tissue space. As this exudate accumulates, it creates a concentration gradient that draws more fluid from the capillaries in an attempt to dilute the concentration of the material. Consequently, swelling stimulates additional swelling.

As the exudate collects and organizes, repair begins. Clots form at the bleeding sites in the lymph and blood vessels to control additional seepage. A hematoma forms within the exudate. Fibrin strands crisscross the tissue space, connecting the wound edges to form the framework for the scab. Capillaries from the surrounding healthy tissue penetrate the site to deliver nutrients and oxygen needed in the repair process. The edges of the wound move closer together to facilitate the closing of the area with the scab. Underneath, granulation tissue slowly fills in the defect as the hematoma is absorbed. Healthy cells on the surface eventually replace the scab. The granulation tissue loses its capillary network and becomes inelastic and fibrous. It is referred to as scar tissue and has none of the properties of the tissue that it replaced.

The time required for healing is determined by the severity of the trauma as well as by the tissues involved. For example, a skin wound requires approximately six to seven days for 90 per cent of the healing to take place, while the remaining 10 per cent requires six to eight weeks. The wound area cannot tolerate stress until approximately the seventh day and is weakest as the hematoma is being absorbed. By approximately the 14th day, the strength of the scar reaches maximum. Although the scar tissue is stronger than the tissue it replaced, it has no elasticity.

Several factors interfere with healing. Swelling not only causes pain but also increases the size of the defect, and it interferes with the approximation of like tissues. Because motion at the wound edges hinders healing by disrupting the healing process, sutures or Steri Strips are frequently used to immobilize the edges. A cast or cloth immobilizer may be required to keep like tissues in approximation and wound edges quiet. If a site becomes infected, healing is delayed as a result of the toxins produced by the invading microorganisms and the infection process. Furthermore, the size of the initial defect enlarges as healthy tissue is destroyed.

Physiology of ice application

The goal in the immediate care of any musculoskeletal injury is to delay or at least minimize swelling. As swelling increases, pain increases because pressure is placed on free nerve endings near the injury site. The sensation of pain causes the muscles to go into spasm to splint the damaged tissue. This is the body's way of protecting an injury against additional trauma. Consequently a pain-spasm-pain cycle is established. Pain causes the initial spasm and the spasm then contributes to the development of more pain by compression of pain fibers. Because of the pain, the individual avoids using the injured part; over a period of a few days, the muscles atrophy. For example, the quadriceps lose up to an inch of girth in the first 48 to 72 hours of immobilization. However, the loss levels off so that some muscle mass is retained. Muscle strength can be regained completely with a thorough rehabilitation program. When immobilization is extended over a prolonged period, structural changes are seen at the cellular level. Consequently, recovery of muscle strength takes longer and may be incomplete— as much as 10 per cent of the structural change within the cell may be irreversible. Atrophy is a common occurrence following a moderate to severe knee injury in which the knee is immobilized and/or the individual is not permitted to bear weight on the injured leg. As the muscles atrophy from lack of use, the joint becomes less stable, particularly if its bony anatomy provides little structural stability in the first place.

This vicious cycle of swelling-pain-atrophy-reinjury can be interrupted at various points to limit its destructive consequence—the development of a chronic condition. First, swelling can be minimized, if not controlled, by the prompt application of ice, compression and elevation of the injured part, and rest. Second, an anesthetic may be injected into the injury site along with an anti-inflammatory agent to reduce the inflammatory reaction and promote healing. Such treatment is strictly the prerogative of the physician and should never be used to deaden pain so that the athlete may return to competition. Third, atrophy from disuse can be minimized by initiating a controlled rehabilitation program consisting of range of motion strength and agility exercises as soon as tolerated. Pain and swelling are used as guidelines; if either increases as a result of activity, the intensity level is reduced. Fourth, athletes are not permitted to return to any activity until they are physiologically and psychologically able to withstand the stress of the activity.

Ice is invaluable in the treatment of any injury, because it affects numerous physiological processes in a beneficial manner. It is a vasoconstrictor and causes a decrease in the circumference of the blood vessels in the area of application. The vasoconstriction is a response to the intense cooling effect of ice—the blood vessels become smaller in an attempt to conserve heat. Moreover, vasoconstriction is also helpful in attempting to control the swelling associated with injury. As the size of the blood vessel becomes smaller, less blood flows through it; hence, less blood seeps through the walls and/or tears in the vessels. Such seepage is further controlled by the cold because vasoconstriction also reduces capillary permeability.

Ice interferes locally with the transmission of impulses from receptors to effectors. Consequently, ice is both an anesthetic and a muscle relaxant. Cooling stops the transmission of impulses along small myelinated pain fibers, and then along the large myelinated fibers. Fortunately, the individual can still experience pain because the unmyelinated fibers are the last to be affected by local cooling. The body's warning system remains intact to relay information about damaging stress imposed on tissues. Muscle relaxation is enhanced because the threshold of the sensory endings in the muscle spindle is increased, and transmission of the impulse from the endings to the spindle is slowed down. Consequently, muscle spindle activity decreases. A decrease of 5°C at the skin reduces motor activity enough to cause a decrease in muscle spasm. Stretching of a muscle in a state of spasm is possible without the consequent shortening of the muscle due to the stretch reflex-firing of the muscle spindle.

Finally, ice decreases cellular metabolism. Such a reduction is important in limiting secondary tissue destruction as a result of oxygen starvation. Cells that survive the initial trauma may not withstand the lack of oxygen imposed by the disruption of the local circulation. Damage to vessels prevents the delivery of oxygen to the cells in the area. Because cooling decreases the metabolic rate, each cell needs less oxygen for metabolic processes. Therefore, immediate application of ice means less destruction will occur.

Prolonged ice application results in vasodilation. This increase in the circumference of the blood vessels is a reflex action to prevent excessive lowering of the skin temperature. It is a safeguard against destruction of tissue. It is referred to as the "hunting response" and may be elicited at temperatures as high as 18°C. In a controlled situation, such as in a training room, skin temperature may approach 0°C with ice application. At this temperature, there is no evidence of tissue destruction (frostbite); destruction usually occurs at subfreezing temperatures—approximately -3 or -4°C.

The vasodilation that occurs with prolonged cooling causes a drop in the hydrostatic pressure within the vessel. Consequently, the exudate diffuses across the membrane into the vessel and swelling diminishes.

When ice is applied, vasoconstriction normally lasts for nine to 16 minutes, followed by intense vasodilation lasting four to six minutes. Thereafter, vasoconstriction and vasodilation alternate, constriction lasting from 15 to 30 minutes and dilation from four to six minutes. When the control of swelling is the major goal, ice should be applied for no longer than 10 minutes at a time.

Following prolonged cooling, the local temperature increases above that of surrounding tissue and reaches a maximum in 15 to 30 minutes. Skin redness and warmth (indicating an increase in circulation) may not subside for several hours after treatment. This reflex vasodilation apparently has a longer-lasting heating effect than that produced by heat application.

The application of an elastic wrap to the injury site provides compression from an external source and assists with the control of swelling. The wrap forces blood back into the capillaries and prevents it from seeping out. The wrap should be wet so that it can conduct the coldness of the ice to the skin. If it were dry, the wrap would act as an insulator. Apply the wrap so it spans an area from several inches below the injury site to several inches above. The distal end should be tighter, with each successive turn of the wrap being looser. In this manner, a pressure gradient is established that may help with venous return. Elevate the part, if possible, so that gravity can assist the return of blood to the heart. Elevation also causes a reduction in blood flow to the distal aspect. When ice is not readily available, immediately apply compression with an elastic wrap and elevate the part.

In the immediate care of injuries, apply ice for periods of no longer than 10 minutes; this prevents reflex vasodilation that would increase swelling. Place the ice on top of the wet elastic wrap at the area of maximum tenderness and elevate the part. After 10 minutes, remove the ice, but keep the injury compressed and elevated. Continue to alternate 10 minutes of ice with 10 minutes without for a total of 60 minutes. This schedule may be repeated several times a day for the next 24 to 48 hours.

Techniques of ice application

Ice application is easy to adapt to home use, and is one of the least expensive forms of therapy. The only disadvantage—other than dripping water—is the discomfort: The initial intense cold is followed by a burning, aching, tingling sensation, and finally by numbness. These sensations are the exact warning signs of frostbite. Fortunately, frostbite is usually not a complication of either short or prolonged icing of the skin. Vasodilation, the body's defense mechanism against temperature extremes, warms the superficial tissue before the temperature drops to the critical level. Evidence of vasodilation is a bright red color to the skin, as vessels beneath the skin open up, allowing an increase in blood flow to the area. In frostbite, on the other hand, the body's attempt at warming is futile against the prolonged cold, and the vessels constrict to conserve heat, so that the once-red skin turns white.

Tissue destruction occurs when the temperature drops to approximately -3 or -4°C and remains there for some time. Water freezes at 0°C, but the temperature of the ice is constantly changing—as indicated by its melting. If the ice continues to melt during the application, the chance of frostbite is minimal. However, if the skin turns unnaturally pale when ice is being applied, it means that the cutaneous vessels have constricted to minimize heat loss, and the treatment should be terminated immediately because the temperature-regulatory mechanism is no longer able to cope with intense cooling. There are other instances in which the application of ice as a therapeutic measure should be avoided or at least done with extreme caution. If the patient has poor circulation, the tissues may not be able to withstand the intense cold. For example, poor circulation to the peripheral extremities may be the consequence of Reynaud's syndrome, which involves occlusion of the peripheral arteries as the vessels go into spasm from the sensation of cold. Impaired sensation is a second contraindication to the therapeutic use of ice. Without the ability to sense extreme changes in tissue temperature, the body may not be able to regulate temperature within its critical range. Therefore, if the area has been frostbitten, it should not be treated with ice. Finally, age is a factor. No one younger than the age of five or older than 70 should undergo either ice or heat treatments.

Ice application is indicated in the following situations so long as the above contraindications are observed:
• Relief of pain
• Relaxation of muscle spasm
• Decrease in local circulation (short cooling—10 minutes)
• Increase in local circulation (prolonged cooling—15 to 30 minutes)
• Increase in edema absorption (prolonged cooling—15 to 30 minutes)

Perhaps the easiest method of applying ice is the ice pack. Chipped or crushed ice is recommended because it conforms to the bony anatomy better than cubes. The ice is placed in either a plastic bag or a towel. The towel should be moistened on one side only, and that side is placed against the individual's skin. The moistness increases the conduction of cold to the skin while the dry layer on top acts as an insulator. The plastic bag is advantageous because it prevents the melting ice from dripping. An English ice cap (a rubberized-cloth container with a wide mouth and screw-on lid) may be used in place of the bag or towel (these caps are available in several different sizes at most drugstores). There is less chance of leakage, and the caps are reusable. However, heavy-duty plastic bags with a ziplock are extremely durable, and the ziplock is convenient for pouring off water as the ice melts.

Ice slush provides uniform cooling for the extremities. Chips or flakes are mixed with water in a large container until the water temperature drops to 55 to 65°F. The involved part is immersed in the water for as long as the individual can tolerate it. As this technique is extremely painful, the first few attempts may last only a few seconds. Between attempts, the extremity should be dried off, allowed to recover momentarily, and then reimmersed. Continue until the part has been immersed five or six times. It should be numb and relaxed at the termination of treatment.

Unfortunately, with the use of ice slush, the injured part cannot be elevated during treatment; however, it should be elevated between periods of immersion, and can still be compressed with a wet elastic wrap applied as previously described. It may enable the individual to withstand or tolerate the extreme coldness of the slush for a longer period of time.

The use of ice slush is contraindicated in persons with peripheral vascular disease or sickle-cell anemia.

Ice massage should not be used to control swelling immediately following an injury. This would forfeit the benefits of compression and elevation. Furthermore, the ice application is restricted to a very small area. However, ice massage may be used the day following the injury as a prelude to the rehabilitation program. An ice cup (water frozen in a Styrofoam cup) is moved slowly over the involved area until sensation is lost. As with the other types of ice application, the individual experiences the coldness, then burning, aching, tingling sensations, and, finally, numbness. The progression usually requires eight to 10 minutes, and the skin may become bright red. When the part is numb it should be exercised; the individual should try normal range of motion without forcing the joint. Simply instruct the athlete to move the joint through its normal movements but to stop when discomfort is experienced. It takes approximately three minutes of exercise before the numbness wears off. The eight-minute ice application with three-minute exercise should be repeated two more times for a total of one set of three—eight-three, eight-three, eight-three; one or two sets a day should be carried out.

Another common method of cooling an extremity during the early stages of rehabilitation is the cold whirlpool. Here, range of motion exercises are executed while the part is being cooled. The buoyancy of the water permits movement of the part with greater ease and less discomfort. The temperature of the water should be the same as that of ice slush, 55 to 65°F. If this temperature can be reached and maintained without the addition of ice, turn the agitator on—the flow prevents a layer of warm water from forming around the part. The stream should not be directed at the injured part lest it irritate the sensitive tissue. Instead, direct the flow elsewhere so the injured part can catch a gentle rebound flow. Treatment should last for no more than 10 minutes, during which time the individual should move the part through its range of motion—again, only to the point of discomfort.

Cold penetrates best (deepest) with ice slush and cold whirlpool treatments, and these are, therefore, the most uncomfortable methods of applying ice. Uniformity of cooling probably accounts for the deep penetration. Next in depth of penetration is ice massage, followed by the ice pack.

As the possibility of additional swelling diminishes, the temperature of the water may be increased slowly. Or heat may be applied when it is evident that swelling has been controlled. One of the common signs of inflammation is an increase in temperature that can be felt even superficially. Compare the surface temperatures of the two corresponding parts; if you can feel a difference in the surface temperature, additional swelling is a distinct possibility. Usually, 24 to 48 hours are required for all bleeding to cease, but it is safer to wait 72 hours. If there is no difference in superficial temperatures, heat may be applied.

Physiology of heat application

Heat assists healing. It facilitates the absorption and removal of the exudate by increasing the permeability of the capillaries. It acts as a vasodilator, increasing the circumference of the blood vessels, so that more blood can flow through the area. The blood brings in oxygen and nutrients needed for repair and healing and carries waste products from cellular metabolism to the kidneys for removal from the body. Cellular metabolism increases in response to heat, but the raw materials required to support this accelerated rate are available.

Heat, like ice, is a muscle relaxant; however, its effect diminishes as soon as the heat source is removed. Ice, on the other hand, has a longer-lasting effect on muscle relaxation because it interferes with the transmission of nerve impulses. Both ice and heat reduce pain. A warm, soothing sensation is associated with the application of heat, and the relief of pain probably has psychological overtones. Because pain relief associated with application of ice involves the blocking of impulse transmission along the small myelinated fibers, relief is prolonged.

The danger of burning tissue is always present when using heat therapy; this does not depend on whether its depth of penetration is superficial or deep. Heat treatment should not be used in any of the following circumstances:

● When fewer than 48 hours have elapsed from the time the athlete sustained the injury.

● When there is circulatory impairment (because the body's adjustment to increased tissue temperature is affected): Replacement of heated blood by cooler blood is slowed down.

● When sensation is absent, because the individual is unable to sense when the tissues are being overheated.

● When metal is embedded at or near the treatment site—the metal may be surgical pins, plates, screws, or even shrapnel. Any metallic object attracts and absorbs heat, causing deep burning of surrounding tissues. The danger is greater with the deep heat modalities—except for ultrasound, which can be used cautiously in areas where metal is present. In this instance, the metal does not attract the ultrasonic energy, but simply transmits it.

● When edema is noninflammatory in origin—such as renal, cardiac, or pulmonary.

● When the eyes or genitals are involved—these are heat-sensitive tissues.

● When the individual is younger than five years of age or older than 70.

The maximum length of time that heat should be applied is 30 minutes; after that, the effect levels off (maximum temperature is reached within 15 to 20 minutes).

Application of heat

Superficial heat modalities that are commonly found in most training rooms, even at the high school level, are the hot pack, infrared lamp, and whirlpool. The analgesic pack may also be considered a form of superficial heat.

With the superficial forms of heat, penetration greater than 1 cm is not to be expected; even so, such modalities can quickly raise the skin temperature to a destructive level (45°C). If the temperature remains at this level for some time, the thermal damage causes tissue death. It is more likely that the individual will suffer burns when treated by a superficial form of heat than with a deep-heat modality. More energy is absorbed by the superficial layers, but they are also more sensitive. There are more sensory receptors in the skin than in the deeper tissues, so the individual may sense the discomfort sooner. Sometimes, however, an individual tolerates the discomfort, firmly believing that "if a little heat is good, then more is better." (Actually, to be therapeutically beneficial, the heat treatment should be warm and soothing.) The first sign of overheating of the tissue is mottling—the appearance of white patches on the bright red surface of the skin. If mottling occurs, discontinue the treatment immediately or decrease the energy output of the machine, or if possible, add more insulation between the heat source and the part being treated.

Heat packs are segmented canvas bags filled with a silicon gel that absorbs heat. They are stored in water in a stainless steel container with a thermostat that maintains the water at 65 to 90°C. A pack must be submerged in water for approximately 24 hours prior to its first heating or heated for at least an hour or two to ensure complete moistening of the silicon and absorption of heat. Thereafter, only 20 to 30 minutes is required for complete reheating. (If the pack is not heated to the proper temperature, the patient won't derive full benefit from it.)

When preparing a hot pack, place sufficient layers of insulation between the individual's skin and the pack to prevent burning. If the commercial pack covers, made of terry cloth with a foam liner, are not available, substitute two bath-size Turkish towels. Fold each one lengthwise and then place one folded towel on top of the other so that they crisscross. Remove the pack from the heat source and let it drip dry for a few seconds. Place the pack in the center of the towels and fold the towels over the pack so there are four double layers of towel on one side. This thicker side is placed on the skin (it should be dry, or the skin may burn). Place another towel on top of the pack to prevent the escape of heat. If the individual lies down on the pack or it is placed underneath the involved part, additional layers of towel are necessary to prevent burning. The athlete should experience a warming sensation within two to three minutes; if not, remove a layer of towel. The skin should be warm to the touch in five minutes whether or not the skin has turned red from dilation of the superficial vessels. The treatment should last for 20 minutes.

Hot packs can easily be used at home and are relatively inexpensive. A variety of sizes is available commercially at most drugstores (along with the special foam-lined terry-cloth covers). The pack can be heated in a pot on the stove, but the pot must be large enough to ensure full immersion of the pack; usually, 20 to 30 minutes is required for thorough heating. Bring the water to a boil, then reduce the setting to low and begin timing.

When the treatment is completed, the pack should be placed back in the water and left submerged until the next treatment. The heat need not be kept on. If the pack will not be used again for some time, place it in an air-tight plastic bag and freeze it. Freezing prevents mold and mildew. Of course, it must be thoroughly thawed before reheating. Try to keep the pack from drying out; that shortens its life.

It has been reported that hot packs relieve pain more effectively than infrared heat lamps—possibly because the packs are in contact with the skin. Thus the heating effect is direct and unaffected by other stimuli such as air currents. Such skin contact, however, may be detrimental. For example, if the involved tissue is extremely sensitive, the patient may not be able to tolerate the weight of the pack.

The infrared heat lamp is the one modality that used to be found in every training room. Today, it has largely been replaced by the hot pack, which is unfortunate, because the heat lamp was useful in the treatment of pressure-sensitive injuries as well as lesions in which even temporary skin hydration was contraindicated. Perhaps the substitution was based on the finding that moist heat permits tolerance of a higher temperature and is more relaxing. Of course, an infrared heat lamp treatment can be converted to a moist-heat treatment by placing a moist towel over the part.

An infrared heat treatment usually lasts for 20 minutes. The involved part is elevated if possible, and depending on the lesion being treated, a moist towel may be placed over the area (it should be checked frequently to see that it remains moist). A luminous lamp is adjusted so that the heating element is 18 to 24 inches above the part while a nonluminous lamp is 24 to 30 inches away. Should the skin become too warm for the individual's tolerance, adjust the lamp. Check the skin for mottling; if it's present, end the treatment.

Both the infrared heat lamp and the hot pack can raise the local skin temperature by five to 10°C. If the athlete's skin temperature normally ranges from 32 to 37°C, this increase could result in tissue destruction.

The whirlpool has its critics as well as its supporters. Some feel that the whirlpool can accomplish nothing more therapeutic than to clean the skin, while others contend that it provides relief of pain and muscle spasm as well as a means of increasing range of motion with less tissue aggravation. The beneficial effect of the unit's massaging action may be more psychological than physiological. Certainly the buoyancy of the water makes the athlete's movements easier, but a similar effect can be acquired by a soak in the swimming pool.

Like other heat modalities, the whirlpool is not without hazards. When half the body (or more) is submerged, the general vasodilation of superficial vessels could affect blood flow to vital areas—if flow to the brain diminishes, the individual could faint, with fatal consequences. Therefore, whirlpool treatment involving such submersion should be constantly supervised.

The temperature of the water should be regulated to avoid irritation or damage to the skin. The maximum temperature that can be tolerated is 113°F (45°C), but this can't be endured for a long period of time. The same therapeutic effects occur at a temperature range of 102 to 104°F, which is soothing, and has less likelihood of causing tissue damage. Even 104°F should not be used until swelling is controlled. If a cold whirlpool is used in the first stage of rehabilitation, slowly increase the water temperature a few degrees every day until the maximum of 104°F is reached. Treatment time for the whirlpool is 20 minutes for extremities and 15 minutes for half-body submersion.

A general rule that must be observed with any of these methods: The therapist or trainer administers the treatment and monitors the machines, but the guideline for intensity is the individual's comfort. Tolerance to heat is individually determined; those with darker skin and hair usually withstand heat applications better than those with lighter coloring.

Analgesic balm, perhaps the most widely used treatment of minor aches and pains among athletes, is readily available in drugstores or sporting good stores, and is one of the least expensive heat modalities. The active ingredient in an external analgesic is usually methyl salicylate or oil of wintergreen.

Actually, an external analgesic is not a direct heating agent but a counterirritant: Its active ingredients irritate the skin, causing a reflex dilation of the superficial blood vessels. As a result, the skin turns red and a sensation of warmth is experienced as more blood flows through the dilated vessels.

A water-soluble external analgesic has several advantages over the oil-based preparation; chief among them is that the water-soluble agent can be removed with cold water should the skin become too hot. But hot water is required to cut the oil-base product; this may intensify the heating effect. Also, the water-soluble analgesic doesn't stain clothing or the elastic wrap of an analgesic pack.

To reduce the danger of burning or blistering of the skin, only a mild analgesic should be used in an analgesic pack. Different materials can be used as the insulating cover—a piece of cotton, part of an old towel, and even a disposable diaper.

To make an analgesic pack, apply a thin layer of analgesic to the tender area. Cover this with the insulator, which is then secured by an elastic wrap. When applying a pack to the thigh, secure it with a figure eight once or twice around the waist and thigh; this prevents the pack from sliding down the leg.

If the individual is sensitive to heat, coat the skin with a thin layer of petroleum jelly before applying the analgesic. Because skin hydration affects the absorption of drugs, an analgesic pack may become occlusive if a disposable diaper is used to cover the analgesic or a sheet of plastic wrap is placed between the insulator and the wrap (to prevent the analgesic from soaking through). With occlusion, skin hydration is increased and absorption of the analgesic through the skin increases. Environmental temperature and humidity also increase hydration of the skin and absorption of the drug. Massaging the analgesic into the skin stimulates local circulation, which in turn results in greater drug uptake.

Alternating hot and cold treatments is a useful technique to try on stubborn swelling in an extremity, but only after bleeding has been controlled. Contrast baths require two large containers, one filled approximately two-thirds full of cold water (55 to 65°F), and the other with water at approximately 104°F. The involved extremity is placed in the hot water first for four minutes; this opens up the blood vessels and increases circulation to the area. At the end of the four minutes the part is switched immediately to the cold water, where it is immersed for one minute. Here, as a result of the intense cooling, the blood vessels constrict. This alternation of vasodilation and vasoconstriction, which should be repeated five or six times, may force swelling out of the area by "massage" action. Always start with the hot water and end with the cold and, if possible, terminate the treatment with local massage.

When treating a musculoskeletal injury, the superficial heat modalities often do not penetrate deeply enough to effect healing. Of the deep-heat modalities, shortwave and microwave diathermy penetrate less deeply than ultrasound, but raise the temperature of tissue 3 cm below the skin—unless the subcutaneous layer of fat interferes with the heating process. Unfortunately, because it is an insulator, superficial fat absorbs heat and partially or completely prevents its penetration to deeper tissues. For example, when the subcutaneous fat layer is 2 cm thick, penetration is completely blocked, and the temperature of the fat layer can rapidly reach the critical level of 45°C. Therefore, when giving such a treatment, one must estimate the depth of the subcutaneous fat layer as well as determine the proximity of the involved tissue to underlying bone. Wave intensity should be modified accordingly. Shortwave diathermy is used to heat a larger surface area than microwave diathermy, which can be used in the treatment of a well-defined localized lesion. With both, the individual should experience a feeling of warmth. The intensity level of shortwave is determined by individual tolerance, as the machine dial does not accurately indicate the energy output of the unit or the amount absorbed by the patient. The energy output gauge of the microwave unit is accurate. Diathermy treatment, either microwave or shortwave, should last no longer than 20 minutes.

Ultrasonic energy can penetrate to a deep joint, causing a rise in tissue temperature at that site. Unlike the diathermies, ultrasound does not raise the temperature of the subcutaneous fat layer, nor does the layer hinder the penetration of ultrasonic energy. Ultrasound should not be used over growth centers (epiphyses) or where a blood clot is suspected, as increased blood flow could cause a clot to break loose and become an embolus.

Tissue temperatures rise more quickly with ultrasound than with the diathermies, with changes occurring within 20 to 30 seconds after starting treatment. Temperatures can rise to a damaging level where different tissue layers come together—such as skin and fat or muscle and bone—because ultrasonic energy is reflected at these junctions. The individual experiences a sudden intense ache when the critical temperature is reached; intensity should be reduced immediately. Treatment time is five minutes. Penetration of ultrasonic energy is increased if the area is first heated with a hot pack or diathermy for 10 minutes.

If the area to be treated is bony, ultrasound may be applied underwater. Ultrasonic energy may also be used to drive a drug through the skin. The technique, referred to as phonophoresis, is used in conditions such as tendinitis, in which an anti-inflammatory agent such as cortisone would be therapeutically beneficial. Injecting the drug directly into the tendon at the site of maximum tenderness may weaken the tendon, eventually causing it to rupture. Therefore, the drug is applied topically, usually in conjunction with an oral anti-inflammatory agent.

The therapies cited in this chapter are used to bring about an optimal environment for repair and healing. But all tissues require a certain time for healing, and overzealous use of these treatments may actually retard healing.

In comparing ice with heat, it is evident that the latter is more expensive as well as more dangerous. The use of heat is restricted to the rehabilitation phase of injury care, while ice can be employed in both immediate care and rehabilitative care.

Factors that affect recovery time

Type and location of injury: Generally speaking, soft-tissue injuries—contusions, strains, sprains, and dislocations—require less time to heal than injuries involving bony structures. Of course, the time required for healing in soft-tissue injuries is dependent on the type of injury, the tissues involved, and the extent of damage. A mild sprain takes a minimum of six to seven days to heal, but the individual may not lose any time from athletics if the function of the joint is not impaired.

In some reconstructive surgeries of the knee in which muscle tendons are transferred, a minimum of nine months is required for complete healing. Both tendons and ligaments are slow to heal; a mild sprain generally keeps an athlete out of activity (or requires a modification of activity) for two to three days, a moderate sprain from one to three weeks, and a severe sprain from six to eight weeks or longer. Some sprains may need surgical repair. For example, because there is a direct blood supply to the outer edge of the tissue, a peripheral cartilage tear may heal. Tears through the body do not heal and the cartilage must be removed surgically if it interferes with the function of the joint.

In a dislocation, the capsule and ligamentous tissue have been disrupted, so the joint must be immobilized to ensure structural stability. The immobilization period usually ranges from two to six weeks, depending on the joint involved and whether the injury is chronic. With few exceptions, the immobilization period for a simple fracture is six to eight weeks, and healing is prolonged if blood supply to the bone is poor or disrupted by the trauma. The blood supply of the navicular bone of the wrist is normally poor, so healing could require many months—if it ever occurs. Finally, if the injury is subject to the stress and strain of repeated movement, the healing process is continually disrupted and requires more time.

Early diagnosis and treatment: The earlier an accurate diagnosis is made, the more favorable the outcome. The longer the delay in diagnosis, the longer the injury may be without proper treatment. Further, there is a chance that the injury could be progressive in nature. For example, if a cartilage tear or ruptured anterior cruciate ligament is missed, it may affect the mechanics of the knee so that other structures are under stress and prone to trauma. Without proper treatment, not only is healing possibly delayed but also the injury may develop into a low-grade inflammation of long duration.

Conservative use vs. *surgical:* The advantages of conservative treatment are that the part is immobilized, resting the tissues and giving them an opportunity to recover; immobilization prevents disruption of healing by keeping the wound edges from moving; and it spares the individual from the stress of surgery. On the negative side, immobilization results in atrophy of the muscles that move the immobilized part; there is a decrease in the normal range of motion when the immobilizing agent is removed; and adhesions may form as a result of restricted movement. Mineral absorption also weakens the bone.

With surgery, there is immediate repair of the tissue, with sutures holding like tissues in apposition, so that there is little chance of the wound edges shifting. However, the possibility of infection increases with the opening of the tissue; the development of scar tissue can be excessive; and adhesions can form between moving tissue.

The decision to operate depends on many factors—the type, severity, and location of the injury, the newness of the injury, the age of the individual, and the sport and position played.

Functional use vs. *immobilization:* An individual is often permitted to use the injured part rather than have it immobilized with a splint or cast. A decision favoring functional use of the part is based primarily on the severity of the injury. Location and type of injury also influence the decision. When the normal function of the part is minimally affected by the injury state, there is little need for immobilization. By allowing function—although movement may be slower than normal—one is avoiding the negative aspects of immobilization. The strength, flexibility, and endurance that are lost during the period of immobilization must be regained before the individual is permitted to return to full activity. As long as functional use does not hinder the healing process, it is advantageous. Where applicable, the cast-brace permits some functional use while still providing immobilization of the injured tissue.

Generally, the rate of healing is directly related to two factors— nutrition and patient compliance. The athlete requires proper nutrients for repair of damaged tissue, and patient compliance with treatment and recommendations is necessary if healing time is to be cut to a minimum and complications avoided.

Concepts of rehabilitation

If an injury affects the athlete's ability to protect her body against further injury, she should not return to activity. The athlete must be restricted from stressful activity until the tissues have time to heal. Unfortunately, the otherwise healthy, well-tuned body reacts negatively to disuse and immobilization. If muscles are not exercised every 48 to 72 hours, the tissue begins to waste away. Consequently, the athlete experiences a loss of flexibility, strength, muscular and cardiorespiratory endurance, and agility and coordination. Each of these components of fitness is a building block for the next one, and the extent of loss determines the period that the individual must remain inactive.

The goals of rehabilitation are to prevent this generalized deconditioning of the body and to return the injured part to normal or near normal function. To accomplish this, the athlete is prescribed a daily exercise program along with therapeutic treatments of cold and/or heat, depending on the stage of healing and physical signs.

The rehabilitation program consists of two parts, general activity and specific exercises for the injured part. General activity is sports-related and maintains total-body fitness and specific sports skills without interfering with the healing process. For example, although crutch-walking is not a sports-related activity, it does maintain strength and cardiorespiratory endurance. An individual with an upper extremity injury can jog on an even surface or bicycle on a stationary machine. Activities that predispose the individual to a fall must be avoided. Specific exercises are prescribed to prevent inflexibility, muscle contractures, muscle atrophy, and healing delays. They are arranged in progressive order, according to intensity as well as purpose.

Passive, assistive, active, and resistive exercises: The least intense type of exercise is a passive one in which the injured part is moved through its range by another person. Such exercise maintains flexibility and range, but is not used very frequently in the treatment of athletic injuries. Second in intensity is an assistive exercise. Here, much of the movement is accomplished by someone else; however, the patient is actively involved by moving the part through whatever range is possible. Assistive exercises develop neurological patterns that may have been "lost" as a result of prolonged disuse as well as add muscle strength and flexibility. An active exercise, as the name implies, is one executed by the athlete without the aid of another person. Such exercise is used to maintain flexibility, improve neuromuscular patterns, and develop strength. In athletics, active exercises are used not only to strengthen the part but, in the early stages of rehabilitation, to regain range of motion. The force of gravity is often used to help regain range when the individual has reached the end point imposed by adhesions, scar tissue, and swelling.

Resistive exercise is performed by the individual against some type of resistance or overload such as disc weights, manual resistance of another person, or resistance of an opposing muscle. Such exercises focus on the development of strength and muscular endurance. There are various types of resistive exercise—isometric, isotonic, isokinetic, and eccentric. An isometric exercise is one in which the muscle contracts maximally so tension increases but there is no shortening of the muscle. Consequently, movement does not occur at the joint as in a quad set or a straight-leg lift. Isometric exercises are used early in the strengthening phase of a sprain when movement of the joint is contraindicated. With isometrics, strength is developed without irritating the joint and healing tissues.

In an isotonic exercise such as a biceps curl, the muscle contracts and shortens to initiate movement at the joint. Tension in the muscle remains constant—unfortunately, so does the resistance as the joint moves through its range. When an extremity moves through its range, the angle of pull of the muscle on its insertion constantly changes, thus affecting the muscle's ability to handle an overload. Therefore, in an isotonic exercise, the maximum overload is the amount of weight the muscle can control at its weakest point. Resistance on a muscle remains at an optimal level throughout the range of motion in an isokinetic exercise. Changes in the amount of resistance are accomplished in several ways—a fulcrum on the movement arm, a cam, a hydraulic clutch, or a cylinder filled with water.

An eccentric exercise makes use of a lengthening contraction of the muscle, as in lowering a weight to the starting position, or a half squat. Muscles can lower more weight than they can lift, but more tension builds up in the muscle while lowering a weight. Consequently, in the initial stages of eccentric exercises, postexercise muscle soreness is greater than with other types of resistive exercises. Isokinetic and eccentric exercises are usually prescribed during the later stages of the rehabilitation program. The individual should always return to the starting position of an exercise in a slow, controlled manner, which takes advantage of eccentric strengthening.

Both parts of the rehabilitation program should be started as soon as possible, with the type, location, and severity of the injury determining the starting time. Above all, the activity should not hinder healing, and time must be allowed for optimal postoperative healing. During immobilization, some maintenance exercise, such as isometrics, is allowed. An exception: If the injury involves a muscle and/or its tendon, no movement—or even increase in muscle tension—is permitted. Certain physiological reactions indicate when the program is too intense for the recovering tissues: Whenever pain and/or swelling increase or the range of motion decreases, the workload has been too great. Cut back the intensity to a level where none of these reactions is apparent.

Guidelines: When rehabilitating an injury, the first step is to regain range of motion. Unless the individual regains normal range before strength, only a small part of the entire range of motion will be strong. In working on range of motion, make use of the buoyancy of water—as in a cold whirlpool—or the anesthetic and muscle relaxant effects of ice massage. Use active exercises and gravity but do not force the joint. Applying force only aggravates the tissue and the resultant swelling may actually decrease the range. Swelling may also cause an increase in ligament laxity as the joint capsule is stretched by accumulation of excess fluid. The exercise should be carried out only to the point of discomfort. Range of motion should not be regained so quickly that the atrophied muscles and weak ligaments are unable to stabilize the joint. With a few exceptions, what strength exists may be maintained and developed at this time by isometrics.

When range is near normal, begin to strengthen the muscles but also continue the range of motion exercises daily until normal. Isometrics may be used predominantly in the initial stages of strength development to ensure adequate muscular stability of the joint before commencing isotonic exercises.

To build muscular strength, the muscle must be subjected to an overload, but not one that causes additional damage to the tissues. The key is to stress the recovering tissues but not strain them. Adaptation does not occur unless demand is placed on the body. Not only must the overload be within the capacity level of the injured tissue, it must also be progressively increased. For, as strength develops, the overload must constantly be increased if stress or a demand is continually to be placed on the body. Muscular strength increases in response to the stress, as does the resistance of the connective tissues in and around the joint—ligaments, capsule, and cartilage.

For each exercise in the program, estimate what weight the individual can lift 10 times in succession. The individual should be slightly fatigued at the completion of the 10th but still be able to execute the exercise. If fewer than eight attempts are possible, the weight is too heavy; more than 12 indicates it is too light.

These starting weights are used according to the formula established by DeLorme, which allows for progressive strengthening of an injury with little danger of straining the sensitive tissue:

1 set of 10 repetitions at 1/2 RM
1 set of 10 repetitions at 3/4 RM
1 set of 10 repetitions at RM

A repetition is the number of times an exercise is executed in succession. They are usually arranged into groups called sets. The RM refers to the "repetitions maximum," or maximum amount of weight the individual can lift properly 10 times in succession. For example, if the RM is 12 pounds, the formula is filled in as follows:

1 set of 10 at 6 lb
1 set of 10 at 9 lb
1 set of 10 at 12 lb

The first two sets serve as a warm-up for the third. A fourth set is often added as a warm-down—1 set of 20 reps at 1/4 RM. The individual may be unable to execute 10 reps at the maximum weight and should never be forced to do so. The goal is to do 10 without pain or an increase in swelling. Once the goal is reached, increase the overload by one to 2½ pounds. When the overload is increased, the number of repetitions the individual is able to complete properly usually drops. Once again, the individual should work toward the goal of 10 repetitions at RM.

The DeLorme program is used throughout the strengthening program, whether the individual is executing isometric exercises, isotonic exercises, or a combination. The overload may be imposed manually, with sandbags, disc weights, or sophisticated exercise machines. The exercise should be executed correctly and slowly. Movements should be smooth, without jerkiness, to avoid pain. Momentum can be eliminated by executing the exercise slowly to a count of seven. Lift the overload to a count of three, hold the intermediate terminal position for one, and then lower the overload to a count of three. Both extremities should be exercised to prevent the uninvolved muscles from becoming weaker as a result of limited use. Furthermore, strength should be as closely symmetrical as possible on the two sides of the body, allowing for a slight difference due to dominance.

Return to normalcy is determined by comparing the strength of the injured part to that of the corresponding part. In addition, preseason physical examination and fitness test records should be consulted if they are available.

Once 60 to 80 per cent of the individual's strength has been regained, the rehabilitation program should shift to include an endurance program. The strengthening program, however, should not be terminated. Alternate it with the endurance program, one day on one program, the next day on the other. Muscular strength is a prerequisite for muscular endurance.

To develop muscular endurance, a light weight is lifted many times. The DeLorme formula is modified as follows:

1 set of 20 to 25 reps at ½ RM
1 set of 20 to 25 reps at ¾ RM
1 set of 20 to 25 reps at RM
1 set of 20 to 25 reps at ¼ RM

The repetitions maximum used for muscular endurance is 60 to 75 per cent of the last RM used in the strengthening program. For example, if the last RM for the strength program is 60 pounds, the RM for the endurance exercises should be 45 pounds.

Dynamic exercises, such as swimming, bicycling, and jogging, are introduced slowly after strength and muscular endurance are developed adequately to support such activity. Pain and an increase in swelling indicate the part is not ready for such activity. Swimming and bicycling are less stressful on a lower extremity injury than is jogging or running. Swimming and bicycling may be introduced when the athlete has adequate range of motion and has started flexion-extension exercises. Jogging should not be started until the athlete can execute a series of six to 10 one-legged squats or lift 80 per cent of the body's weight with the involved leg. When introduced, jogging should be done on level ground. Distance should be built up before increasing speed. Eventually, the individual is allowed to run on uneven terrain, but straight ahead with gradual changes of direction. The athlete's speed is slowly increased. Such activities are used for the development of cardio-respiratory endurance.

The final phase of the rehabilitation program focuses on the development of agility and coordination. Agility involves quick changes of directions as well as starts and stops. When running, the individual progresses from gradual changes in directions (such as circles or figure eights) to sharper cuts, like zig-zags, and finally to quick right-angle turns. If at any time the individual limps during any of these activities, the level should be decreased. Coordination involves the correct execution of isolated skills in the individual's particular sport. The isolated skills are eventually put together so the individual must perform the movement patterns required by the sport.

Objective measures can be made to determine when range of motion, strength, muscular endurance, and agility are back to normal so the athlete can return to activity. Range of motion should be pain-free. The individual should continue the strengthening program at least three days a week throughout the season. Prior to any strenuous activity, some form of superficial heat should be applied to the area to stimulate the circulation. After activity, ice should be applied to control any swelling.

After complete recovery, if the individual desires to increase overall general body strength beyond its normal level and the physician approves, the program should focus on heavy weight. However, it should be lifted only a few times, such as one set of eight. Such an intense program should be executed on alternate days because approximately 48 to 72 hours are required for muscle tissue to recover. Otherwise little progress is seen and the outcome could even be negative—the overstressed muscle tissue may actually break down.

Exercise programs

Ankle exercises*: The first stage of ankle exercises consists of simple flexion, extension, inversion, and eversion to full range of motion:
- Flex foot as far as possible, point toes upward.
- Extend foot as far as possible, point toes downward.
- Turn sole of foot inward.
- Turn sole of foot outward.

If the above exercises can be done in full range of motion and without pain, do the following exercises:
- Foot circles—foot circumscribes a small circle. Ball of foot down first, then in, up, and finally out.
- Alphabet—sitting on table with knee straight and only ankle extended over the end of the table, print in capital letters the entire alphabet with your foot.

If the above exercises can be done in full range of motion and without pain, do the following exercises:
- Towel exercise—sitting on a chair with foot on a towel, pick towel up with toes. After completing the above successfully, secure a weight on the other end of the towel to offer resistance to the lifting movement.
- Pickup exercise—pick up marbles, small pieces of sponge rubber, or partly used roller bandage. Alternate placing the object in the hand opposite knee of good leg and in the hand behind buttocks of the injured leg.

---

*This section on the ankle is printed with permission from Sayers Miller of the Sports Research Institute of Penn State University.

• Toe rises—stand with feet one foot apart and toeing in. Rise on the toes as high as possible without pain. Repeat this exercise with toes pointed straight ahead and pointed out.

If the above exercises can be done in full range of motion and without pain, do the following exercises:

• Repeat flexion, extension, inversion, eversion exercises with the trainer giving resistance with his hand.

• Hopping exercise—first standing on the good leg hop as high as possible. Then repeat on the injured leg.

When the athlete can perform the hopping exercise equally as well on his injured leg and without pain, do the following exercises:

• Active jogging and walking in a straight path with the ankle strapped—1. Walk 25 yards, jog 25 yards; 2. Walk 25 yards, jog 50 yards; 3. Walk 25 yards, jog 75 yards. Note: Anytime the athlete limps, stop all running. Repeat walk and jog exercise, except at half of athlete's top speed. Repeat walk and jog exercise, except at three-quarter speed. Repeat, except at full speed.

• When the athlete is able to do sprints at full speed and without a limp, then have her run circles both clockwise and counterclockwise. Start with large circles and work down gradually to smaller sizes.
without pain, then have her run figure eights.

• When the athlete can run figure eights at full speed without a limp and without pain, then have her run a zig-zag course the length of a football/soccer field.

• Finally, test the athlete on right angle quick cuts both to the right and left. When she can do this, she is ready for practice and competition.

All exercises should be repeated 10 or more times daily. When the athlete starts jogging with her ankle strapped, she can do all the previous exercises at home and on her own with the trainer checking twice a week on these exercises.

Knee exercises: The first phase of knee exercises consists of simple range of motion and muscle-strengthening exercises. Do not force motion in a hinge joint, for it usually results in tissue aggravation and decreased range. Sit on the edge of a table with the injured leg extended and use gravity as a force. Do not add any external weight.

Go on to strengthening exercises. When exercising the quadriceps—the anterior thigh muscles—work on the good leg as well as the injured one.

• Quad set—sitting with the leg straight, pull the kneecap upward by tightening the muscles on the front of the thigh. Hold for five seconds, then relax. Do the exercise five minutes of every waking hour.

• Straight-leg lifts—on your back or sitting with legs straight, tighten the muscles on the front of the thigh and lift the leg six to eight inches off the floor. Hold the position for five seconds. Lower the leg slowly and repeat.

Progress to exercises with an external weight. Start with a light weight placed on the lower leg immediately below the kneecap. As the muscles on the front of the thigh become stronger, move the weight toward the ankle. In strengthening these thigh muscles, the leg must be held completely straight so that the muscle on the medial side is tightened. When more weight is added, move the overload back to the area just below the kneecap.

Pain and swelling are the guidelines to determine if the workout is too strenuous. If swelling around the joint is evident the day after the workout, or if the athlete experiences pain while executing an exercise, the overload is too great. The athlete should start with three sets of 10 reps. As soon as she can easily handle this weight, increase to three sets of 15 reps. The final step is three sets of 20 reps. When the athlete can execute this workout program with no pain or swelling, move the weight down the leg and repeat the progression.

When working on the hamstrings, exercise the good leg as well as the injured one:

• Hip hyperextension—on your stomach with legs straight, tighten the muscles on the back of the thigh and buttocks. Lift the leg 10 to 15° off the floor, keeping it straight. Hold for five seconds, relax, and repeat.

Again, progress to exercises with an external weight. Start with a light weight placed on the heel. The weight should be lighter than that lifted by the muscles on the front of the thigh. As the muscles on the back of the thigh and buttocks become stronger, either increase the number of times you lift the weight or add more weight.

● Hamstrings set—on your back with knees bent and feet flat on the floor, attempt to bend the knee against the resistance of the floor (push the heel into the floor without moving the leg). Hold for five seconds, relax, and repeat. The muscles on the back of the thigh should tighten.

● Hamstrings isometric—on your stomach with legs straight, attempt to bend the leg against the resistance of a partner's hand. These posterior thigh muscles (hamstrings) may not be used to the overload, so be cautious of the development of muscle cramps.

● Knee flexion. On your stomach with the legs straight, place a light weight on the heel. Tighten the posterior thigh muscles and bend the knee through its entire range of motion. Hold for five seconds, relax, and repeat.

For the abductors:

● Sitting with the legs hanging over the edge of a table and crossed, attempt to pull them apart. Hold for five seconds, relax, and repeat.

● On your back with the knees bent and feet flat on the floor, attempt to pull the legs apart against the resistance of a partner (the partner encircles the athlete's knees). You can use a padded loop of ankle wrap to provide the resistance. Slip your legs within the loop and then attempt to pull them apart. With either method, hold for five seconds, relax, and repeat.

● On your side with legs straight, attempt to spread the legs apart with a partner applying resistance. If you do not have a partner, substitute the padded loop of ankle wrap or external weight.

For the adductors:

● Sitting with your legs hanging over the edge of a table, place your fists between the knees. Attempt to pull your knees together. Or place an empty tennis-ball can with padded ends between your knees to provide resistance. Hold for five seconds, relax, and repeat the exercise.

● On your back with the legs straight and spread apart, attempt to pull the legs together against the resistance of a partner.

With the calf muscles, work on the good leg as well as the injured one:

● Point your foot against the resistance of a partner.

● Stand on the edge of a stair and stabilize the body by holding onto the wall. Tighten the calf muscles and raise the body weight,

FIGURE 16-1

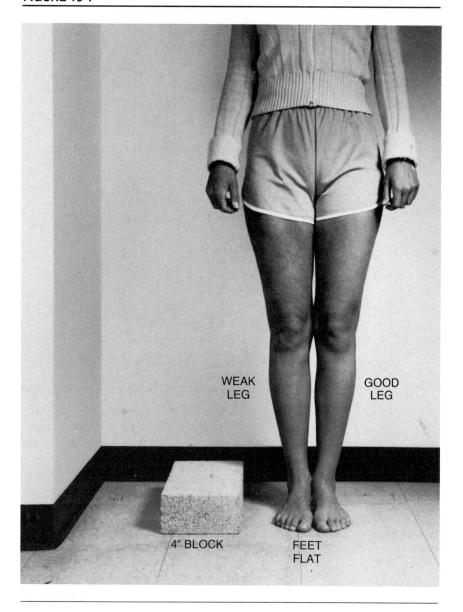

Begin step-up exercises standing with foot of weak leg 4 inches away from a 4-inch block.

so you are standing on your toes. Hold for five seconds, relax, and lower the body so the heels are below the edge of the stair. Slight discomfort should be felt in the calf muscles. Hold for 20 seconds and return to the starting position. Repeat. Initially, the athlete may need to execute the exercise on the floor without stretching the calf muscle.

Later, as the calf muscles become stronger, add external weights. Initially the weights can be held at the side of the body in the hands. As the external weight increases, use a barbell placed on the shoulders.

Phase 2 of knee exercises consists of step-ups, flexion and extension exercises, and jogging. The step-up exercise (see Figures 16-1 to 16-4) should not be started until the individual can flex the knee to at least 90° and execute successfully a one-legged squat on the involved leg. A four-inch block or a stair step is required in the initial phase of the exercise.

The individual should stand with the feet together with the weak leg next to the block, approximately four inches away. The foot of the weak leg is placed on the block. The body weight is lifted by straightening the knee of the weak leg. Do not put the foot of the good leg on the block; it remains suspended.

When lifting the body weight, the individual should avoid pushing off the floor with the toes. This can be accomplished by touching only the heel to the floor.

The body weight should be lifted to a count of two and held to a count of five. Then it should be lowered to a count of two, and the individual allowed to rest for a count of one. The exercise should be repeated at this cadence until the individual is fatigued. The goal is five minutes of continuous exercise. Repeat the exercise six to eight times a day.

As strength is regained, the individual should stand farther away from the block. When approximately 10 to 12 inches away, the height of the block should be increased to at least 10 inches. Fourteen inches is the maximum. Also the number should be increased to eight to 10 a day.

Flexion-extension exercises are prescribed when the athlete can execute three sets of 20 reps of the straight-leg lift exercise with an overload of 25 to 30 pounds and if no increase in pain or swelling occurs. If the athlete complains of a painful grating sensation when

FIGURE 16-2

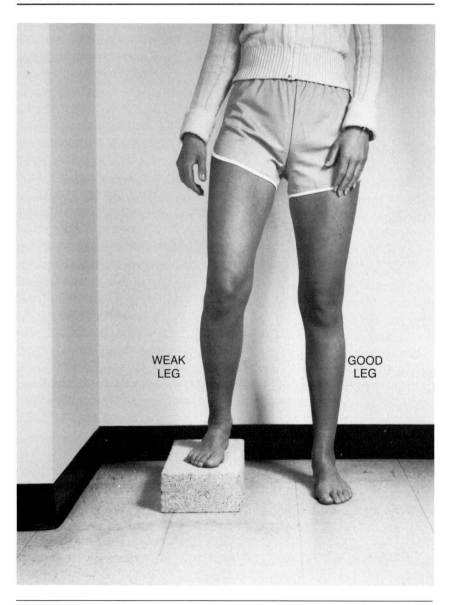

WEAK
LEG

GOOD
LEG

Place foot of weak leg flat on block, keeping weight
mainly on heels.

executing flexion-extension exercises, the exercise should be terminated immediately. The athlete in all probability has developed chondromalacia patellae. Substitute straight-leg lifts to gain quadriceps strength. Adequate quadriceps strength, particularly of the muscle on the medial side, is necessary for the patella to track smoothly.

If the athlete uses an iron boot for an overload during the flexion-extension exercises, the involved leg should be supported on a bench. Limit the overload to approximately 20 pounds, especially when exercising the hamstrings. The athlete may not have sufficient strength to control rotation at the joint when the knee is flexed. As the overload increases in weight, switch to the De-Lorme program.

Phase 3 adds running to the flexion and extension exercises, and phase 4 adds agility drills.

In phase 1 of an athlete's program, she should work toward three sets of 10 repetitions of each exercise (3×10). When she can successfully execute 3×10 of the particular exercise with no pain or swelling (swelling may not be evident until the following day) increase the weight but decrease the repetitions. Work up toward 3×10 again.

When working on strength in phases 2 and 3, aim toward three sets of six. For endurance exercises in phase 3, work toward three sets of 15. In combination strength and endurance exercises in phases 3 and 4, do three sets of 10 to 12.

Supplementary exercises may be added only during the later stages of rehabilitation and only on the recommendation of a physician and/or trainer.

- Swimming is O.K., but avoid the whip and frog kicks.
- Bleacher runs—run up and *walk* down. Either toe in or straight ahead. Toeing out introduces outward (external) rotation beyond that which normally occurs during extension of the knee and may result in a torn cartilage. Toeing in introduces some stability to those athletes who have rotational instability. It is also beneficial in cases of chondromalacia patellae and for those who experience recurrent patellar dislocations.
- Bicycling—use a bicycle ergometer or a nongear bicycle. Adjust the height of the seat so you can almost completely straighten your leg while pedaling.

FIGURE 16-3

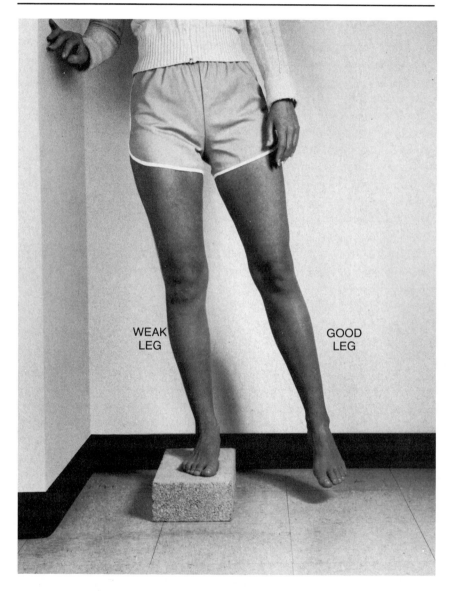

WEAK
LEG

GOOD
LEG

Body weight is lifted by straightening the knee of the weak leg.
Athlete should not push off the floor with toes. This is avoided
by keeping weight on heel.

Principles of taping

First and foremost, it must be realized that taping a joint or muscle group is no substitute for complete rehabilitation of the injured part. There is no way that a few layers of tape can stabilize a joint if the muscles fail to do so. In fact, the effectiveness of taping has yet to be proven scientifically. A small group of medical practitioners contend that tape may even predispose an individual to a sprain rather than prevent it or minimize its severity.

Obviously, tape is no panacea, but it does have a role in athletics. When properly applied, it can be used to restrict a painful movement or support irritated tissues. However, before tape can be properly applied, the underlying anatomy must be clearly understood, as well as the mechanism of injury. The injury must be accurately diagnosed as to the extent and severity of tissue damage. Finally, the individual must have a knowledge of kinesiology (the science of movement) to determine whether a strip of tape actually fulfills its purpose of restriction or support.

Tape can be applied in dozens of patterns, but each strip making up a specific pattern has a purpose. If the purpose of each is understood, then any number of patterns can be developed to provide optimum support for injured tissue or resistance of a painful movement. Every injury is different because different tissues are damaged and to a different extent. Consequently, all sprains of the same joint are not alike and must be treated individually. For example, not all inversion ankle sprains should be taped using the same pattern.

Tape should not be applied if it does not have a purpose either physiological or psychological. Even when the application of tape is justified, the possibility of secondary complications, such as folliculitis, tape burns or blisters, and contact dermatitis, is still present. There are a few guidelines, however, that may help reduce the likelihood of such complications:

• Apply the tape so that it conforms to the body part, but never stretch the tape to make it do so. If a body part tapers, the tape must be angled slightly upward to avoid wrinkling or puckering of the tape—such imperfections can cause irritation of the skin. Use narrower tape or elastic tape to strap the smaller body parts and those with acute angles. In the adolescent female, some body parts

FIGURE 16-4

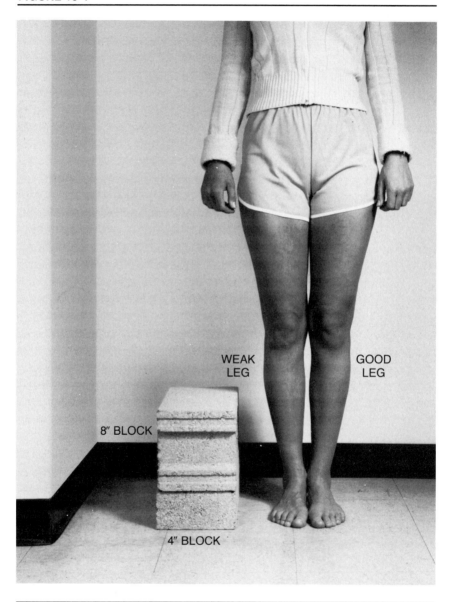

Progression in step-up exercises is to height of 10 to 14 inches, with athlete standing 10 to 12 inches away from block.

may not be amenable to taping, such as the shoulder. The breast interferes with the application of tape and the skin in the area is extremely sensitive.

• Use white tape to restrict a movement and elastic tape to assist a movement. Keep white tape wound close to the roll during application. Elastic tape should be unwound and only slightly stretched where applied; otherwise, the tape's elasticity could interfere with circulation.

• Place the part to be taped in a position directly opposite the motion that is to be restricted. For example, if hyperextension of the elbow is painful, tape the joint in a slightly flexed position.

• Protect existing skin lesions from irritation imposed by the tape. Apply a protective dressing over each lesion and cover with an underwrap prior to taping. Pad with gauze sponges areas that are subject to stress, extremely sensitive, or in close proximity to underlying nerves and arteries. Remove a strapping immediately after the activity so the skin can recover from its temporary semiocclusive environment. Although maximum support is achieved by taping directly to the skin, the resulting skin trauma does not justify the practice in most cases.

• Compress a new injury with a wet elastic wrap rather than tape. As there is little indication of the amount of swelling to expect, the tape could have a tourniquet-like effect if swelling is excessive. It is easy to adjust the amount of compression provided by an elastic wrap. The tape must be completely removed if it interferes with blood flow or nerve function as indicated by numbness, tingling, coldness, or cyanosis distal to the tape. If removed, compression against swelling is lost.

• Do not tape continuously with white tape as it has a tendency to hinder circulation. Never encircle a muscle mass with white tape because the muscle must have space to relax as well as contract. If expansion of the muscle is not permitted, it may go into spasm. If elastic tape is used, the muscle may be enclosed, provided the tape is not applied too tightly.

• Overlap tape one-third to one-half the width of the previous piece to ensure maximum stability. Do not allow any gaps between the layers of tape.

• Learn to tear tape without tugging against the tissue.

Further reading

Downer AH: *Physical Therapy Procedures Selected Techniques.* Springfield, Ill: Thomas, 1974

Downey JA and Darling RC: *Physiological Basis of Rehabilitation Medicine.* Philadelphia: Saunders, 1971

Griffin JE and Karselis TC: *Physical Agents for Physical Therapists.* Springfield, Ill: Thomas, 1978

Klafs CE and Arnheim DD: *Modern Principles of Athletic Training.* St. Louis: Mosby, 1977

Riley DP, ed: *Strength Training by the Experts.* West Point, NY: Leisure Press, 1977

Stone WJ and Kroll WA: *Sports Conditioning and Weight Training.* Boston: Allyn and Bacon, 1978

EAR, NOSE, AND THROAT PROBLEMS

John W. Cavo Jr., M.D.

CHAPTER

17

T
he human ear is divided into three parts: the external ear, including the pinna and ear canal; the middle ear, including structures between the eardrum and the oval window; and the inner ear, including structures between the oval window and the internal auditory meatus.

Ear pain

It is not uncommon for fairly significant degrees of discomfort in the ear to originate in other areas. The most common source of ear pain in an adolescent female, for example, is not the ear but the adjacent temporomandibular joint. Many of the victims of temporomandibular joint syndrome (Costen's syndrome) happen to be brace-wearers or chronic gum-chewers. The constant trauma to the jaw joint sets up an arthralgia, which the patient experiences as ear pain. The diagnosis of this syndrome usually can be made by eliciting the discomfort experimentally: Press your fingers firmly in the patient's ear while she slowly and fully opens and closes her mouth.

Tonsillar irritation can also be the source of referred ear pain. The diagnosis is made by the characteristic findings of tonsillitis. Other possible sources of referred pain are third-molar problems, elongated styloid processes, and mucosal lesions of the pharynx, hypopharynx, and larynx.

246

The external ear

The skin-lined cavities of the external ear canal are not subject to the normal sloughing and discarding of exfoliated layers. Therefore, normal hygiene of the external ear canal depends upon the consistent presence and slow lateral migration of a thin layer of cerumen. Mechanical factors such as ear-cleaning with cotton-tipped applicators or washcloth-tipped fingers are the most frequent causes of ear-canal skin irritation, wax impactions, and bacterial external otitis. Nevertheless, an anatomic factor such as narrow ear canals, osteomata, or "collapsing ear canals" can also play a role.

External otitis: Water-sport participants are frequently the victims of external otitis—swimmer's ear. This condition is characterized by edema and inflammation of the external ear-canal skin. Exposure of the ear to water and breakdown of the standard cerumen barrier are the customary causes. The condition is often accompanied by a surprising degree of pain, and the skin of the ear canal is edematous and erythematous. Often it is impossible to clearly visualize the drum. This leads to confusion—is the otitis primary or secondary to irritating drainage through an underlying drum perforation? Therefore, it is prudent to follow a patient with external otitis carefully in order to thoroughly examine the drum when the external otitis has cleared.

Swelling of the canal-wall skin is often so severe that the prescribed topical medications cannot get into the ear. Under these circumstances it becomes necessary to place a vehicle such as a cotton wick into the canal, so that the drops will get to where they're needed. While initial insertion can be traumatic to all concerned, a wick is desirable when there is doubt as to the patency of the ear canal.

Each episode of external otitis scars and partially destroys some cerumen glands, making the victim vulnerable to further episodes. Therefore, a person who has had external otitis should be encouraged in prevention. Judicious use of alcohol-and-vinegar ear drops (90 per cent isopropyl alcohol, 10 per cent vinegar) after swimming, for example, can be an excellent preventive measure. Commercially available preparations containing acetic acid, benzethonium chloride, and propylene glycol are also effective.

External canal osteomata: Benign bony tumors of the external ear canals are apt to occur primarily in the superior aspect of the canal just lateral to the pars flaccida of the drum. For obscure reasons, such tumors are particularly prevalent in cold-water swimming enthusiasts. Rarely do these asymptomatic growths occupy enough of the canal to cause complete blockage, but they can obstruct the normal passage of cerumen and may therefore contribute to repeated wax impactions and bouts of external otitis. X-rays can detect these tumors, which may be surgically removed, if necessary.

Collapsing canals: A relaxation of soft-tissue suspension and support is the most common cause of collapsing canals. In this entity the medial end of the conchal cartilage falls forward and literally tends to narrow the lateral end of the external ear to a slit. The canal can easily be opened to insert an ear speculum, but the narrowing at the lateral end of the canal can result in retarded wax migration, poor natural cleansing of the external canal, and infection.

Pinna trauma: Fibrocartilaginous structures of the pinna are covered by tightly bound perichondrium, making the ear particularly vulnerable to the development of painful and potentially mutilating hematomata. These develop as a result of rather severe trauma to the ear and require drainage and the application of a molded pressure-dressing. Otherwise, a cauliflower ear could develop.

Frostbite: Cold-weather sports enthusiasts frequently are victims of frostbite. Slow warming of the ear with loosely applied, lukewarm, moist cloths should be instituted without using unnecessary pressure. If tissue destruction has occurred, antibiotics should be administered to avoid secondary infections. The victim must be warned of her particular vulnerability to further episodes of frostbite, and care must be taken to protect the ears from future exposure.

Burns: These are treated with the same local measures used for burns elsewhere. Efforts must be made to limit tissue destruction from secondary infections.

Lacerations: An attempt should be made to surgically restore a completely severed ear, although the chances of success are not good. Time is of the essence and pre- and postoperative antibiotic coverage is appropriate. The prospect for ear survival is significantly improved if a pedicle of tissue remains between the intact ear and the severed portion.

In caring for lacerations of the external ear canal, the principal objectives are avoiding infection and being certain that the drum itself has been spared. Frequently, the presence of swelling, dried blood, clots, and wax within the canal prevent an adequate initial assessment of the drum. The patient should be treated with systemic antibiotics and topical ear drops, and the ear should be kept dry until a more thorough examination can be made (usually in about two weeks).

The middle ear

The transmission of sound from the environment to the inner ear depends upon an intact eardrum, an air-filled middle-ear space, and an intact, mobile chain of ossicles. Modification of these factors can result in a conductive hearing loss of up to 60 dB.

Otitis media: This problem arises as an expression of inadequate eustachian tube function, with fluid collection in the middle-ear cleft. The classic history is a cold followed by a sudden feeling of fullness in the ear. Shortly thereafter the ear becomes painful, and the drum appears red and thick. Comparison with the appearance of the uninvolved drum helps to establish the diagnosis. If appropriate treatment—antibiotics, topical and systemic decongestants, and a warning to avoid abrupt changes in environmental pressure—isn't instituted, the drum may rupture, and the victim experiences sudden drainage with dramatic relief of pain.

Serous otitis: The presence of uninfected serous fluid or mucus behind an intact drum can be difficult to detect. It helps to compare the appearance of the involved ear with the normal ear. A yellowish or amber-colored eardrum, diminished movement of the drum as seen with the pneumatic otoscope, and tuning fork test results compatible with a conductive hearing loss are the signs of serous otitis. This condition should be treated with decongestants and antibiotics.

Drum perforations: A sudden blow to the ear can result in traumatic perforation of the drum. Such trauma can also cause ossicular damage and hearing loss. These can be detected by careful audiometric testing, but often are not evident until re-evaluation when the ruptured drum is healed.

A ruptured drum usually heals spontaneously and leaves only a small scar. However, until healing is complete, the victim must keep her ear dry and avoid flying and violent noseblowing.

Repeated examinations: Careful follow-up is obligatory in treating inflammatory and traumatic middle-ear infections. Otitis media is not controlled until the serous otitis has cleared. Perforated drums can't be assumed to have healed on the subjective basis of symptomatic improvement and cessation of drainage. Adequate care requires repeated examinations and appropriate audiometric re-evaluations until proper middle-ear function has been restored.

The inner ear

Tinnitus, sensorineural hearing loss, and vertigo are the hallmarks of inner-ear disorders. In addition to careful examination, the evaluation of suspected inner-ear disorders requires audiometric testing, caloric testing, and appropriate radiographic examinations. An early distinction must be made between actual dizziness and lightheadedness or syncope, so that unnecessary, time-consuming, and expensive evaluations can be avoided.

Trauma: Encased in a capsule of very dense bone, the cochlea and labyrinthine apparatus are generally well protected from all but the most severe forms of direct trauma. Indirect trauma in the form of violent Valsalva maneuvers or exposure to pressure changes can cause perilymphatic fistulae, characterized by sudden severe vertigo, hearing loss, and tinnitus. Suspected fistulae should be surgically explored relatively early. Oval-window fistulae are much more common than round-window fistulae and both are usually repaired using autogenous tissue.

Viral labyrinthitis: This acute and sometimes disabling dizziness is characteristically preceded by other viral symptoms such as coryza or gastroenteritis. It is self-limiting, lasting for only a week or two, and is not associated with a hearing loss.

Meniere's syndrome: Endolymphatic hydrops results from pressure changes in the inner-ear fluids. A number of underlying disease states are recognized as causes of Meniere's syndrome (hypothyroidism, syphilis, diabetes, allergic diatheses, and pituitary-adrenal imbalances). Although pure cochlear and pure labyrinthine forms of the syndrome are recognized, most Meniere's victims have both a hearing disorder and evidence of labyrinthine dysfunction. The syndrome occurs as a paroxysm of dizziness—usually preceded by a feeling of fullness in one ear—tinnitus, and hearing loss. There is often a fluctuating but progressive hearing loss. Between 15 and 20 per cent of victims eventually develop bilateral symptoms.

Benign paroxysmal postural vertigo (BPPV): True spinning vertigo that is provoked by postural change and whose paroxysms last for only a few seconds may be benign paroxysmal postural vertigo. In this interesting condition, there is usually a short latent period between the provoking stimulus and the onset of subjective vertigo and objective nystagmus. The response of vertigo can be exhausted by repeatedly trying to elicit the symptom. It is wise not to make this diagnosis until other possible sources of vertigo, such as Meniere's syndrome and an acoustic neuroma, have been ruled out. BPPV is probably a reflex. The afferent limb of the reflex derives from cervical spine proprioceptors. A useful technique in treating this disorder is a series of exercises in which the patient deliberately tries to provoke the vertigo by putting her head and neck into positions known to cause dizziness.

CNS vertigo: Central nervous system disorders can also be the source of dizziness. One of the early manifestations of multiple sclerosis, for example, is intermittent vertigo. Other CNS signs and symptoms are usually the clue that central problems are the source of vertigo.

The nose and sinuses

The nose, nature's own air conditioner, is the most frequently traumatized facial structure. Its function largely determines the temperature and relative humidity of air reaching the bronchopulmonary system during quiet respiration. It has been suggested that nose-breathing protects a susceptible individual from asthmatic symptoms, but there is a price. Air moving through the nose encounters more flow resistance than air moving through the mouth. Furthermore, because of turbulence, this flow resistance increases exponentially as the rate of flow increases. Thus, at some

point during the development of heavy breathing, a person uncon-
sciously decides that the effort of nose-breathing is too great and
resorts to mouth-breathing. In so doing, she trades her ability to
adequately warm and humidify the inspired air for a higher volume
of flow at lower resistance.

The lateral wall of the nose is endowed with three baffles or
turbinates that allow a large surface area of nasal mucosa to contact the inspired and expired air. This permits greater efficiency in
warming and humidifying inspired air. The turbinates also serve to
keep the air-flow pattern reasonably laminar.

Epistaxis: Although rarely a life-threatening problem, nosebleeds can be a source of significant frustration and stress to victim
and physician. Few clinical problems are as ineffectively treated
with folk remedies—many with no known basis—as nosebleeds.
Even a few professional remedies are employed despite an unknown mechanism of action and unproven efficacy.

Epistaxis can be the expression of underlying disorders such as
hypertension, coagulopathy, or Weber-Rendu-Osler syndrome.
However, nosebleeds are most often a primary problem, caused by
the cracking of dry nasal mucous membranes, and therefore most
prevalent during the dry winter months. If bleeding is scanty and
infrequent, bleeds are best treated by wetting agents—a mineral-
oil spray or saline nose drops and sprays—and home vaporizers
and humidifiers.

Cauterization is sometimes needed to control brisk nasal bleeding. Fortunately, most of the bleeding sites are located on the
easily accessible anterior portion of the nasal septum. Good illumi-
nation, topical anesthesia, silver nitrate sticks, and above all, a
cooperative patient, are the keys to success in treating epistaxis
with cautery. Anterior nasal packing is occasionally successful but
commits the subject to two or three days of discomfort with no
assurance that the bleeding won't start again when the packs are
removed.

The rare unfortunate person with a posterior bleeding site that
can't be controlled with cauterization or anterior packing is a can-
didate for posterior nasal packing or arterial ligation.

Nasal obstruction: This condition is usually the result of several
factors. The relative contributions of anatomic problems (most often a deviated septum) and mucosal thickening (related to inflam-

matory conditions and allergic reactions) differ in individuals.

The deviated septum is exceedingly common and rarely causes symptoms. The individual's tolerance to septal deviation is the key factor in weighing the significance of the deformity.

Upper respiratory infections, local irritants, and inhalant allergens are frequent factors in nasal obstruction because of the associated mucosal swelling. Judicious use of topical and systemic decongestants, antihistamines, topical steroid sprays, and allergic hyposensitization will often solve the problem.

Polyps: Mucosal thickening carried to its extreme results in polyposis of the nasal passages and paranasal sinuses. In adults, nasal polyps are most often the manifestation of severe allergic disease; in children, they are among the earliest signs of cystic fibrosis. Control usually involves a combination of allergic management and periodic surgical removal. Occasionally, a short course of a steroid-containing nasal spray can achieve polyp shrinkage and symptomatic relief.

Probably the greatest hazard in dealing with nasal polyps is the possibility of missing other diagnoses. Meningoceles in children and a host of bizarre pathological entities in adults, such as inverting papillomata and esthesioneuroblastomas, can be the true source of nasal polyps. The best chance of controlling these problems lies in early detection. Taking indiscriminate biopsies, however, can be dangerous, and appropriate radiographic studies should be done before one attempts to make a tissue diagnosis.

Sinusitis: This disorder is high on the list of erroneous diagnoses made by unskilled but aggressive self-diagnosticians. The condition is marked by localized tenderness, pain, pus in the nose, low-grade fever, and impaired vocal resonance. One often finds a history of previous sinus infections or of a recent upper respiratory infection.

Chronic sinusitis can be nearly asymptomatic, or it may be the source of impaired vocal resonance, headaches, or mild facial tenderness. Unchecked progressive chronic sinusitis can develop into osteomyelitis, especially in the area of the frontal bone. Local pressure from chronic sphenoid sinusitis can cause deficient eye movements and visual loss.

The headaches associated with sinusitis are typically present when the victims awaken in the morning and seem to diminish as the day progresses. This provides an occasionally useful distinction between headaches caused by sinusitis and those related to tension. Tension headaches usually worsen as the day progresses. Nearly all headaches become more severe as the subject lowers her head, but this is especially true of sinus headaches.

Sinus infections are the result of blockage of the normal channels of communication with the nose. Polyps, a deviated nasal septum, foreign bodies, tumors, and even thick mucus can cause the obstruction. The usual causative organisms are alpha- and beta-hemolytic streptococcus, Diplococcus pneumoniae, Staphylococcus aureus, and Hemophilus influenzae. The infections should initially be treated with antibiotics, decongestants (both topical and systemic), analgesics, and humidification. Eventually, a search should be made for a possible precipitating cause of the infection.

Trauma

Fractures: One of the most deceptive X-rays is the radiograph of the injured nose. Because of the significant contributions made to the nasal skeleton by cartilaginous elements in the nose, rather severe injuries can be present despite normal-appearing X-rays. Conversely, the tendency of nasal fractures to heal by forming fibrous union between the fractured fragments can result in permanent positive findings on nasal films.

There simply is no substitute for the careful and thorough clinical evaluation of an injured nose. The best time for evaluation is about four days following the injury, when the swelling has subsided. If 10 to 14 days have elapsed, the deformity is virtually impossible to correct without refracturing.

Septal hematoma: An acute hematoma of the nasal septum is fortunately rare. In this condition, the blood collects between the perichondrium and the cartilage. Prompt evacuation of the hematoma is required, and should be followed by application of a snug anterior nasal pack. The hematoma can cause enzymatic and ischemic chondral necrosis and a collapse of the cartilaginous support of the nose. Repairing the resulting saddle deformity is a challenge to the most creative and resourceful nasal surgeon.

Infections: Nasal infections should be treated with minimal mechanical manipulation, because these infections are associated with cavernous sinus thrombosis, a potentially life-threatening catastrophe. Topical heat and high doses of broad-spectrum antibiotics should be promptly instituted when cellulitis develops in the nose or in the surrounding tissues.

The oral cavity, pharynx, larynx, and neck

Inflammatory conditions: Inflammation of the salivary glands can be either a general or a local condition. Isolated inflammation of a major salivary gland (the submaxillary or parotid) is usually attributable to ductal obstruction, with stones and strictures the most common source. Accurate diagnosis of a recurrent inflammatory condition requires sialography to localize the site and cause of obstruction. Stones, which are usually radiopaque, are frequently related to strictures in the salivary ducts. Appropriate early treatment is analgesics, local heat, antibiotics, and the maintenance of proper hydration.

Ultimate management of salivary gland inflammation depends upon the location and nature of the obstruction. Easily accessible stones in Wharton's duct, for example, can be removed. Some Wharton's duct strictures can be dilated or surgically opened. Unfortunately, the course of Stensen's duct makes it less amenable to these procedures.

Alternative therapeutic methods include surgical excision of the gland, parasympathetic denervation procedures, or low-dose radiation to destroy the secretory capacity of the gland.

Canker sores: One of the most common—and almost unquestionably the most difficult—inflammatory problems of the oral and pharyngeal area is canker sores. These exquisitely painful areas of inflammation are characterized by a well-demarcated central whitish exudate surrounded by a halo of erythema. They are somewhat more prevalent during periods of stress, menstrual periods, and during episodes of various viral illnesses. They may respond favorably to topically applied steroids and to bland mouthwashes. It also has been empirically noted that modifications in the body's immune response can reduce the severity of canker sores.

Mycotic infections: Mycotic mouth infections are usually related to systemic antibiotic therapy and respond satisfactorily (if a bit slowly) to an oral suspension of nystatin.

Tonsillitis: Beta-hemolytic streptococcus is the usual cause of tonsillitis. As such, it is responsive to penicillin and should be given for a full 10-day course. Throat cultures are taken prior to institution of treatment and are helpful in confirming the diagnosis. Infectious mononucleosis often presents in adolescents as tonsillitis. It certainly can lower an individual's resistance, making her easy prey to repeated streptococcal infections. Various adenoviruses, leukemia, and diphtheria can mimic the appearance of streptococcal tonsillitis.

Peritonsillar abscesses: A peritonsillar abscess (quinsy) must be vigorously treated. It appears as unilateral tonsillar swelling and fullness in the surrounding tissues. Trismus is often present, and the uvula is usually swollen, edematous, and pushed to the opposite side of the pharynx. In the view of most specialists, this is one of the few absolute indications for tonsillectomy. Initially, the abscess should be treated with high doses of antibiotics and surgical drainage—drainage can be accomplished by an immediate tonsillectomy. Undrained pus in the peritonsillar space has potential access to the parapharyngeal space, the retropharyngeal space, and the mediastinum.

Unerupted or partially erupted third molars can become infected and cause local swelling, trismus, and a mimicking peritonsillar abscess.

Angioneurotic edema: Acute swelling of the uvula and tongue are usually the result of allergic reactions and should be treated with antihistamines, epinephrine, or steroids.

Epiglottiditis: Acute epiglottiditis can be life-threatening because of its potential threat to the airway. It is usually caused by an H. influenzae infection and is characterized by an extremely sore throat, fever, and inspiratory stridor. The definitive diagnosis is made by directly or indirectly (with a mirror) visualizing the swollen and inflamed epiglottis. Because a paroxysm of gagging can quickly obstruct a marginal airway, it is advisable to examine a suspected victim of epiglottiditis under carefully controlled conditions with easy access to a laryngoscope, endotracheal tube, and tracheotomy instruments.

Although an immediate tracheotomy was once among treatments of choice, a number of recent reports have advocated treating epiglottiditis with high doses of parenteral antibiotics, hydration, and extremely close observation. Progressive airway obstruction is then treated by placement of an endotracheal tube or by a tracheotomy.

Neck trauma: Airway adequacy is the prime matter of concern in caring for any victim of facial or neck trauma. Relatively innocent-appearing injuries may be associated with significant edema, and apparently adequate airways can suddenly be rendered grossly inadequate.

Oral lacerations: Simple lacerations of the mouth, tongue, pharynx, and larynx are generally best left untreated. The tissues in these areas have a superb blood supply, and healing is rapid. Associated injuries of the underlying skeletal structures must be sought and appropriate measures taken.

Fractures and dislocations: Airway inadequacy, local pain, hoarseness, swelling, absence of customary skeletal landmarks, and crepitus (signifying the presence of free air in the soft tissues) indicate a potentially serious laryngeal injury.

Cricothyroid fractures: Two cartilages of the larynx, the cricoid and the thyroid, are vulnerable to direct trauma to the neck. The cricoid, forming the midline prominence in the average neck, directly below the Adam's apple, is the only skeletal structure completely encircling the airway. As such, it is a critical component of the competent airway. Displaced fractures of the cricoid must be openly reduced. Associated mucosal tears or lacerations should be carefully reapproximated in order to avoid long-term subglottic stenosis.

The keel of the thyroid cartilage is the most prominent skeletal structure of the airway in the neck. Like the cricoid, the Adam's apple is usually injured by direct trauma and should be explored early when displaced fractures are suspected.

Tracheal injuries: Isolated tracheal fractures are very rare because of the relatively protected location of the trachea in the neck. Isolated cricotracheal separations are also rare, but can occur as a result of a "clothesline" type of injury. Suspected injuries of this type, like other serious laryngeal injuries, should be promptly explored.

Hyoid injuries: The hyoid bone, the highest skeletal landmark in the cervical airway, is rarely the site of an isolated injury. The bone makes little contribution to the structural integrity of the airway, and aside from the immediate concern of potential edema development, isolated hyoid injuries should be no major problem.

Mandibular fractures: Next to nasal fractures, the most common injury to the facial skeleton is a fractured mandible. The fractures are often multiple and are classified according to where they occur.

The most frequent (and probably the most often overlooked) mandibular fracture involves the condyle. It is often the result of a blow to the chin and should be suspected when a victim of jaw trauma complains of ear pain.

An early tracheotomy may be necessary if soft-tissue swelling

FIGURE 17-1

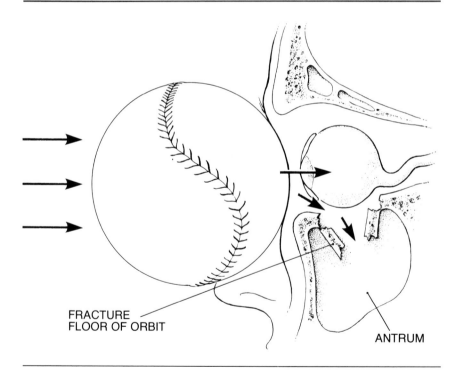

Schematic drawing of baseball striking the eye directly, causing a blow-out fracture of the orbit.

threatens the airway after a severe mandibular fracture. Certainly, an oral airway should be kept handy. Pain, swelling, and instability are common in fractures of the ramus, angle, body, and symphyseal region. The instability and displacement of these fractures depends on their orientation and the expected vectorial forces from various attached muscle groups. They are treated by immobilization for four to six weeks; open reduction is sometimes necessary.

Following immobilization, caution must be taken to avoid vomiting. The danger of aspiration dictates that the wires or elastic bands holding the jaws together should be immediately divided if nausea occurs.

Zygomatic fractures: Fractures of the zygomatic arch are often caused by a direct blow to the cheek. The collapsed zygoma can mechanically impinge upon the coronoid process of the mandible, causing trismus as the victim tries to open her mouth. The initial swelling of these fractures makes them deceptively innocuous. With the resolution of swelling, the unreduced fractured zygoma may become evident as a sunken cheek. Internal fixation of these fractures is rarely necessary, but they should be reduced.

Blow-out fractures: A direct blow to the eye can result in a blow-out fracture of the orbit (see Figure 17-1). In this fracture, the orbital rim is intact and substantial associated periorbital swelling is present. Trauma can occur to the infraorbital nerve in its course through the orbital floor, resulting in cheek anesthesia. Diplopia may be caused by either entrapment of extraocular muscles in the fracture or by injury to the nerve supply to one of the muscles. Enophthalamos and muscle entrapment are the principal indications for exploration of a blow-out fracture. As with other facial fractures, blow-out should be explored and reduced before 10 days, if possible, and certainly before two weeks.

Tri-malar fractures: Like the simple zygomatic arch fractures, tri-malar fractures occur as the result of a direct blow to the cheek. They involve fracture lines through the infraorbital rim (usually in the vicinity of the infraorbital foramen), the lateral orbital rim in the region of the frontozygomatic suture line, and the zygomatic arch. Inferior or superior displacement depends upon the direction of the inflicted blow. Early assessment of displacement is hindered by swelling. The fractures can be associated with severe intraocular injuries, infraorbital anesthesia, and diplopia. They usually require exploration and fixation.

Hairline sinus fractures: A blow to the anterior portion of the face can occasionally cause a small hairline fracture of the thin membranous bone of the maxillary or ethmoid sinus. Aside from the occasional fluid noted in associated sinuses, the fractures are essentially invisible on customary X-ray studies. They may become clinically apparent by the development of free air in the soft tissues of the cheek when the victim blows her nose. No treatment is indicated but decongestants and antibiotics. The patient should avoid further trauma to the cheek for a few weeks.

FIGURE 17-2

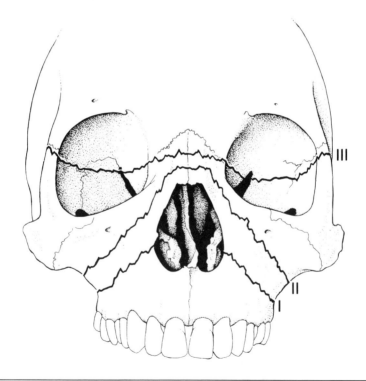

Schematic presentation of LaForte I, II, and III fractures.

LaForte fractures: Major fractures of the maxilla are marked by instability of the upper jaw. These are classed as LaForte I, II, or III fractures (see Figure 17-2). This distinction is based on the path of the fracture through the maxilla. The fractures are the result of very significant trauma to the face and are often associated with intracranial injuries. Severe mandibular and ocular injuries may be present. Soft-tissue swelling may represent a very real threat to the airway and early tracheotomy should be considered. Dural tears occur reasonably commonly with LaForte III fractures and should be suspected when cerebrospinal fluid rhinorrhea is detected.

When the patient has stabilized and the swelling has subsided, these injuries are treated with open reduction and fixation.

EYE PROBLEMS

**William F. Grant, M.D., and
Alfonse A. Cinotti, M.D.**

CHAPTER

18

As they become more active in sports, women become susceptible to the same ocular injuries that beset male athletes. The chance of incurring an eye injury is greatly increased in such fast-moving and/or contact sports as racquetball, volleyball, basketball, field hockey, wrestling, and even boxing. The use of protective goggles, when indicated, is the best way to prevent possibly permanent damage to the eyes. However, despite precautions, there is always a possibility of an injured eye.

Of 890 eyes removed at our hospital, 40 per cent were from women; 39 per cent of the eyes were removed following ocular injuries. Trauma from everyday objects such as screwdrivers, mopsticks, exploding glass bottles, eye-glasses, and flying foreign bodies from lawn mowers accounted for 13 per cent of the enucleations; 4 per cent resulted from direct injury with a fist. Many injuries are not serious enough to result in loss of the eye, but up to 15 per cent may result in legal blindness.

General principles

It is very important to find out how, where, and when the injury occurred, and to know what type of object struck the eye, how fast it may have been going, and the exact circumstances. Once the history is obtained, the first eye examination should determine visual acuity and, if a previous record is available, whether there have been any changes as a result of the injury. If there is no previous record, the athlete herself might report changes she has noticed and how well she is seeing now as compared with before.

An inspection of both the eyelids and eyeballs, using a hand light, preferably with a magnifying lens, should then be carefully carried out to note any swellings, ecchymoses, tearing or other discharge, lacerations, abrasions, or foreign material. Observations of the pupil, cornea, and iris may reveal deviation from normal. Blurred vision, redness, pain, or abnormal appearance of the eye suggests a need to consult an ophthalmologist.

The physician doing the initial exam would want to carry out an ophthalmoscopic examination to determine if there has been any intraocular damage—vitreous or retinal hemorrhage or retinal detachment. The athlete herself might note a marked decrease in visual acuity or the loss of a part of her side vision. An exception to these precepts of first-aid care is the treatment of chemical burns, discussed later on.

There are essentially three types of eye injury: those that arise from blunt, sharp, and/or burn trauma. Each is covered in order.

Blunt trauma

Subconjunctival hemorrhage: This occurs when the athlete is struck in the eye by an object larger than the eyeball itself—by a fist, elbow, hockey stick or puck, tennis ball. Swelling and ecchymoses of the eyelids are frequently associated with subconjunctival hemorrhage. There is no pain in the eyeball itself, nor is any change in visual acuity noticed. The blunt trauma has caused a rupture in one of the tiny conjunctival blood vessels, which then bleeds under the conjunctiva and appears as a localized patch of conjunctival redness surrounded by white sclera. A subconjunctival hemorrhage may arise spontaneously, usually with no apparent cause, or it may be associated with high blood pressure.

Other ocular injury—abrasion, hyphema, blow-out fracture, and intraocular damage—should be ruled out. Despite its frightening appearance, the subconjunctival hemorrhage is treated mainly by reassuring the patient that the condition is benign and will disappear within two weeks. An immediate method of reducing the spread of the hemorrhage is the application of an ice pack followed by warm compresses to help speed the absorption of the hemorrhage. No specific medication is required.

Corneal abrasion: This occurs when the athlete's eyeball is scratched by an object, such as a fingernail, ball, or piece of equipment. This is associated with tremendous pain in the eye, blurred vision, sensitivity to light, and increased tearing. The front of the eye may appear scraped.

A person with a corneal abrasion should be referred to a physician who can confirm the diagnosis by topical use of a dye. The doctor will administer eye drops and may apply a pressure patch. The patch should remain in place for 12 to 24 hours before removal for follow-up treatment by the ophthalmologist. Most abrasions, depending on their extent, heal within 24 to 48 hours. In some cases, there will be a spontaneous recurrence weeks or months later; it is treated in the same way as the initial injury.

Hyphema: This can occur if the eye is struck by an object of any size, but usually larger than the eyeball. The athlete will complain of pain in the eye and fuzzy vision, and her eye will show either red or black blood obscuring the lower part or all of the iris and pupil, giving them a hazy appearance.

Immediate treatment is to try to relax the athlete. A simple patch should be applied over the injured eye, and the athlete should have an immediate referral to an ophthalmologist, who will probably hospitalize and sedate her, and keep her in bed until the hemorrhage clears completely. This takes from five to 10 days.

Blow-out fracture: The force of a direct blow to the eye may cause a fracture in the floor of the bony orbit. The athlete will complain of pain and double vision, and teammates may notice that there is a restriction of motion in the affected eye. Because these fractures open the orbit into the sinuses, the possibility of infection must be kept in mind. Rule out other possible eye injuries, apply cold compresses, and refer the patient to an ophthalmologist. Surgical repair may be necessary.

Sharp trauma

Lid lacerations: Although listed under "sharp trauma," many lid lacerations arise from severe blunt trauma, especially in persons playing contact sports such as field hockey and basketball. Cuts about the eyes will be obvious. Apply a nonstick sterile gauze dressing with pressure—to stop any bleeding—and refer the patient to an ophthalmologist for surgical repair.

Corneal lacerations: Lacerations of the eyeball are most likely to occur in activities in which contact with sharp or pointed articles is a possibility. The athlete will complain of pain in the eye and a decrease in vision. The cornea appears cut, with an irregular corneal reflex. The pupil may appear tear-shaped, with a black tip at the apex of the tear. The iris might show a hole torn through it. A protective shield should be placed over a loose patch and the athlete referred to an ophthalmologist immediately.

Superficial foreign bodies (conjunctival or corneal): The athlete will complain that "something is in my eye." There will be pain, blurred vision, increased tearing, and conjunctival redness. It may be necessary to evert the upper and lower lids to locate the foreign body, or it may be seen either grossly or with a magnifying lens to lie on the conjunctiva or cornea.

If the foreign body is located, a topical ophthalmic anesthetic should be instilled and an attempt made to remove the foreign body with an ophthalmic irrigating solution or moistened cotton-tipped applicator. If the foreign body is successfully removed, the eye should then be treated as for a corneal abrasion. If the foreign body cannot be removed or cannot be located, the athlete should have a light patch applied to the injured eye with immediate referral to an ophthalmologist.

Burn trauma

Of the three types of burns, only chemical and ultraviolet burns are discussed here. The first aid for thermal burns of the eye does not differ from that rendered to another part of the body, as the eyeball itself is rarely directly involved.

Chemical burns: The athlete could become the victim of an acid burn (battery explosion) or alkali (lye) burn during the preparation for or participation in a sport activity. The victim will complain of pain and blurred vision. The conjunctiva will appear red and the cornea may appear hazy.

Chemical burns are the only true ocular emergencies that do not require a detailed history to be taken, visual acuity to be recorded, or careful examination completed before treatment is rendered. All that is necessary to initiate treatment is the chief complaint that "something has splashed into my eyes." Copious irrigation of the eyes should be instituted immediately with whatever source of water is available—hose, faucet, swimming pool, bucket, ophthalmic irrigating solution, or intravenous solutions. This irrigation should be continued for at least 15 minutes, after which time the patient should be transported quickly to an ophthalmologist for more definitive treatment. Remember, it is the first person to attend the victim with a chemical burn who plays the most important role in preventing serious eye damage, and simple irrigation with water is all that is required.

Ultraviolet burns: Long-distance skiers who fail to wear protective goggles can suffer ultraviolet burns or "snow blindness." The burn results from sun reflections off the snow. The symptoms of this type of burn do not occur immediately, as in a chemical burn. Instead, it is usually a number of hours later that the athlete complains of severe pain, inability to tolerate any light (photophobia), excessive tearing, and possibly even a headache. The patient requires the aid of another person for transportation to a hospital or physician for definitive treatment.

Cold compresses may alleviate some of the discomfort before definitive treatment is rendered. If a topical ophthalmic anesthetic is available, one drop should be placed in each eye (this will markedly reduce the discomfort), and the patient should be transported immediately to an ophthalmologist. The ophthalmologist will treat this patient in the same manner he treats a patient with a corneal abrasion. As painful and frightening as ultraviolet burns appear, they are in reality superficial burns and most totally heal within 24 hours.

Nontraumatic disorders

There are other ocular conditions that may be alarming to the athlete or her coaches and trainers. These usually involve a red eye not associated with any known trauma. These can be broken down into conjunctivitis, blepharitis, and iritis.

Conjunctivitis: There are three essential types of conjunctivitis or "pink-eye." Bacterial infections are associated with matting of the lids upon waking, sticky purulent discharge, no change in vision, and no pain or sensitivity to light. These usually respond to an antibacterial regimen in three to five days.

Viral infections are associated with a recent upper respiratory infection, watery discharge, bumps (follicles) on the palpebral conjunctiva, tender preauricular nodes, no change in vision, and no pain. There is no specific treatment for viral conjunctivitis except an antibiotic regimen to prevent secondary bacterial infection. Most cases resolve in 10 to 14 days.

Allergic conditions are associated with a history of allergy, itching, increased tearing, swollen lids, no change in vision, and no pain. Treatment consists of removal of the allergen (if possible), local vasoconstrictors, and systemic antihistamines. Resolution usually occurs in one to two days, but recurrences are not uncommon and treatment must be reinstituted.

Blepharitis: An inflammation of the lid margin is usually caused by either staphylococci or seborrhea.

Staphylococcus blepharitis is more severe than that caused by seborrhea and presents with matting and loss of lid lashes. The lids appear swollen and inflamed, are tender, and may also present with styes. Treatment consists of scrupulous cleansing with soap and water to remove the particles and discharge from the lashes and lid margin, followed by the application of ophthalmic antibiotic ointment.

Seborrhea blepharitis is associated with a seborrhea of the scalp, nose, or ears. The lashes present with dandruff-like particles. The lids are not usually swollen or inflamed but may become "itchy." Treatment consists of the use of a good antidandruff shampoo for the scalp, scrupulous cleansing of the lashes, and the application of an ophthalmic ointment (ammoniated mercury) to the lashes.

Iritis: Inflammation of the iris is a more serious condition and should be referred immediately to an ophthalmologist for treatment. Iritis presents with a history of severe pain and photophobia and often with blurred vision. There is conjunctival injection, especially surrounding the cornea (ciliary flush), no discharge, a small pupil, and the cornea itself may appear cloudy.

Two pre-existing conditions, cross eyes and color deficiency (not true color blindness), usually do not handicap the adult athlete to any great degree. During their formative years and throughout their training for a particular sport, these athletes develop their own clues and guides and adapt well to circumstances to perform proficiently.

The first step in providing protection from injury to the eyes is a preseason ocular examination for every athlete. This examination should consist of more than a visual acuity test and correction. An external and slit lamp examination should be done, and the peripheral vision of each eye should be recorded. Loss of side vision can be devastating to an athlete. A thorough examination of the retina should be made, especially if the athlete is near-sighted or intends to engage in a contact sport. If these examinations reveal any condition that might lead to a serious eye problem, such as retinal detachment or vitreous hemorrhage, then the athlete should be discouraged from participating in contact sports or at least told to wear protective goggles if she insists on taking part. If the athlete happens to have but one good eye, she should be strongly discouraged from participating in a contact sport and should shift her interest to a sport in which injury to the eye is unlikely.

A complete postseason eye examination should also be mandatory, as some asymptomatic injury, such as a hole in the retina, which may in the future lead to a serious problem, could be discovered and preventive measures initiated.

One additional examination should be conducted, both pre- and postseason, and yearly after retiring, especially for women engaged in contact sports: the test for glaucoma. The onset of secondary glaucoma due to trauma is insidious and usually cannot be detected without this test.

The best safety measure to prevent eye injury is the wearing of glasses. Government regulations require all lenses dispensed to be impact-resistant. However, plastic lenses with a center thickness of at least 3 mm in a sturdy frame are the most reliable. Special sports goggles are also useful.

Contact lenses offer little protection and in some instances may cause serious injury. A contact lens might prevent a corneal abrasion by shielding the cornea from a fingernail, but a cracked hard contact lens might also be responsible for causing a laceration of the cornea. Of the two types of contact lenses, the soft lens is preferred in contact sports. Soft lenses are more comfortable, do not pop out as easily as hard lenses, and give very good vision.

But because of the limited protection contact lenses provide, spectacle glasses or one of the types of goggles should be considered for wear along with the contact lens.

Contestants engaged in winter sports should have sunglasses available to protect the eyes from the tremendous glare reflecting from the snow. Metal frames, because they conduct cold, may be dangerous in extreme cold, as they may freeze to the skin.

DENTAL PROBLEMS

John C. Loomis, D.D.S.

CHAPTER

19

Injuries to the dental structure are an inevitable part of contact sports. As women's participation in hockey, lacrosse, rugby, basketball, football, and similar sports has increased, so have their dental injuries. In recognizing these injuries, it is helpful to think in terms of dental problems involving three types of structures: the teeth, the periodontium or tooth-supporting tissues, and the bone.

Injury to the crown of a tooth

Cracking or "crazing" of the enamel of one or more teeth, without loss of tooth structure, is termed a crown infraction. The tooth or teeth may be slightly loose and sensitive to cold. They will almost certainly be tender to biting pressure. They will not be displaced from their normal position in the arch, however, and the dental arches should fit together in normal occlusion. Crown infraction does not require treatment, and symptoms disappear in time. Enamel that is crazed in this way is still tightly bonded to the underlying dentin and does not come apart at a later time. The athlete should be assured that the tooth will not later "fall apart."

If a tooth sustains a blow of sufficient force to fracture the crown, it is important to discover whether that fracture involves the tooth pulp. A fracture of the enamel alone (see Figure 19-1, A) or of enamel and dentin (see Figure 19-1, B) is uncomplicated and requires only cosmetic treatment within a few days. If significant dentin surface is exposed, the tooth will be temperature-sensitive and should be covered by a restoration (filling or crown). If left untreated, a small percentage of these injuries result in pulpal degeneration and necrosis. If the fracture penetrates the pulp or "nerve" of a tooth, a pink or red spot will be visible in the center of the fractured surface (see Figure 19-1, C). Frank hemorrhage from the pulpal tissues may be seen but this should not be confused with gingival bleeding.

When the pulp is directly involved in the line of fracture, the injury deserves immediate attention by a dentist. Depending on the amount of time elapsed since the injury was sustained, and also the extent of the pulp exposure, the dentist either medicates the remaining pulp and covers it with a temporary restoration, or removes the pulp in preparation for future root canal treatment.

Injury to the root of a tooth

A fracture that begins in the crown of a tooth and extends below the attached gumline is called a crown-root fracture (see Figure 19-1, D). Here, the fractured portion of the tooth is still present, held in place by the gingival tissue to which it is still attached. One segment of the tooth may be extremely mobile. This type of injury should be seen by a dentist as soon as possible, especially if the tooth is very painful. Pain may indicate that the fracture has exposed the pulp.

The dentist may determine the course of the fracture by clinical examination or by radiographic means. If the fracture extends through pulp tissue, a root canal is required; if the fracture extends more than 2 to 3 mm below attached gingiva, the tooth is not treatable, and extraction and replacement are advisable.

The root fractures of a tooth are more difficult to pinpoint (see Figure 19-1, E). Examination usually reveals a slightly extended tooth displaced toward the tongue or palate. The tooth is mobile to varying degrees. If you place a finger on the alveolus and move the tooth, you will feel movement only in the crown portion. The fracture may or may not be evident on X-ray. Sometimes a fracture line is not evident immediately after the injury, but will appear on a radiograph taken a few weeks later.

An athlete with a suspected root fracture should be seen by a dentist. This condition does not constitute an emergency, and extraordinary haste is not essential unless pain is severe. A fracture that does not extend to the surface may be treated by immobilization of the crown (splinting) for two months, together with radiographic follow-up for one year.

Between 20 and 44 per cent of all root fractures undergo pulpal necrosis. Less frequent problems include resorption of the root from within, obliteration of the pulp canal by the cells lining the pulp chamber, and loss of surrounding bone through cyst or granuloma formation. In spite of these possible complications, it is worthwhile to attempt to save an otherwise healthy tooth with a fractured root.

FIGURE 19-1

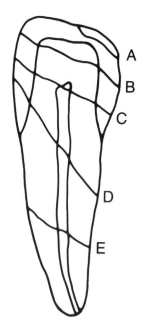

Schematic drawing of various fractures of the tooth.

Injury to periodontal tissues

The tissues that secure the teeth to their places consist of the fibers of the gingival connective tissues—either tooth-to-tooth or tooth-to-gingiva—and periodontal ligament, which extends from the tooth root into the alveolar bone. Both these structures can absorb a certain amount of force. When that force is exceeded, damage to the tissues will occur. This may be in addition to fracture of the tooth, or it may occur without damage to the tooth.

When a tooth receives a blow but doesn't show abnormal loosening or displacement, it's termed a concussion. Sensitivity to biting or temperature may be present for a short time afterward. If the tooth is loosened but returns to its normal position, the condition is called a subluxation. No immediate treatment is needed in this case, unless there is discomfort in biting.

Luxation is the condition of actual displacement of a tooth. This can be intrusive, extrusive, or lateral displacement. Intrusive luxation, or displacement of the tooth into the socket, involves comminution or fracture of the socket. Treatment consists of simply letting the tooth re-erupt. When a tooth has been partially extruded from its socket, or if it has been laterally displaced, the dentist forces the tooth back into position and splints it to uninjured teeth for three to six weeks. Follow-up lasts a year, to look for signs of pulpal necrosis, internal root resorption, pulp canal obliteration, or bone loss.

Exarticulation or complete avulsion of a tooth requires immediate action. The tooth is quickly placed in normal saline—or at least washed in clear water and wrapped in gauze. The time of the accident is noted, and the injured player and the tooth are brought to the dentist as soon as possible. The dentist irrigates the socket to remove the clot and then implants and splints the tooth. If the elapsed time between injury and reimplantation is less than an hour or two, chances for success are great.

Injury to facial bones

Possible injuries to the facial bones must not be overlooked, whether or not teeth have been displaced. A fracture of the zygoma (cheekbone), the maxilla (upper jaw), or mandible (lower

jaw) may be suspected if bimanual palpation discloses motion between two parts of a bone, or if the teeth do not fit together in
proper occlusion. Another suspicious sign is tissue tenderness over
a particular point of a bone when it is pressed lightly. Fractures of
the subcondylar region are a common type of mandibular injury
(see Figure 19-2, A). With a fracture of the subcondylar area of the
lower jaw, the jaw deviates toward the affected side upon opening.
Other areas most often fractured are the angle (third molar region)
and cuspid area of the mandible (see Figure 19-2, B and C, respectively).

Suspected or known fractures of jawbones are generally treated
by oral surgeons. It is not necessary to treat immediately, but
suspected fractures should be seen within 24 hours.

FIGURE 19-2

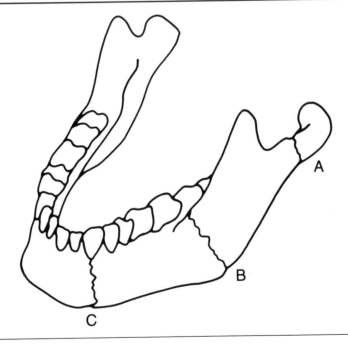

Schematic drawing of mandibular fractures.

When individual teeth are displaced, a fracture of the alveolus or bone surrounding the roots of teeth may be suspected. There are essentially three types of alveolar fractures: comminution of the socket, which occurs as a result of intrusive luxation and which heals spontaneously when the tooth re-erupts; fracture of the socket wall secondary to tooth luxation, which is treated by reduction and follow-up; and fracture of the alveolar process, which may occur when a group of teeth have been displaced in a body. This is most commonly seen in the upper anterior region. This injury should be treated as soon as possible with the reduction of the fracture, splinting, and follow-up for one year.

Mouthguards

There is now no question that the use of mouthguards reduces injuries to the teeth and supporting structures. A blow that would otherwise be received by a single tooth is dissipated over a wider area by the mouthguard. Thus, a much greater force can be resisted by the dental structures without damage to them.

Three types of mouthguards are available. The type custom-made by a dentist or dental technician is formed over plaster models of the athlete's jaws; thus, accurate fit is assured. The material is cured under pressure and at a fairly high temperature, assuring a very dense, strong consistency. The relatively low porosity attained has the added advantages of cleanliness, lack of taste and odor, durability, and comfort. Due to its high cost, it should not be recommended for growing athletes.

The most widely used in school programs is the mouth-formed variety. This is softened in boiling water for a few seconds and then placed in the mouth while still warm. The mouth is chilled with cold water and the guard is removed and trimmed.

Stock mouthguards are not formed to the individual athlete's teeth but come in various sizes and may be trimmed at the borders for a more comfortable fit. This type offers the least protection.

Care of the teeth

A lifetime of healthy teeth and gums is not possible without a sensible diet. It is well known that intake of sugar, especially refined sugar, has been causally linked to dental caries. The frequency with which one consumes sugar, more than the quantity eaten, is what affects the decay rate. Eating foods that supply nutrients, vitamins, and minerals in optimal amounts is also important in developing resistance to gingivitis and other chronic destructive diseases of the oral tissues.

The control of dental plaque assures cleanliness and also lowers chances of caries development. Plaque is visible as a sticky white film that forms on the teeth. It is composed of countless bacteria and other microorganisms that have the ability to adhere to tooth enamel and form "colonies" many millions thick. These destructive bacterial colonies use sugars taken into the mouth as nutrients in their own metabolic processes. It is the waste products of this metabolism, primarily organic acids and other substances toxic to gum tissue, which cause dental caries and gum diseases.

For most people, plaque control consists of daily brushing and flossing. Brushing should be done with a soft, flat-topped toothbrush, the narrow, flexible bristles of which fit easily into the crevice or "sulcus" that surrounds the healthy tooth at the gumline. This sulcus is the primary locus of organisms that damage gum tissue and cause decay between the teeth.

The objective of flossing is to wrap the floss around the tooth as completely as possible and clean the surfaces between the teeth—which are missed by the brush—from the level of gingival attachment to the biting surface. This is accomplished by positioning the floss as far "under" the gums as it will go, wrapping tightly, and scraping the tooth surface.

SKIN PROBLEMS

Roger H. Brodkin, M.D.

CHAPTER

20

Dermatologic problems are a common cause of disability and performance impairment in all athletes. In general, there are few dermatologic problems confined exclusively to the female athlete.

Trauma

Trauma, a common cause of dermatologic problems, may be physical or mechanical, thermal, and actinic. Physical and mechanical trauma can produce abrasions, lacerations, and puncture wounds of the skin.

Frictional injuries, depending on the amount of friction, may induce calluses, blisters, erosions, and fissures. These are generally painful and tender and occur in areas where firm contact is made with equipment or clothing, such as the feet and hands. Treatment consists of proper protection and cleanliness to prevent infection, as well as the removal of fluid from large, painful blisters. In general, the skin accommodates, after a period of time, to this trauma; it tends to be a problem at the beginning of the athletic season.

Thermal injuries in athletes are usually not the result of local burns but of vigorous physical activity in an environment where the ambient temperature and humidity are high. The skin functions as a thermoregulator for the body; in order to accomplish its task, heat is dissipated by the production of sweat, which then evaporates, producing a cooling effect. When the temperature is high, sweating is increased. In order for evaporation to occur, the air must not be fully saturated with water; therefore, the lower the humidity, the more easily sweat is evaporated. When the temperature and humidity are relatively high, the athlete pours off sweat but is not efficiently cooled, and heat exhaustion or failure of the thermoregulatory mechanism may result, with profound systemic effects, including collapse and even death. In other situations, the intense production of sweat by the sweat glands may not be accommodated by the sweat ducts, and sweat may be retained within the ducts, producing a condition known as miliaria. In this condition, one sees innumerable small vesicles over the areas where sweating is most intense. These sweat-filled vesicles eventually become infected, producing pustules that may cause pain and itching. In general, this also is a disease of accommodation—it occurs either early in the season, before the sweat apparatus has developed its capacity to handle increased sweating, or when environmental conditions of temperature and humidity are particularly severe. Miliaria may be treated and prevented by frequent cold compresses and showers as well as with topical preparations such as rubbing alcohol and mentholated calamine lotion or those that dissolve the outermost layer of the skin, thus preventing obstruction of the sweat ducts.

The final type of traumatic dermatosis is actinic injury. Actinic injury may be acute or chronic. With the acute form, the result is sunburn. Depending on the severity of the sunburn, there are varying degrees of pain and tenderness and of redness, blistering, and crusting. The best treatment of sunburn is its prevention through the use of hats, protective clothing, and sunscreens. It should be remembered that intense and prolonged sweating may wash away the sunscreen. Eventually, the skin accommodates to actinic exposure by thickening of the outermost layer and hyperpigmentation. Longer periods of sun exposure may then be tolerated. Chronic actinic injury may result in more serious consequences: premature wrinkling, and lentigines—hyperpigmented spots scattered over the exposed areas, particularly the face, neck, and upper torso. More serious, however, is the development of actinic keratoses—red, warty, and scaly tumors—and basal-cell and squamous-cell carcinomas.

Basal-cell carcinomas lack the capacity to spread into the body by metastasis but can invade neighboring tissues and organs very deeply, producing substantial disfigurement around the eye, ear, or nose. They generally start as small and insignificant sores or lumps that may bleed and heal, only to bleed again. Early lesions are treated by removal or destruction, with good cosmetic results and a high cure rate. Squamous-cell carcinomas usually appear on the face, back of the hands, or lips. They do not bleed as readily as basal-cell tumors, but grow somewhat more rapidly. This tumor can spread into the body by metastasis and requires more aggressive treatment. Inadequate treatment may result in recurrence and further spread with substantial disfigurement, disability, or death.

Infections

Infections of the skin may be caused by bacteria, fungi, and viruses. Insects also may injure the skin. Bacterial infections of the skin include impetigo, folliculitis, furuncles and abscesses, and cellulitis. These are caused by staphylococci and streptococci, often after marked exposure to dirt and sweat as well as from minor or severe injuries to the skin. These infections may cause itching or pain. Impetigo usually starts as a pustule on an exposed area and produces crusted lesions confined to a particular area of the skin. Folliculitis is a pustular eruption, generally on the hairy areas of the body. Furuncles and abscesses consist of one or more painful and tender nodular, red, hard, lesions. Cellulitis is an area of redness and induration of the skin. Not only does it produce local pain and itching, but it is often accompanied by chills and fever.

Treatment of these lesions consists of drainage of pus along with proper hygiene. Systemic and topical antibiotics may be required for the more severe and extensive infections.

Fungal infections of the skin are caused by several species of dermatophytic fungi and also by the yeast Candida albicans. The areas most frequently affected are the feet and groin, but the area beneath the breasts is uniquely susceptible in females. These diseases are accompanied by itching, burning, and pain, which may at times produce severe discomfort and interfere with running. Therapy consists of topical application of a fungicide or, if necessary, systemic use of griseofulvin. A measure of prevention may be achieved by scrupulous cleansing of the intertriginous areas, drying thoroughly after showering, and using powder to keep the areas dry and clean.

Viruses produce skin infections that may interfere with performance. Plantar warts are a particular problem, as pressure on the wart can produce intense pain that may markedly interfere with running. Mollusca contagiosa infections are also seen in female athletes, not only as a result of body-contact sports but acquired from swimming pools, benches, and the like. Herpes produces a cluster of blisters or pustules on a red, swollen base, whereas mollusca infections generally occur over a larger area of the body and consist of discrete, pearl-like papulas with a smooth surface and central umbilication. There is no consistently effective treatment for herpes simplex.

Mosquito bites produce scattered, itching, hive-like areas. The same is true of certain biting flies; these and wasps cause painful stings. Crab lice may be transmitted by athletic equipment and clothing or by common toilet seats. Water sports also expose the athlete to dermatologic injury: Certain forms of schistosomes, algae, and jellyfish may produce intensely itching lesions.

Allergic diseases of the skin are generally represented by contact allergy, which may develop to a variety of athletic equipment and clothing. In particular, clothing dyes and the formalin in wash-and-wear and drip-dry clothing may produce allergic contact dermatitis. The antioxidants in rubber and elastomers in synthetic elastic garments may also produce this dermatitis. Metal allergy results from exposure to the nickel in many metal alloys. Leather allergy is not rare. Plants such as poison ivy, sumac, and oak may also produce allergic contact dermatitis. Treatment consists of cool compresses and, in the more severe cases, topical and systemic administration of steroids.

Pre-existing dermatologic problems may be aggravated by athletics. Inflammatory dermatoses such as atopic dermatitis and various infections may be aggravated by the trauma of athletic participation. Sweating and heat may further aggravate these diseases as well as decrease the efficacy of medication. Also, numerous drugs sensitize the user to sunlight; among these are antibiotics, tranquilizers, sleeping pills, and diuretics. These drugs enhance sun injury, and even the amount and duration of exposure that is normal for an individual may cause extremely severe, disabling sunburn.

Another potential problem is aggravation of certain hereditary and metabolic diseases. Epidermolysis bullosa is a genetic disease in which the surface layer of the skin is not firmly attached to the underlying layers, resulting in large and severe blisters after relatively minor injury. There are several photosensitivity diseases, such as xeroderma pigmentosum, porphyria cutanea tarda, and Darier's disease. These are rather rare, but would certainly limit the performance of the female athlete by preventing her from sunlight exposure. However, sun exposure from athletic participation may benefit certain diseases such as psoriasis and acne.

Finally, there are a number of dermatologic problems unique to the female athlete. There may be some limitations and constraints on the way the hair is worn. In the athlete, it is best pulled out of the way or worn short, as tight braiding and pulling into buns and ponytails may result in traction alopecia; this generally is not of sufficient degree to cause concern. Another conceivable problem is the need for short fingernails. The minor injuries of athletic competition tend to traumatize the fingernails, resulting in splitting and breaking of the ends. Another problem is the wearing of external sanitary napkins during menstruation. If these are sufficiently large or bulky, they rub and irritate the inner thighs during long and vigorous athletic competition.

In general, the dermatologic problems of the female athlete can easily be minimized by simple preventive and active-treatment measures. At the beginning of the season, it is wise to start slowly and build up participation. This allows the skin to accommodate to the demands of sweating and cooling as well as to the mild injuries that beset it during the course of athletic training and competition. If a dermatologic problem does arise, it would be wise to care for it promptly and to seek the help of a dermatologist if it persists.

HEAD INJURIES

Harry A. Kaplan, M.D.

CHAPTER

21

H
ead injuries occurring during a sporting event fortunately are usually of less severity than those associated with a vehicular accident. The speed of contact and size of the object striking the head determine the type of injury. Being struck by a fist does not, as a rule, produce a severe brain injury, but falling back and striking the head on the floor may. Wearing a football-type helmet may prevent brain injury.

Initial examination

When examining a patient at the site of the injury, a relatively superficial examination is carried out. Yet, it should be systematic, with overall observation of the state of the injured person. The state of awareness should be noted: Is the patient moving, does she respond to your voice, is breathing normal? If the patient remains unresponsive for more than a minute or two, vital signs should be checked. The pulse should be regular, but a slow or rapid pulse immediately after an injury may be of no diagnostic value; however, a rising blood pressure and slowing pulse sometime later may indicate development of an intracranial hematoma. Signs of surgical shock point to a nonhead injury, unless the patient is terminal. Always look for bleeding into a large body cavity or fracture of large bones when the patient is in a shock state with a low blood pressure and rapid pulse.

The examination should begin at the top of the head. Check the scalp for lacerations or a depressed skull fracture. Look into the nose and ears for the presence of blood or spinal fluid. Palpate the cervical and thoracolumbar spine for any tenderness or deformity. Look at the back for an object that might have been driven in and for bleeding sites. Palpate the chest and abdomen for deformity or tenderness. Examine the extremities for tenderness or deformity.

If the individual had been unconscious and has regained a state of awareness, do a brief neurological examination. If the person is only moderately responsive, tap the side of the face lightly to see if a more responsive state can be brought about. Check the cranial nerves: Look at the pupils and see whether they are the same size and respond to light; check the movement of the eye muscles. To see if the injured person has full control of her facial muscles, have her open and close her eyelids and mouth. Make a clicking noise in each ear to see if she has any problem with hearing. Inspect her tongue. Have her say a few words to check speech. After checking the cranial nerves, see if the patient is able to move all extremities equally. Touch the skin on both sides of the body superficially to grossly check sensation. If the injured person is alert, check her ability to walk.

This gross examination can be executed in two to three minutes. If the injured athlete appears slightly groggy or complains of any injury, removal from the game should be suggested.

Types of head injuries

Injuries to the head are of various types: The skin may be lacerated, the skull may be fractured, and the intracranial contents may be damaged. Each of these injuries must be taken seriously and treated accordingly.

Damage to the scalp is usually not of serious consequence unless excessive bleeding occurs or, with improper treatment, a scalp infection develops. The laceration should be cleaned and covered with sterile bandages; repair of the laceration should be carried out in an emergency room.

A simple fracture of the skull is of no great consequence, although it indicates that a severe head injury has been sustained; the athlete should be admitted to the hospital. A depressed or compound skull fracture requires immediate hospital treatment. The presence of a clear fluid (subarachnoid fluid) in the nares or ear canals indicates a basal skull fracture that requires hospital treatment.

Involvement of the brain varies according to the type of injury sustained: The patient may have brain dysfunction secondary to a concussion; brain contusion or compression by a mass such as in a depressed skull fracture; or an intracerebral, subdural, or extradural hematoma.

Changes in the brain secondary to a head blow may be categorized as pathophysiologic—without morphologic changes in the tissue—or pathologic—with changes in the tissue structure.

A pathophysiologic alteration in brain function is that of cerebral concussion. The dysfunction consists of a loss of consciousness immediately following the head blow and lasting for seconds. With recovery, no residual changes are demonstrable in the neurologic state. This is a completely reversible situation. Pathologic changes in the tissue structure occur with a cerebral contusion. When secondary to a fall, cerebral contusion is usually found at the base of the frontal and temporal lobes of the brain; loss of awareness may persist for hours or days or, if severe enough, be incompatible with recovery.

Central nervous system

In order to understand the problem, we have to look at the anatomy and physiology of the central nervous system. The brain, an extremely complex device, consists of thousands of neurons, with each neuron a complex system in itself. Chemical and physical changes are constantly going on in the cell and through the cell wall. The cell functions through its axon. The brain receives a constant input of stimuli from its environment and digests this information through a cooperative cell effort that includes the part of the system dealing with memory.

In order for the central nervous system to properly function, the cells must be constantly alerted. There is an area in the brain stem—the upper midbrain and caudal diencephalon—that receives a constant inflow of stimuli and transmits these stimuli to all parts of the nervous system. Should this alerting mechanism be affected either pathophysiologically or by morphologic changes in its cells, then unconsciousness follows; the length of time depends on the type and severity of pathology involved.

A certain number of cells may receive a stimulus and respond in an orderly fashion. This presupposes a specific number and speed of impulse transmission. Should the number of impulses enter the central nervous system in sufficient magnitude to overwhelm the cell groups, then the system blocks and the individual does not respond. It is this mechanism that appears to be the basis for loss of consciousness accompanying a head blow. When the head is struck, it swivels and receives a sudden tremendous inflow of impulses from the vestibular and neck-righting reflexes as well as impulses from the skin, muscle, and jaw. In the normally functioning state, the brain has the ability to block out some impulses, but when it is overwhelmed by a sudden tremendous inflow of stimuli, the block may lead to unconsciousness. A blow on the side of the face, because it causes the head to swivel, much more readily produces loss of consciousness than a blow landing on the front of the head. That cerebral concussion is reversible is readily demonstrated in the boxing arena. A boxer will always tell you that, when he has put his opponent into a dazed state, the next blow should be thrown to the abdomen so that the opponent will drop his gloves. The following blow is then thrown directly to the head to produce a knockout. If the boxer aims a blow at the reflexly guarded head of his dazed opponent, he may inadvertently reduce the force of the blow by striking his opponent's glove and alerting the opponent with this lesser blow. We are all aware that a slight tap on the face of a dazed person will arouse him. The lesser impulse flow to the brain may stimulate the brain cells to proper function.

The cerebral concussion of a head-injured person is not the major problem; the real danger is that the individual will fall backward, striking her head on the ground. Then, a cerebral contusion may occur—with dire consequences. The force of the boxer's gloved hand striking the head is not extreme; the force of the head striking the floor is great. The human skull has a very rough base, with its sphenoid ridges and sella turcica. It must be remembered that the alerting mechanism of the brain—the caudal diencephalon and the midbrain—lies right at the site of the clivus and sellar region and will strike these areas when thrown forward. Furthermore, other vital areas of the brain at the base may become contused by being thrust across the rough base of the skull. The mesial inferior part of the base of the frontal lobes and the mesial aspect of the tips of the temporal lobes of the brain may be injured, and these areas are related to autonomic function. Prolonged alteration in the state of consciousness and in metabolic regulatory mechanisms may result. An individual who has had a head injury and remains unresponsive for a period of more than a few minutes must be presumed to have sustained a severe head injury with cerebral contusion. The longer the period of unresponsiveness, the poorer the prognosis. However, as long as a patient is able to breathe on her own, there is a chance for recovery. Cessation of respiration with dilated fixed pupils, even though the heartbeat continues, carries a poor prognosis.

A simple skull fracture, implying a rather severe injury to the head, may at first be associated with rapidly clearing brain dysfunction. The injured person should be carefully followed for several days, as the force of the blow may have produced a stripping of the dura underneath the injury site. The fracture of the skull may have caused a laceration of an underlying artery. The stripping of the underlying dura leads to a free space for accumulation of arterial blood from the lacerated artery in the vicinity. This epidural hematoma then begins to compress the underlying brain, with the development of cerebral edema and compression of the brain stem. We are all aware of the athlete who goes home after having received a seemingly mild head injury and within several hours becomes lethargic and then stuporous. When examined shortly thereafter, a dilated pupil from brain-stem compression is noted. Surgical removal of the epidural hematoma must be rapidly carried out before a decerebrate rigidity state develops. If there is any delay in treatment, the developing blood pressure rise may be followed by a fatal brain-stem hemorrhage.

The average physician's experience with head trauma is obtained from duty in an active emergency room or the neurosurgical service of a large city hospital. These observations are usually made many minutes or hours after trauma has been sustained. And although a number of animal studies on the immediate effect of head trauma have been reported, one must remember that the animal has been anesthetized before being struck on the head. To overcome these problems, I worked as a ringside physician for several years and was able to make direct observations on the effects of head trauma in humans. I also have been the electroencephalographer for the New York State Athletic Commission for a number of years. This gave me an opportunity to see EEG patterns immediately after an individual sustained a number of head blows, as well as to follow his EEG patterns for a long period after the trauma. Furthermore, studies of boxers at ringside allowed me to observe head trauma unassociated with other bodily injury—which is seen less often in the hospital emergency room.

A well-trained boxer does not sustain severe multiple blows to the head; they are either deflected by the upper extremities, or the head is removed from the path of the blow. An alert, well-trained boxer can probably set himself for a blow almost at the moment it arrives. It is well known that a blow to a head held rigid by the neck muscles is not very effective in disabling a boxer. Of the approximately 1,000 blows thrown during a match, not more than one or two land solidly on their mark—most matches are not ended by physical knockouts.

That head blows in boxing are relatively nondamaging to the brain was shown by the EEG studies. A review of more than 6,000 EEG records made on boxers—many of them repeat recordings over a number of years—showed no changes suggestive of alteration in brain electrical activity. EEGs taken immediately after a boxer lost a fight failed to show any changes from prefight recordings. Repeat recordings over a period of years failed to demonstrate anything suggestive of the diffuse petechial brain hemorrhage so often described in the literature. The so-called punch-drunk syndrome seems to be a myth.

SPINE AND NERVE INJURIES

Roger W. Countee, M.D.

CHAPTER

22

T he spine and associated soft tissues—neural structures as well as ligamentous and muscular supporting structures—are vulnerable to injury in a variety of athletic activities. Although publicity about injuries to professional athletes has served to highlight the tragic consequences that may result from contact sports, the pernicious potential of such high-velocity non-contact sports as skiing, diving, surfing, horseback riding, and gymnastics should be recognized. Unfortunately, data on the incidence of spine injuries—by sex, severity, or exposure—are quite limited, and estimates have had to be extrapolated from isolated reports and surmise.[1] Leader has estimated that athletic injuries account for 4 to 7 per cent of all cases of spinal cord trauma resulting in permanent paralysis.[2] Although this low incidence of permanent paralysis may seem unimpressive, for the injured athlete it is indeed a catastrophe. Moreover, the much more frequent injuries to the spine (and/or associated structures) that result in less than permanent paralysis but in restrictive disabilities should also be recognized as a cause for concern.

Principles of emergency management

Injuries to the spine carry a serious risk of major disability. Consequently, if there is any question about the presence of a spine injury, it is safest to assume that the most severe injury has occurred. Proper care is the immediate institution of medical treatment at the site of the accident. Under no circumstances should the patient be asked to sit or stand. If she is lying on the ground, she should not be moved until an evaluation has been made. Although this may require some time, delay of the contest is of no consequence in such circumstances, and the physician must not be hurried in the evaluation, inadvertently permitting what may be fatal movement.

Every athlete who sustains a head injury severe enough to render her unconscious may have a cervical spine injury and should be managed accordingly. If the patient is conscious, she should be queried about her subjective feelings about her neck and back and about any localized pain. Determine if she has normal sensation and movement of the hands and feet. This doesn't require a detailed neurological examination but only a sensible gross evaluation. The spinous processes can be palpated by placing your hand—carefully—under the neck and spine to detect any localized deformity or tenderness. If there are no subjective complaints or obvious defects in limb function, a voluntary range of motion of the neck should be evaluated. The athlete is asked to nod her head and touch her chin to her chest and then to each shoulder. She is then asked to touch each shoulder with the ipsilateral ear. If she is unwilling or unable to perform these maneuvers voluntarily, proceed no further.

The athlete with less than a full and pain-free range of neck motion, and/or complaints of paresthesis, and/or weakness of the limbs should be protected immediately. Using an adequate number of assistants, carefully lift the athlete onto a flat, hard (usually plywood) board, placing her on her back. This must be done without any motion between the head and trunk and with efforts to minimize postural changes as well. Hand traction to the chin and occiput can be applied during this transfer to a carrying board. Once on the board, the head can be stabilized with sand bags on either side of the neck. The head and trunk should be secured to the board by belts, straps, or tape. The patient can then be moved to where a more detailed evaluation can be made. Although, on occasion, these measures overdramatize what is later proved to be a minor injury, they may serve to save a life or prevent lifetime paralysis.

As soon as the athlete is carried to a suitable location for a more detailed examination of her condition, attention must be directed to determining the adequacy of respiratory exchange, blood pressure, pulse, and temperature. Associated trauma to the athlete's other organ systems must be ascertained. If ventilatory exchange is less than adequate after judicious nasal-oral-pharyngeal toilet, nasotracheal intubation or emergency tracheostomy should be done expeditiously and *without moving the head.* The examiner must keep in mind that cervical- and high thoracic-cord injuries invariably present with mild to moderate hypotension, bradycardia, and a lowered body temperature. Consequently, such a state in athletes with these injuries is not necessarily indicative of hemorrhagic shock.

Although it is often suggested that vasopressor medications are indicated in the treatment of hypotension secondary to cervical or high dorsal-spinal cord injuries, experience has shown that they may predispose patients to acute pulmonary edema.[3] Consequently, I prefer to treat systemic arterial hypotension in these patients with intravenous infusions of lactated Ringer's solution, or a 5 per cent dextrose solution in 0.45 per cent saline, and careful monitoring of central venous pressure measurements. The degree of elevation of blood pressure required in the individual patient is determined by what systemic pressure is necessary to keep the patient fully alert and conscious and provide adequate systemic perfusion, as evidenced by a normal urinary output and the absence of metabolic acidosis on arterial blood gas evaluations. Using these parameters, systolic blood pressures of 80 to 100 mm Hg may be entirely adequate.

Typically, in the "sympathectomized" individual who has a spinal cord injury, the skin is warm and dry and, therefore, not a good indicator of the adequacy of systemic arterial perfusion. Minor depressions in body-core temperature require no active treatment if the temperature is above 96 to 97. However, body temperatures that are lower must be avoided. Low body-core temperatures are particularly prone to develop in athletes who are outdoors in cold or inclement weather.

After assurance that the respiratory and circulatory states are adequate, the physician should proceed to a more detailed neurological evaluation in an attempt to determine the level and severity of spinal cord injury. This assessment of cord involvement serves as a baseline for future examinations and is invaluable in documenting the course of the injury and the adequacy of management. In addition to the neurological and general physical baseline examinations, other parameters should be included in the "flow-sheet" concept of serial recordings—blood pressure, pulse, respiratory rate and pattern, temperature, urinary output, type and amount of intravenous fluids administered, medications. It is strongly recommended that all individuals suspected of having sustained serious spinal trauma be transported to properly equipped and staffed emergency medical facilities initially, if possible, rather than simply to the first available medical institution. The patient should be accompanied by trained personnel who recognize the paramount importance of protecting the spine with consistent immobilization and maintenance of adequate respiratory and circulatory function.

If there are no obvious neurological deficits, no evidence of osseous or ligamentous spinal injury on physical examination or X-ray, the decision as to whether the athlete can continue in the contest should be made by the physician in attendance. The judgment is best made if one understands the anatomical structures that are involved in the injury as well as the severity of the injury and its implications.

Cervical spine injuries

Free flexibility of the head demands much more mobility of the cervical spine than that necessary anywhere else in the vertebral column. The demand for extreme flexibility is met at the expense of compromising some of the protective features of the osseous and neural elements, which are better preserved in less mobile regions of the spinal column. Consequently, the cervical spine is the most frequent site of severe skeletal and neural injury and, therefore, commands the major focus of this chapter. Athletic injuries to the cervical spine can involve the bony elements, intervertebral discs, ligamentous and muscular structures, elements of the brachial plexus, nerve roots, and/or the spinal cord itself. Torg has outlined a useful classification of cervical injuries based on the severity of the injury.[4]

Mild injuries (stable vertebral column)

Contusions: Blows to the back of the neck may result in bruising of the cervical musculature and, less often, the spinous processes of the vertebrae. Such injuries are quite painful, and tenderness on palpation is frequently elicited, especially when the head is flexed. Occasionally, the spinous processes of the more prominent 6th and 7th cervical vertebrae may be fractured as well. Treatment of these fractures, as well as the more common consequences of a contusion—hematoma formation, muscle spasm, stiffness, pain—should be treated with cervical-collar immobilization and exclusion from athletic activity. Symptomatic relief may be achieved with the local application of heat, massage, analgesic balms, and the like, as well as mild analgesic medications and muscle relaxants.

Strains and sprains: Muscle strain is caused by overuse of the muscle(s). A sprain is caused by forcing a joint through an abnormal range of motion with consequent damage to the ligament designed to prevent this motion. Sprains and strains are very common injuries to the neck and, indeed, may coexist. They both result from violent head-on neck movements or forcible extension of the neck against resistance. Such injuries vary in severity. The mild injury is of little significance and requires only symptomatic treatment (as with neck contusion). Exclusion from vigorous activities until the symptoms have abated is warranted, and a well-implemented program of neck-strengthening exercises is the most effective method of preventing recurrences.

Moderate injuries (stable vertebral column)

Occult fractures and degenerative changes: This group includes the occult fractures of the posterior elements (including the spinous processes), vertebral-body compression fractures, intervertebral disc space narrowing, or other degenerative changes. Although clinical signs and symptoms in these cases are frequently absent, the radiographic findings are presumed to have resulted from repetitive trauma to the cervical spine. Management of the athlete with this type of injury is not so much concerned with treatment per se as with the determination of guidelines for exclusion from participation. If the spine is stable, and if there is full and painless motion of the neck, participation may be permitted at the discretion of the child's parents or after the adult athlete has been fully informed of the potential for further accelerated degenerative changes and associated problems.

Pinch/stretch neuropraxias of cervical nerve roots: This is a frequent and poorly understood consequence of cervical injury to one side of the head and neck or shoulder. It is characterized by a sharp burning pain on one side of the neck, with pain commonly radiating into the ipsilateral shoulder, arm, and hand. There may be weakness and paresthesia of the involved extremity; it may last from several seconds to at most a few minutes. Full and painless neck motion is conspicuously preserved. If spine X-rays are normal and neurological function quickly returns to normal, athletic participation may be continued. Episodes may recur, and if so, sports participation should be discontinued, detailed neurological and radiological assessment should be done, and a neck-strengthening exercise program should be implemented. Persistent neurological deficit suggests a brachial plexus injury, and exclusion from athletic activity is mandatory.

Severe injuries

This category of injury includes unstable spinal lesions without neurological deficit, and brachial plexus injuries with neurological deficit but no significant skeletal injury.

Subluxations, dislocations, fractures without neurological deficit: These frequently occur with head injuries and should be presumed in any athlete who has been rendered unconscious. In awake athletes who cannot voluntarily perform a full range of cervical spine motion without pain or spasm, these lesions can be excluded only after detailed radiographic evaluation. Although neurological impairment may not be evident initially, there is great potential for spinal cord injury by ill-advised manipulation of the spine during transportation or examination of these patients. Consequently, spine trauma precautions as outlined earlier should be instituted immediately and absolute immobilization of the spine must be maintained until appropriate X-rays are taken. Definitive management of unstable spine lesions should be dictated by the neurosurgeon and/or orthopedist.

Brachial plexus injury (axonotmesis): This lesion involves loss of axon and myelin continuity of the nerve fiber with preservation of the supportive connective-tissue framework of the nerve. The epineurium, the perineurium, and the endoneurial tubes are preserved. Brachial plexus axonotmesis has been defined clinically by Clancy as a stretch injury resulting in weakness of the upper extremity, with or without sensory changes, which lasts for at least two weeks.[5] There is usually demonstrable weakness of shoulder abduction and external rotation, and elbow flexion, suggesting upper plexus or nerve root involvement. A pain-free and full range of motion of the neck is conspicuously preserved. Athletes with this injury must be immediately excluded from competition. When recovery has been complete and endurance of the involved muscles approximates those on the normal side, return to vigorous activity may be permitted. This may take several weeks to several months.

Very severe injuries (acute spinal cord injuries)

Fracture/dislocation: These lesions are manifested by obvious tetra- or paraparesis. The exact type and extent of the skeletal lesion can be determined only by appropriate radiographic examinations. The cord injury may be partial or complete. A partial neurological deficit may stabilize and subsequently improve. With a complete cord injury, however, the prognosis is usually hopeless. Emergency management is immediate protection of the spinal cord by immobilization and the prompt institution of life-support measures. Definitive management is in the province of the neurological and orthopedic surgical team.

Spinal cord injury with "normal" X-rays: Infrequently, profound cord injuries may occur with what appears at first to be normal spine X-rays showing no evidence of fracture or dislocation of vertebral elements. Acutely ruptured cervical discs may account for this injury and may be evidenced radiographically only by diminished height in the intervertebral disc space at the affected level. A congenitally stenotic or narrowed osseous cervical canal may also account for a profound spinal cord injury after relatively minor trauma and with seemingly normal spinal X-rays.[6] This uncommon condition occurs in women but at a lower rate than in men. The radiographic diagnosis is made by measuring the sagittal diameter of the cervical canal from a lateral roentgenograph and finding a diameter of 14 mm or less at one or more vertebral segments.

Decisions regarding additional radiographic evaluations and definitive treatment of these patients is made by the neurosurgeon-orthopedic team. Emergency measures by the physician in attendance are as previously outlined.

Catastrophic injuries

Spinal injuries that result in permanent paraplegia or tetraplegia are nothing short of a catastrophe. Although such injuries are infrequent, they must be carefully considered from the standpoint of cause and prevention. They usually occur in the person who accidentally falls, receives an unexpected blow to the head or neck, or poorly executes a physical act. Treatment of these as well as other injuries is best done by vigorous and intelligent efforts toward preventing their occurrence. This entails marshaling strong medical and financial support for good coaching and training, programmed exercise and physical conditioning, and improved facilities and protective equipment for athletes.

Thoracic spine injuries

As a result of its intrinsic architecture as well as its attachment to the ribs and thorax, the dorsal spine is the most stable section of the vertebral column and is the least frequent site of fractures, ligamentous sprains, dislocations, or herniated discs. Because of the many muscles which attach to it, as well as the subcutaneous position of the spinous processes of the thoracic vertebrae, contusion of these processes and/or muscles is not uncommon after blows to the back. Muscular strains may likewise occur. These conditions are of little neurological consequence, though they may result in severe discomfort. Local measures for symptomatic relief and protective padding may be sufficient treatment to allow continued competition. Severe discomfort or recurrent symptoms demand exclusion from athletic participation and rehabilitative measures to avoid intractable and painful sequelae.

Compression fracture of the dorsal spine with collapse of a vertebral body is the most common fracture in this region and is extremely unusual in ordinary athletic competition. It generally occurs with violent falls onto the buttocks or after the head is forcibly pushed between the knees. Neurological injury is infrequent, and the patient may walk away from the site of injury in spite of his back complaint. X-ray evaluation is imperative to determine the extent of the injury and to choose treatment.

Lumbar spine injuries

The lumbar spine is designed to provide more mobility than the dorsal spine, but offers inherently much more stability than the cervical spine. The vertebrae and musculature in this area are massive. Muscular contusions are common but usually not severe. Muscular strains may, likewise, occur but should be infrequent in the physically conditioned athlete. Frank dislocations and fractures are extremely uncommon in ordinary athletic activities and occur only after severe violence, such as a fall from a height. This lesion most frequently occurs at the T_{11}, T_{12} to L_1 region and is indeed a serious injury that requires operative management. Although a profound neurological deficit may result, the ultimate outcome depends on whether the neural damage is a consequence of injury to the conus medullaris (the terminal part of the spinal cord) or the cauda equina (intraspinal peripheral nerves). In this type of injury, particular attention should be paid to excluding associated injuries to thoracic and abdominal viscera.

The intervertebral discs are interposed between each vertebral body and act as shock absorbers or cushions between these bony blocks. Herniation of these discs posteriorly or laterally to impinge upon lumbar nerve roots is usually a result of chronic degenerative changes within the spine. Consequently, they occur most frequently during and after the fourth decade of life. In younger and physically fit individuals, they are much less common. When they occur in adolescence or early adulthood, they are almost invariably related to acute back trauma, as from a blow or from a fall.

The syndrome of low back pain that radiates into the leg(s) in the distribution of a lumbar nerve root is well known and needs no deliberation here. Acute urinary retention as the only manifestation of an acutely ruptured disc in women is less commonly appreciated, however.[7] Acutely ruptured or recurrent disc protrusions can most often be relieved by cessation of vigorous physical activity and strict bedrest for at least 10 to 14 days. Afterwards, a well-implemented program of muscle-strengthening exercises for back and abdominal musculature should be carried out.

Neurological deficit, loss of voluntary sphincter control of bladder and/or bowel, and/or severe intractable pain demand immediate neurosurgical or orthopedic evaluation. Decisions as to whether the athlete may be allowed subsequent sports participation must be individualized. Fortunately, because a splendid muscular condition reduces a geat deal of the strain on intervertebral discs, ruptured lumbar discs are an infrequent problem in athletes.

Although one usually assumes that women's athletic activities are confined to noncontact sports, it seems evident that female participation in any form of vigorous athletic activity is restricted mostly, if not solely, by social traditions rather than by biological limitations.[8] These social restrictions are rapidly disappearing. As seemingly absolute barriers continue to fall, experience has shown that, with few exceptions, men and women experience the same kinds of injuries when they participate in the same kind of sport under similar conditions. The risk of injury and the severity of injury appear to be a function principally of the strength, the skill, and the physical conditioning of the participant, as well as how well the rules of the particular sport are constructed and enforced to promote the safety of play. Consequently, I believe that the medical community has the responsibility of not only assuring the equality of medical care for female athletes but of also providing the leadership for gathering the necessary financial and social support to insure that women's athletic activities are encouraged and that their sports injuries are kept to the fewest possible.

References

1. Clarke KS: A survey of sports-related spinal cord injuries in schools and colleges, 1973-1975. *J Safety Res* 9:140, 1977

2. Leader WF (ed): Statistical reports for traumatic spinal cord injury (1975-1976). Florida Central Registry for the Severely Disabled, 1976

3. Brisman R, Kouach RM, Johnson DO, et al: Pulmonary edema in acute transection of the cervical spinal cord. *Surg Gynecol Obstet* 139:363, 1974

4. Torg JS: Athletic injuries to the cervical spine. *Surg Rounds* 1:40, 1978

5. Clancy WG Jr, Brand RL, and Bergfield, JA: Upper trunk brachial plexus injuries in contact sports. *J Sports Med* 5:209, 1977

6. Countee RW and Vijayanathan T: Congenital stenosis of the cervical spine: Diagnosis and management. *J Natl Med Assoc* 71:257, 1979

7. Emmett JL and Love JG: Urinary retention in women caused by asymptomatic protruded lumbar disk: Report of five cases. *J Urol* 99:597, 1968

8. Thomas CL: Special problems of the female athlete. In *Sports Medicine* (Ryan AJ and Allman FL Jr, eds), pp 347-373. New York: Academic Press, 1974

NEUROPSYCHIATRIC ASPECTS

Chester M. Pierce, M.D., and
Kristen J. Kuehnle, Ed.D.

CHAPTER

23

Coaches, trainers, teachers, parents, and doctors must be acquainted with significant psychosocial trends in order to advise females about exercise and athletics. Crucial to their understanding is an awareness of the far-reaching effects of the progressive emancipation of women. Our entire society is altering its views and expectations of female behavior. As more women demand and receive freedom to define their own route to happiness, the number of women who choose to exercise and/or compete in all kinds of sports rapidly increases.

Psychosocial factors

In 1970, 294,000 high school girls participated in interscholastic sports. By 1977, 1.6 million high school girls were participating in school sports. At about the same time, the Association for Intercollegiate Athletics for Women (A.I.A.W.), the counterpart of the male National Collegiate Athletic Association (N.C.A.A.), grew from 278 member schools to 825. Even casual observation shows an impressive number of female joggers. Very few people can recall seeing even one female jogger as recently as 1960. Yet, it is now considered unremarkable to have nearly 5,000 female competitors in a single 10,000-meter (6.2-mile) minimarathon. Television's success in luring audiences to watch female gymnasts, swimmers, runners, golfers, and tennis players indicates an increasing and genuine acceptance. At last, females are earning a living as professionals in a variety of sports. Some of these livelihoods are handsome by any standard.

The old belief that females should not be too active in sports seems to have been modified. Liberated women insist that the physical and emotional benefits of athletics should not be denied to them. They argue that exercise and/or sports participation will help them live longer, better, and more meaningful lives. Sports activity leads to self-esteem, self-confidence, self-fulfillment, and a sense of mastery—traits that men have long insisted their sons learn on the playing fields.

Sport training and/or competition teaches the athlete about herself and the limits of her abilities, but it also teaches her to strive for ever higher goals. Such an value, when fixed into the character, should make anyone happier.

Similarly, participation in exercise or sports shows that there are multiple ways of coping with problems, thus reducing feelings of helplessness and dependency. Being free to pursue athletics allows more women to feel better about themselves in terms of independence and assertiveness.

Another advantage of sports participation is that using energy and emotions in such channels reduces feelings of tension, anger, envy, or dissatisfaction. Having more socially accepted means of expressing hostility and frustration offers, according to current thinking, both psychological and physiological advantages.

Some have thought that sports are a peerless vehicle to teach self-discipline, courage, and diligence. Other valuable attributes historically assumed to be taught by the sacrifices involved in training are loyalty, teamwork, and appreciation of careful preparation and strategic planning. Whereas nearly all able-bodied boys have participated in contests in which these factors were emphasized, until recently few girls had a similar opportunity.

For 50 years, educators have known that, in general, athletic school and college youth get better grades than nonathletes. This was thought to be due not so much to the versatility of the athlete but to the necessity, imposed by training and competition, of being more organized and more goal-directed. Theoretically, the same benefits should obtain for female athletes.

From the viewpoint of the sports-medicine specialist, the new emphasis on exercise and sports is interesting because it may contribute to upgrading the nation's health. If, as some believe, the major health problem in our country is obesity, earlier, wider, and more general exercise by females should help. In general, people who exercise as adults were exposed to exercise early in life. Therefore, it is hoped that females introduced early to exercise will continue to exercise and thereby contribute to the reduction of our major public-health problem.

Whether continued exercise reduces a public-health problem and permits increased longevity is of less importance than whether people who exercise feel better and thus live better, if not longer. In addition, the person who exercises believes that she is contributing to her own well-being. In this sense, the individual believes that she is directing and controlling her own destiny.

There are a few more reasons for physicians to applaud a more active life for females. First, in selected clinical circumstances such as in therapy for lameness, burn disfigurement, or susceptibility to actinic injury, it is often useful to get a patient involved in exercise and/or sports. Previously, such possibilities were not as readily available for females.

Secondly, during pregnancy, the psychological advantages of being able to exercise and of being accustomed to exercise are thought to be considerable. The pregnant woman, who has been used to exercise might be better prepared to become a mother. This is because she believes she has done her best to prepare for the dangers of childbirth and to withstand possible untoward happenings during pregnancy. In this belief she is similiar to the high school male whose football letter attests that he is tough and able to care for himself.

The woman who has exercised or been involved in sports is likely to have a mental attitude that can help her through pregnancy. Such women can overcome relatively minor concerns such as fear of falling—"I won't fall because I'm strong, nimble, and agile." More profound concerns such as changes in body image can be lessened, too—"After as the baby is born I'll regain my figure because I've kept myself in good condition and my muscles are tight."

For all these reasons, it is commendable that more women are taking part in exercise and sports. It is especially felicitous that this interest is being started early in life and continuing throughout life. The psychological benefits will accumulate and succeeding generations of women, happier and more content and confident about themselves, will make even more contributions to society. And they will, in all likelihood, offer a different quality of mothering, in part because of the impact that exercise and sports activity have on the development of their personalities and character structure.

Mental health

Whether the female is to exercise for recreation or by prescription, whether she is to be a competitor or not, whether she will be in an individual or group activity, and whether she will be in coeducational or all-female activities, she may welcome some basic reassurance. The favorable psychosocial climate permits the advisor to tell the athlete and her parents that:
• Exercise and sports are not exclusively masculine activities. A female athlete does not necessarily become more masculine in appearance or interest.
• Exercise and sports do not alter sex drive or preference.
• Exercise and sports can be used to maximize physical attractiveness, while at the same time helping the participant to gain poise and charm.
• Exercise and sports can be a means to rewards and status for those sufficiently dedicated and talented to earn athletic scholarships or to compete on a national or international level.
In rendering this sort of assurance, the advisor should communicate explicitly and implicitly that, from a psychological or physiological view, there is no reason to disapprove of athletic activity in a female. The advisor must be prepared, depending on the specific situations, to counsel about such emotionally charged areas as preparing a young swimmer to use tampons instead of sanitary napkins. The advisor must also be sensitive to the adolescent's concern over a changing body image, especially in terms of becoming too muscular.
Psychosis: Psychotics should be in the care of specialists who treat such major mental illnesses as schizophrenia, manic-depression, or psychotic depression. In general, if a coach or trainer is

asked to help in such situations, the important consideration is to provide structure via exercise or games for the patient. Such patients may be overwhelmed by their illness. Usually they are no danger to others.

The care-giver should insist upon reality and deal firmly but evenly with patients. Young female patients may be flagrantly seductive. A care-giver, especially a male, should be careful about being alone with such patients, and not touch them, lest the gesture be misinterpreted.

Neurosis and character disorder: Neurotics are people with anxiety symptoms such as irrational fears, hypochondriasis, and depression. Character disorders are habitual, lifelong, patterned responses revolving about expressions of aggression. A person with a character disorder might show such symptoms as sudden swings in mood or frustrating procrastination.

In a setting in which the diagnosis of one of these illnesses is important, specialists would presumably be on hand to give precise guidance and to elaborate the role of the trainer or coach. In general, a trainer/coach might work as a team member with a physical therapist and occupational therapist. The team's assignment might be to channel or increase mobility, to get the patient to use energy to combat and deflect suicidal preoccupations, and to observe, measure, and record the patient's progress in interpersonal actions and motor skills.

Other illnesses

It is possible that a coach, trainer, or general physician will have to deal—without the aid of a psychiatrist—with an athlete who has a psychosomatic illness or is mentally retarded, epileptic, or handicapped. In these instances, the general support, interest, and reassurance that the advisor can give would be critical. Accepting the athlete's performance, gently helping her to achieve what she wants to achieve, assuring her that any physical troubles can be managed, and emphasizing the certainty that the exercise will be helpful and healthful are the overall psychological tasks.

The epileptic: We take a conservative view of epilepsy, and believe that some sports activities should be prohibited to the epileptic. She should be counseled against aquatic sports and those involving operation of a vehicle. Despite nearly perfect control of convulsions by medication, an epileptic, by definition, could have unpredictable paroxysms. If the person were in water, drowning could result.

If the athlete is in an aquatic activity, the advisor may have to summon skill and acumen to counsel her into another, more appropriate, less dangerous exercise or activity. Awareness of other possibilities and available facilities, of course, is crucial. Yet more important may be the tact, empathy, respect, and patience that the advisor must display. Such a test can be especially severe when dealing with an adolescent, who, by virtue of her age, is very sensitive about being different. To be steered away from something she wants to do because she *is*, in fact, different, can be painful for her.

No less difficulty is encountered in dealing with an epileptic who happens to have a seizure in the gym or on the playing field in front of peers—or, indeed, in front of a large crowd. The advisor must deal with her shame and embarrassment, which could be monumental enough to make her quit a sport. At the same time, the advisor must deal with the fears, ignorance, and possible insensitivity of the athlete's peers. This requires the ventilation of feelings by the group and at least some reinforcing education about the nature of epilepsy and the grip it has on the unfortunate teammate. The group must be shown the importance of reaching out and "normalizing" their relationship with the epileptic.

An advisor may be asked to discuss the young-adult epileptic's courtship and marriage problems. Unless the advisor is a physician he or she should be cautious in discussing heritability of the disease or its likely evolution.

Thus, one is left with the not inconsiderable role of being a supportive, nonjudgmental confidant.

The mentally retarded: Mental retardation can be classified as severe, moderate, or mild. Its causes are diverse, but all mentally retarded people can benefit from exercise and should be encouraged to exercise. In addition, exercise is most important in keeping weight down, encouraging a sense of mastery, and augmenting body image.

Group activities and the emotional support and attention given by care-givers during exercise and sports, may be especially beneficial to the mentally retarded. Perhaps the major task of the care-givers is to try to provide "normalcy" in terms of how the individual is regarded and perceived. Such attitudinal communications help to dilute the loneliness and alienation that characterize the lives of many mildly and moderately retarded individuals. To this end, over the last decade, "Special Olympics" have been held for the retarded.

The sports advisor must reassure and reward the individual for her participation. Mental first-aid to reduce stress from competitive pressures must be available. She should not feel compelled to perform or feel that she is on display. Protection from overzealous and callous fans (including parents) must be provided.

Another matter of concern is the sexual life of the mentally retarded female. Traditionally, doctors and family members have been concerned about the consequences of chance solicitation. This general concern is no less real in an exercise or sports program. The advisor must be certain—without puritanical zeal—that the retarded female is not exposed to gratuitous dangers of pregnancy or venereal disease.

The disabled: It is useful to distinguish between the handicapped and the disabled individual. A disability is a condition that can be described by a physician. A handicap, on the other hand, is the result of the obstacles that the disability has interposed between the individual and her maximum functional level.

There are, of course, all sorts of disabilities. Disabling conditions differ in type, location, and degree. Hence, the problem of the gifted athlete who suffers a burn is different from that of a young girl whose progressive rheumatoid arthritis demands an exercise prescription. Therefore, it is not possible here to attend to the various specific needs occasioned by disabilities. When a disability has become a handicap, however, the aim of exercise or sports should be to promote a sense of health, self-sufficiency, and a more positive body image. Psychological intervention should underlie this aim. The exact intervention is determined by such considerations as amount of disability, severity of handicap, age of the patient, types of facilities available, past athletic interest and experience, and the quality of family support.

GYNECOLOGICAL AND ENDOCRINOLOGICAL FACTORS

Mona M. Shangold, M.D.

CHAPTER

24

Much attention has been paid to the relationship between sports participation and female reproductive function. The reasons: Many more women are now engaging in athletic activities; both men and women now openly discuss topics that were previously considered too personal; and advancements in scientific understanding and laboratory technology now permit a more critical analysis of reproductive physiology and pathology.

This discussion is intended as an overview of gynecology as it pertains to the athlete, but is not meant as a comprehensive review of gynecology or endocrinology.

Female reproductive physiology

The events leading to ovulation and menstruation involve production and secretion of hormones by the hypothalamus, the pituitary, and the ovaries. The dynamic relationship between these structures includes positive and negative feedback mechanisms in a complex sequence of carefully timed events. In view of the delicate balance required to effect this sophisticated program, it is much more surprising that women generally ovulate and menstruate regularly than that they sometimes do not.

The hypothalamus and the pituitary: The hypothalamus, located at the base of the brain, secretes releasing and inhibiting factors that cause the pituitary gland to produce and/or release specific hormones. The hypothalamic-pituitary-ovarian axis is affected by its own internal dynamics and also by external influences, including higher brain centers. Thus, the endocrine system is inseparable from the nervous system and its activity.

The hypothalamus produces gonadotropin-releasing hormone (GnRH), which is also referred to as luteinizing hormone-releasing hormone (LHRH) or luteinizing hormone-releasing factor (LHRF); this decapeptide causes the pituitary gland to release follicle-stimulating hormone (FSH) and luteinizing hormone (LH). These glycoproteins promote development of ovarian follicles and production of ovarian steroids.

The ovary: The ovary is composed of three steroid-producing structures: the follicle, the corpus luteum, and the stroma. The ovarian cycle is more easily visualized in two phases, the follicular phase (prior to ovulation) and the luteal phase (after ovulation). Estrogen is produced by the ovary throughout the menstrual cycle; its plasma concentration is highest in the late follicular phase, just prior to ovulation. Production of estrogen by the developing ovarian follicles (in the follicular phase) leads to increased sensitivity of each follicle to FSH. Thus, in any cycle, the most mature follicle, which is the most efficient estrogen-producer, selectively binds FSH better than its peers and is therefore destined to ovulate next. The high estrogen signal sent by this most mature follicle to the hypothalamus and pituitary leads to the sudden pituitary release of large amounts of gonadotropins. This great "LH surge," accompanied by a smaller FSH surge, triggers ovulation. After ovulation, the corpus luteum (which is what remains of the most mature follicle after expulsion of the ovum) produces progesterone as well as estrogen. The ovarian stroma (the fibrous and supporting connective tissue) continues to produce androgens and estrogens throughout the menstrual cycle and even after the menopause, when no functioning follicles remain.

The endometrium: The endometrium, which is the inner lining of the uterus, is shed during menstruation. Its cycle is more easily visualized in two phases: the proliferative phase, which relates temporally to the ovarian follicular phase and results hormonally from it, and the secretory phase, which relates temporally to the ovarian luteal phase and results hormonally from it. Thus, estrogen causes proliferation of the endometrium, and progesterone

317

causes maturation of the estrogen-primed endometrium. It is the declining production of these two hormones by the corpus luteum of the ovary that causes menstruation at the end of the luteal phase of the menstrual cycle.

Regular and irregular menstrual intervals: The menstrual "interval" is defined as the number of days from the beginning of one period to the beginning of the next. In the classic 28-day cycle, the follicular and luteal phases are each approximately 14 days. However, very few bodies are that precise—the normal stresses of everyday life affect hormone production by the hypothalamic-pituitary-ovarian axis. The length of the follicular phase is determined by how long it takes one follicle to produce enough estrogen to induce the LH surge that triggers ovulation. In some women, this almost always requires 14 days and is rarely affected by outside influences. In others, follicular maturation may require three to six months, and menstruation occurs only two to four times a year. The life-span of the corpus luteum is generally about 14 days. The duration of the luteal phase is much less variable than that of the follicular phase.

Endocrine problems

Anovulation with normal estrogen levels: If follicles are being stimulated and are producing estrogen at the same time that there is either abnormal androgen metabolism (as is seen in polycystic ovary disease) or immature development of the hypothalamic-pituitary-ovarian axis, ovulation may not be triggered. In such a situation, follicular ovarian cysts develop, and estrogen levels are normal or slightly elevated. These anovulatory women have continuous, unopposed estrogen stimulation of the endometrium without the protective effect of progesterone. Occasional shedding of the endometrium may occur and may be either incomplete or profuse. These women are at increased risk of developing endometrial hyperplasia and endometrial adenocarcinoma, and should be treated with exogenous progesterone every two or three months to protect the endometrium. This condition is commonly seen at the beginning and end of reproductive life. Abnormal bleeding patterns in adolescents are usually due to anovulation and can be treated hormonally. But abnormal bleeding patterns in peri- and postmenopausal women are often related to anatomic or neoplastic pathology and should be evaluated by microscopic examination of the endometrium before initiating hormone therapy.

Polycystic ovary syndrome: The term polycystic ovary syndrome is often used synonymously with "Stein-Leventhal syndrome," but the latter is responsible for only a small fraction of cases. In polycystic disease, excessive androgen production by the ovaries and/or adrenals leads to a self-perpetuating cycle of chronic anovulation (with or without palpable cyst formation), continuous production of androgens and estrogens by the ovaries, and continuous production of LH by the pituitary. Following thorough diagnostic evaluation, treatment of these women by a gynecologist-endocrinologist should be goal-oriented. Appropriate therapy is: clomiphene citrate for the patient with anovulatory infertility; bimonthly progesterone for the patient with anovulatory amenorrhea who does not wish to become pregnant right then; oral contraceptives for the patient whose prime concern is hirsutism; and prednisone for the patient with demonstrable dexamethasone-induced suppressibility of androgen overproduction.

Stress-related anovulatory amenorrhea: Chronic stress may produce a syndrome similar to that seen in polycystic ovary syndrome, with resultant anovulation. This entity is not completely understood but involves absence of the LH surge due to neurologic-endocrine input. This type of stress-related anovulatory amenorrhea is seen in athletes, but it is not clear whether the etiology involves the exercise itself, the physical stress of training, the emotional stress of training or competing, or a combination of these. In amenorrheic athletes of normal weight, normal body fat composition, and normal plasma-estrogen concentrations, this type of anovulatory amenorrhea should be evaluated and treated in the same manner as described for polycystic ovary syndrome. There is no known risk associated with anovulatory amenorrhea in an estrogen-producing athlete—provided her endometrium is protected by periodic administration of progesterone.

Obesity: Very obese women tend to have high estrogen levels, largely due to fat-cell conversion of androgens to estrogens. Such women are often anovulatory, with the same underlying mechanism as is seen in polycystic ovary syndrome. This problem also warrants evaluation by a gynecologist-endocrinologist. Induction of ovulation in an obese woman should be undertaken only with great caution. Therapy should include a program for weight loss.

Any medical or endocrine problem is a potential cause of anovulation in a woman with normal estrogen production. Thus, a general history and physical examination are essential in the evaluation of an amenorrheic patient and should be supplemented by a complete blood count, urinalysis, SMA-6, SMA-12, VDRL, and thyroid-function tests. Any abnormal test result should be evaluated and appropriate treatment given. If these studies are normal in a well-estrogenized woman with amenorrhea or oligomenorrhea, she should be referred to a gynecologist-endocrinologist for individualized evaluation and treatment.

Pituitary insufficiency: In some women, no follicle ever matures sufficiently to trigger ovulation. This may result from inadequate gonadotropin stimulation (primary or secondary hypogonadotropism, which is primary pituitary insufficiency in producing FSH and/or LH, or pituitary insufficiency secondary to inadequate hypothalamic stimulation).

Post-Pill amenorrhea: The gonadotropin suppression that produces the contraceptive effect of an oral contraceptive occasionally continues after the drug has been discontinued. This leads to the same picture of low estrogen production by the ovaries as is seen in other instances of hypopituitarism. The situation is usually temporary and resolves spontaneously.

Hyperprolactinemia: Some cases of amenorrhea are caused by overproduction of prolactin, a protein hormone produced by the pituitary gland under the control of releasing and inhibiting factors. Increased prolactin levels are seen acutely after stress, exercise, or administration of a variety of drugs. Modern radiologic and laboratory techniques now permit recognition of very small groups of pituitary cells—pituitary microadenomas—that consistently produce excessive amounts of prolactin. These should be evaluated by an endocrinologist. Galactorrhea is a diagnostically useful finding, but is often absent in hyperprolactinemia. Treatment, which should be individualized, may include close observation through repeated radiographic studies and hormonal measurements, drug therapy to lower prolactin levels, or microsurgical resection (transsphenoidal hypophysectomy). Such tumors are slow-growing and can be detected at early stages.

Low weight/poor nutrition: Very low weight women and/or those with low body fat or poor nutritional status may be subject to hypoestrogenic amenorrhea resulting from inadequate gonadotropin stimulation. This is somewhat similar to what is seen in anorexia nervosa, in which pre- and midpubertal gonadotropin secretion patterns develop.[1] (LH levels are normally very low in prepubertal girls because their pituitary is very sensitive to negative feedback from the very low levels of estrogen secreted by prepubertal ovaries. During puberty, LH secretion increases at night and decreases during the day. After puberty, LH concentrations remain within the normal adult range during both day and night.)[2] This entity is not completely understood but often resolves with weight gain and/or improved nutrition.

Frisch, studying a group of healthy white American girls, found body weights at puberty to be similar, even though puberty occurred at different ages.[3] She examined lean body mass in this group and proposed that a minimum of 17 per cent body fat is necessary for the onset of menstrual cycles. She also concluded that a minimum of 22 per cent body fat is necessary for the restoration and maintenance of menstrual cycles in women who are over the age of 16.

Amenorrheic athletes of very low weight and/or low body fat composition often demonstrate this picture of low estrogen levels. It is not clear whether—as with stress-related anovulatory amenorrhea—the etiology involves the exercise itself, the physical stress of training, the emotional stress of training or competing, or a combination of all of these.

These women should undergo pituitary evaluation by an endocrinologist. The hypogonadotropic/ hypoestrogenic state is not known to be dangerous to an athlete with no other hormone deficiencies—except, possibly, for the lack of estrogen's protective effects on the cardiovascular and skeletal systems.

There is no conclusive evidence that sports participation causes amenorrhea. While some investigators have reported a higher incidence of amenorrhea among athletes than nonathletes, careful analysis of prior menstrual histories was lacking. (If an athlete had irregular menses prior to athletic training, the training cannot be blamed for her menstrual irregularity.) It is true that many athletes have irregular periods—but many nonathletes also have irregular periods. In any event, association does not prove causality. More research in this field is necessary.

A distinction should be made between primary amenorrhea—describing a woman older than 18 who has never menstruated—and secondary amenorrhea—describing the woman who previously menstruated but no longer does so. Both require endocrinologic evaluation, but primary amenorrhea is more likely to be associated with chromosomal abnormalities. Thus, a karyotype should be included in the diagnostic evaluation of all women with primary amenorrhea; those with secondary amenorrhea warrant routine chromosomal studies only when there is premature ovarian failure.

Ovarian failure: The menopause is heralded by cessation of ovarian cycles, cessation of menstruation, exhaustion of ovarian follicles, marked reduction in estrogen production by the ovaries, and marked elevation in plasma gonadotropin concentrations. Because of the absence of follicles, failing ovaries are incapable of responding normally to high levels of gonadotropins. The low amounts of estrogen produced by these ovaries decrease pituitary feedback, leading to enhanced production of FSH and LH.

Ovarian failure is expected between the ages of 40 and 55. Any woman who develops ovarian failure prior to age 40 warrants chromosomal evaluation, just as any woman who continues menstruating after the age of 50 to 55 should consult a gynecologist.

The perimenopausal syndrome includes hot flushes, which may be related to marked or sudden fluctuations in LH concentration. These can be extremely distressing and disruptive. Not all women experience them, and, of those who do, not all find them intolerable. Low-dose estrogen therapy is often effective in women who request symptomatic relief from vasomotor symptoms. Of course, such risks of estrogen therapy as endometrial cancer and thromboembolic complications must be considered before instituting treatment. Some women are satisfied by the reassurance that vasomotor symptoms are probably temporary and short-lived. Others find successful relief with tranquilizers or placebos. Again, optimal therapy must be individualized.

The postmenopausal syndrome includes dryness of the genitourinary tract, most commonly presenting as atrophic vaginitis. This may be treated with topical application of an estrogen cream or a combination estrogen-androgen cream.

In a healthy woman, there is no absolute contraindication to athletic participation during or after the menopause. Certainly, anyone undertaking a training program after the age of 40 should first have a thorough physical examination that includes a stress electrocardiogram.

Anyone who develops light-headedness, dizziness, chest pain, nausea or vomiting, diarrhea, excessive weight loss, or insomnia in the course of training should seek medical attention—no matter whether she's pre- or postmenopausal. The postmenopausal absence of the beneficial effect of estrogen on bones may increase the risk of orthopedic injuries, especially fractures. However, conclusive evidence of such a risk in athletes is lacking. In addition, the cardiovascular, psychological, and other benefits of exercise probably outweigh this potential hazard in postmenopausal women.

Inappropriateness of routine treatment with birth control pills: Administration of estrogen and progesterone, the hormones normally produced by the ovaries, can induce cyclic bleeding in any woman with a responsive endometrium and patent outflow tract. Many abnormalities of hypothalamic, pituitary, or ovarian function are therefore camouflaged by ingestion of birth control pills, as women with pituitary tumors, ovarian failure, panhypopituitarism, and immature hypothalamic-pituitary-ovarian axes can all be made to bleed regularly. Thus, the practice of giving oral contraceptive pills to regulate periods is to be strongly denounced, for it merely confirms the presence of a functioning endometrium and patent outflow tract and may mask or worsen significant pathology. A specific cause for the amenorrhea should be sought and treated appropriately.

Menometrorrhagia: Heavy bleeding at the time of menstruation (menorrhagia) and bleeding between menstrual periods (metrorrhagia) warrant evaluation by a gynecologist. Endometrial sampling for microscopic examination will probably be necessary.

Other common gynecologic problems

Dysmenorrhea: This problem has received much attention during the last few years. While the causes of primary, functional dysmenorrhea may be complex, they are probably related to release of prostaglandins at the myometrial and/or endometrial level. The pain and gastrointestinal symptoms are often effectively relieved by administration of prostaglandin inhibitors (aspirin, indomethacin, mefenamic acid, ibuprofen, flufenamic acid, and sodium naproxen). Many athletes and gynecologists have reported relief of pain with exercise; the explanation for this remains conjectural. Some authors have reported a higher incidence of dysmenorrhea among athletes, while others have reported a lower incidence. It has also been reported that the incidence of dysmenorrhea among swimmers is higher than among other athletes. No explanation is offered.

Premenstrual tension syndrome: This syndrome, described as including anxiety, edema, carbohydrate intolerance, and depression, has been attributed to hormone imbalances and other causes. Some have reported relief with administration of pyridoxine, which enhances liver metabolism of estrogen.[4] Specific therapy aimed at each symptom—e.g., a diuretic for edema—also seems reasonable. This syndrome continues to be poorly understood.

Pain is very subjective, and its perception varies greatly among individuals. The experience of pain is intimately dependent upon both the physical stimulus delivered and the emotional milieu in which it is received, with reciprocal causality—people who experience much pain often develop certain personality traits, and certain personality traits influence perception of pain.

In general, athletic, professional, and other active women seem to be less incapacitated by pain than more sedentary women. It is not clear whether the self-discipline and pain tolerance they have developed during training enables them to tolerate more pain, their innate resistance to pain or diminished perception of it permits them to be more active, the distraction of other activities diminishes awareness of pain, or if the answer is a combination of these. In any event, exercise may have acute and chronic therapeutic effects on some types of pain for many women. Its role in dysmenorrhea seems particularly striking.

Pelvic infection: Acute salpingitis (infection of the fallopian tubes) causes fever, abdominal pain, signs of pelvic peritonitis, and leukocytosis. This condition is often caused by the gonococcus, which can be identified by Gram's stain of the cervical mucus and culture on appropriate bacteriological medium. Acute gonococcal salpingitis is best treated by antibiotics.

Chronic salpingo-oophoritis often causes pelvic pain, typically with a postmenstrual exacerbation. Fever may or may not be present. Pelvic examination may reveal adnexal masses (tubo-ovarian abscesses) without signs of peritonitis. Leukocytosis is usually slight. Because multiple bacteria are usually involved, treatment should begin with high-dose, broad-spectrum antibiotic coverage for both aerobic and anaerobic organisms. If drug therapy is unsuccessful, surgical intervention—abscess drainage or removal or abdominal hysterectomy and bilateral salpingo-oophorectomy may be necessary.

Abdominal pain of unknown etiology should not be loosely labeled "pelvic inflammatory disease," unless there is evidence to support the diagnosis. Pelvic pain, in the absence of fever or leukocytosis, warrants further diagnostic evaluation. Pain, with or without an infection, can certainly impair the training or performance of an athlete.

Vaginitis: Vaginal pruritus and/or discharge warrant microscopic examination in the form of a "wet preparation" in normal saline. The most common causes are Candida albicans, Trichomonas vaginalis, and Hemophilus vaginalis, which can usually be treated effectively with nystatin vaginal suppositories, oral metronidazole, and oral metronidazole or ampicillin, respectively. The irritation from such an infection could hinder the training or performance of an athlete.

Urinary incontinence: Stress urinary incontinence is a symptom of pelvic relaxation resulting from loss of the posterior urethro-vesical angle, with or without alteration in the urethral angle. This problem is more common in multiparous women and may be especially bothersome in athletes, who are both more likely to strain during participation and more likely to be inconvenienced by urine leakage during activity. Some improvement may follow practice of Kegel exercises, which serve to strengthen ancillary perineal muscles.

There is no evidence that any athletic activity produces or aggravates the basic anatomic defect responsible for the problem. However, active women may have more symptoms than sedentary women. The anatomic defect responsible for this problem is often amenable to surgical correction by the vaginal and/or abdominal routes. A gynecologist should be consulted.

Infertility: Both partners, and their interaction, must be evaluated. Investigation must include the following: male factor, tubal patency, ovulation, cervical mucus, corpus luteum adequacy, mycoplasma infection, immunologic factors, mechanical problems, uterine abnormalities, and endometriosis. Treatment by the infertility specialist must be individualized.

There is no evidence that athletes have a higher incidence of infertility than the general population. However, several alterations in concentrations of reproductive hormones that have been shown in association with exercise might represent potential causes of infertility in both men and women. Further investigation is certainly needed.

Other considerations

Contraception: Any couple, athletic or nonathletic, must find the contraceptive mode best suited to them. There are no contraindications to the use of any type of contraceptive for athletes. A few considerations are worthy of mention, though. Some women who wear intrauterine devices experience pelvic pain, which might impair performance in an athlete. The increased menstrual flow noted by some IUD-wearers might predispose a woman toward development of iron-deficiency anemia. It is reasonable for all women of reproductive age—both athletes and nonathletes—to ingest supplementary iron as replacement for iron lost in menstruation. It is wise for athletes, in particular, to follow this practice, as the added oxygen-carrying capacity of higher hemoglobin concentrations should benefit athletic performance. A diaphragm might prove inconvenient to an athlete who has to wear it during training or competition a few hours after coitus. Oral contraceptive agents have been thought to impair athletic performance, based on findings by several investigators that poorer performances occurred premenstrually in naturally cycling women. (Endogenous estrogen and progesterone concentrations are high in the naturally occurring late luteal phase, and levels would be even higher throughout three weeks of Pill ingestion.)

Myths: It should be unnecessary to review old myths, but for the sake of completeness and final denouncement, they are aired again. There is no reason to avoid athletic participation—including aquatic activities—during menstruation. Coitus during menstruation is also medically acceptable. Most athletes find tampons more comfortable and esthetic than sanitary napkins, but both are medically acceptable during exercise.

Anabolic steroids: These have received much publicity and are reportedly used in the training of athletes in some countries. There is now no conclusive evidence that their use is beneficial, while there is some evidence that their use may be harmful. Administration of androgens to women may produce masculinizing and defeminizing effects; administration of androgens to men may inhibit endogenous androgen production and lead to testicular atrophy and oligospermia.

Postoperative training: It is reasonable to permit pain to guide the resumption of training following abdominal or pelvic surgery. It is probably safe to perform most activities that cause no pain (including stair-climbing, automobile-driving, hair-washing, running, and throwing). Activities that produce pain should probably be postponed until they produce none, which represents a rough indication of more complete healing. Similarly, coitus can probably be practiced postoperatively in the absence of pain, unless the cervix is open (as after an abortion or D&C), which would provide a route for ascending bacterial infection into the uterus. After an abortion or D&C, all vaginal entry, whether by penis, tampon, or douche, should be put off until the cervix has closed (probably by two weeks after the procedure).

Effects of exercise on reproductive hormones

A number of investigators have reported the acute effects of exercise upon peripheral concentrations of LH and androgens in men. Sutton and others found increased serum androgen levels following brief maximal exertion and unchanged serum androgen levels following submaximal effort; LH concentrations remained unchanged after both.[5] Dessypris and others reported increased plasma androstenedione levels, decreased plasma testosterone levels, and unchanged plasma LH levels following a noncompetitive marathon run.[6] Kuoppasalmi and colleagues found increased plasma concentrations of LH, androstenedione, and testosterone after brief maximal exertion.[7]

There have been fewer reports of acute changes in hormone concentrations in exercising women. Sutton reported increased serum concentrations of androgens and unchanged concentrations of LH in women after brief maximal exertion. Jurkowski and coworkers described increased plasma levels of FSH, estradiol, and progesterone following light or heavy endurance exercise during the follicular and luteal phases.[8]

Little is known about the chronic effects of exercise upon gonadotropin and ovarian steroid concentrations in women athletes. My colleagues and I studied a long-distance runner through 18 menstrual cycles and found shorter luteal phases in cycles of greater running and lower midluteal phase plasma progesterone concentrations during training.[9] More investigation is clearly needed in this area.

Recommendations

Women athletes should be reassured that a menstrual interval between 25 and 32 days probably reflects normal function. A menstrual interval between 20 and 60 days probably warrants no attention in the absence of infertility. An infertile couple should consult a specialist. A woman should consult her gynecologist if her menstrual interval is shorter than 20 days or longer than 60 days or if she has galactorrhea or bleeding between periods. Attention is also warranted if menstrual irregularity developed in association with increased training. It should be pointed out that, while these conditions all deserve evaluation, none necessarily represents a contraindication to continued training.

References

1. Boyar R, Katz J, Finkelstein J, et al: Anorexia nervosa: Immaturity of the 24-hour luteinizing hormone secretory pattern. *N Engl J Med* 291:861, 1974

2. Boyar R, Finkelstein J, Roffwarg H, et al: Synchronization of augmented luteinizing hormone secretion with sleep during puberty. *N Engl J Med* 287:582, 1972

3. Frisch RE and McArthur JW: Menstrual cycles: Fatness as a determinant of minimum weight for height necessary for their maintenance or onset. *Science* 185:949, 1974

4. Abraham G: Personal communication.

5. Sutton J, Coleman M, Casey J, et al: Androgen responses during physical exercise. *Br Med J* 1:520, 1973

6. Dessypris A, Kuoppasalmi K, and Adlercreutz H: Plasma cortisol, testosterone, androstenedione and luteinizing hormone (LH) in a noncompetitive marathon run. *J Steroid Biochem* 7:33, 1976

7. Kuoppasalmi K, Naveri H, Rehunen S, et al: Effect of strenuous anaerobic running exercise on plasma growth hormone, cortisol, luteinizing hormone, testosterone, androstenedione, estrone and estradiol. *J Steroid Biochem* 7:823, 1976

8. Jurkowski J, Jones N, Walker W, et al: Ovarian hormonal responses to exercise. *J Appl Physiol* 44:109, 1978

9. Shangold M, Freeman R, Thysen B, et al: The relationship between long-distance running, plasma progesterone, and luteal phase length. *Fertil Steril* 31:130, 1979

PREGNANCY

Mona M. Shangold, M.D.

$\mathbf{A}$s women of reproductive age have become more interested and involved in sports, it is not surprising that many questions have arisen about athletic activity during pregnancy. Most women who have appreciated the benefits of exercise in the nonpregnant state are reluctant to accept a nine-month sedentary interval. Highly trained athletes are even more fearful of the effects of a prolonged layoff on future athletic performance.

There is very little information on the effect of training during pregnancy. Obstetricians and pregnant athletes would welcome such data but it is difficult to obtain from human subjects because there is no control population—for each exercising woman, how the pregnancy would have turned out in the absence of exercise remains unknown—and it is unethical to suggest a potentially dangerous activity when a human life is involved.

The following discussion is intended as an overview of obstetrics as it pertains to the athlete, not as a comprehensive review of obstetrics per se.

Normal obstetrical physiology

Cardiovascular: Normal pregnancy is accompanied by increases in heart rate, cardiac output, stroke volume, and maximal oxygen consumption. Heart rate is greatest at 34 to 36 weeks and then decreases toward normal by term. Maximal oxygen consumption increases progressively throughout pregnancy. Cardiac output is greatest at 25 to 28 weeks. Total blood volume increases as a result of a significantly greater plasma volume and a somewhat greater red cell mass; total blood volume reaches a maximum at 32 to 34 weeks and plateaus at that level until term. The augmented cardiac output of pregnancy results from the increased metabolic demands of the fetoplacental unit, the hypervolemia, and the increased vascularity with arteriovenous shunting. The rise in cardiac output exceeds the rise in pulse rate because stroke volume is also augmented. The increase in cardiac output exceeds the increase in maximal oxygen consumption, leading to a reduction in the arteriovenous oxygen difference. The greater magnitude of the plasma volume expansion compared to that of the red cell mass creates a physiologic hemodilution (or "physiologic anemia of pregnancy") at 28 to 32 weeks. Blood viscosity and circulation time are decreased as a result of the increased plasma volume. Mean blood pressure and peripheral vascular resistance are decreased, especially in the second trimester. Increased venous pressure develops in the lower extremities as a result of greater pressure from the uterus on the inferior vena cava and pelvic veins. In late pregnancy, cardiac output becomes exquisitely sensitive to changes in maternal position. When the woman is supine, the enlarged uterus rests on the inferior vena cava, leading to decreased venous return and decreased cardiac output. Lateral recumbency removes the impediment to venous return, thus increasing cardiac output.

Uterine blood flow is tremendously enhanced in pregnancy, providing oxygen and nutrients to the growing fetus and placenta. Skin blood flow is also greater during pregnancy, allowing for greater dissipation of the heat that results from the increased metabolism of the pregnant body. Renal blood flow and glomerular filtration rate are increased throughout most of pregnancy, but both decline to normal near term.

Pulmonary: Normal pregnancy is accompanied by increases in the tidal volume and the respiratory minute volume ("hyperventilation of pregnancy"). Uterine enlargement causes decreases in the inspiratory reserve volume, the expiratory reserve volume, and the residual volume. Bronchial dilatation produces less resistance in the tracheobronchial tree, thereby increasing the physiologic dead space. Because of these changes, vital capacity and respiratory rate remain essentially constant throughout pregnancy. Alveolar oxygen tension tends to remain normal; the hyperventilation leads to a decrease in alveolar carbon dioxide tension.

Musculoskeletal: Bones develop increased vascularity, especially in the red marrow. Changes in the center of gravity lead to exaggerated lordosis, which increases strain on lower back muscles. Pelvic joints demonstrate edema, capsular thickening, increased synovia, increased vascularity, and relaxation. These changes make the joints somewhat more susceptible to injury.

Effects of sports on pregnancy and labor

The fetus is well protected during early pregnancy by the bones and muscles of the mother's pelvis and during later pregnancy by the cushion of amniotic fluid. The jarring movements involved in strenuous athletic endeavors probably affect it very little. However, many women find it physically uncomfortable to continue training after the fifth month because of the size of the pregnant uterus and the bouncing around of the baby inside, but many have continued strenuous activity throughout pregnancy and have had no adverse effects. There is certainly no evidence to suggest that athletes have any more complications than the general population. Many obstetricians find that their athletic patients have less backache and fatigue. Some have even suggested that athletes might have shorter labor than nonathletes. It has also been suggested that the improved pain tolerance shown by many athletes permits better endurance of pain during labor and delivery. While some investigators have reported a lower incidence of cesarean sections among athletes, such statistics were compiled prior to the modern age of obstetrics and its accompanying techniques for fetal monitoring and different indications for cesarean section.

Pregnancy increases the workload imposed on a woman's body both at rest and during exercise. In addition to supplying the caloric needs of the growing fetus, a pregnant woman works harder by carrying more weight. Physically fit subjects can perform a standardized workload with less of a decrease in blood pH than physically unfit subjects. Thus, it is reasonable to expect a woman entering pregnancy or labor in a state of physical fitness to be better able to handle this added workload than a less-fit woman.

Erkkola and Rauramo studied the physical fitness of 120 primigravidas before and after delivery.[1] They measured pH and lactic acid in the maternal radial artery, the umbilical artery, and the umbilical vein. Higher maternal and fetal pHs were found in women of better physical fitness. These women had lower lactic acid levels after a standard workload and lower lactic acid levels in the umbilical vessels after delivery. Women of greater fitness performed at least as much anaerobic work during labor as did women of lesser fitness; lactic acid accumulation and metabolic acidosis in the former group were averted by high oxygenative capacity. Better-fit women were less likely to have asphyxiated infants than their less-fit counterparts.

Dressendorfer looked at the effects of a strenuous jogging program during two pregnancies and lactation in a healthy, nonathletic woman.[2] Training included running approximately 15 miles a week throughout pregnancy until delivery. Both pregnancies were uncomplicated; both labors and deliveries were uncomplicated; both infants were normal and weighed about 3.5 kg each. Milk production was normal during both lactation-training periods.

During exercise, more blood flows to muscles and skin and less flows to the liver and kidneys. It is not known how strenuously a pregnant woman can exercise before the blood supply to the uterus becomes compromised. Emmanouilides and colleagues found that maternal exercise in sheep caused a decrease in fetal arterial oxygen tension.[3] Morris and coworkers found a decrease in effective uterine blood flow with moderate maternal exercise.[4] Women who have prolonged inadequate blood flow to the pregnant uterus tend to have smaller infants with intrauterine growth retardation. It is probably reasonable for a pregnant woman to continue any activity she practiced before pregnancy at the same level of exertion. It is also probably reasonable for pregnant women to avoid exercising to the point of exhaustion, in order to avoid potential risk to the fetus.

Excessive heat (sustained above 39°C) should be avoided during pregnancy because of a demonstrated association between such exposure and birth defects. This is especially true during neural-groove closure. Women who are distance runners and others exercising in hot environments should check their temperatures immediately after exertion.

While pregnant women with enthusiastic appetites might benefit from the caloric expenditure of vigorous athletic activity, others might find that regular exercise expends too many calories. A woman should gain about 25 pounds during the course of her pregnancy. Weight loss or weight maintenance during pregnancy is not advisable because nourishment will be inadequate for the developing baby. Gaining more than 25 pounds does not provide any additional benefit to the fetus and adds undesirable fat to the mother. Thus, it is important for a pregnant woman to find the precise balance between food intake and exercise to permit gradual weight gain throughout pregnancy.

Effects of pregnancy on sports and fitness

Dressendorfer found improvements in both maximal oxygen uptake and endurance performance associated with running approximately 15 miles a week throughout pregnancy until delivery.[2]

The scientific and lay literatures abound with anecdotal reports of highly competitive athletes who are mothers. Many women find that childbirth did not hinder their athletic performance; others claim that the experience of labor and delivery promoted development of greater stamina. Most such reports are based on questionnaires and subjective findings. Objective data are scarce.

Recommendations

The main determinant of the type of training appropriate for a particular pregnant woman is her prepregnancy fitness and activity level. While the average woman generally can continue any activity at the same level of exertion, extremely active or inactive women might best be advised to follow slightly different guidelines. World-class athletes might consider a reduction in intense training because of the potential adverse effect of exhaustion on uterine blood flow and the high caloric cost of strenuous exercise on a woman who should be gaining weight. (It must be emphasized that these are only potential, as yet unproven, dangers. A physically fit woman probably suffers less of a decrease in uterine blood flow during exercise than one who is physically unfit.) Extremely sedentary individuals will probably benefit from mild and gradual exercise, such as walking and calisthenics. On the other hand, women who are professionally active might not require as much additional exercise for weight control and general well-being during pregnancy as women who are professionally sedentary. There is no evidence to suggest racial differences or age limitations in exercise needs, although women older than 40 should certainly have a stress electrocardiogram before undertaking a training program. It should be noted that the larger breasts of the pregnant woman are in need of particularly good support in order to protect the heavier and more glandular breast tissue from becoming stretched and injured.

In a normal, uncomplicated pregnancy, swimming and jogging can provide excellent cardiovascular and psychological benefits throughout the entire pregnancy, in addition to aiding food-lovers in weight control. Activities that involve sudden starts and stops such as tennis or basketball might be more uncomfortable, although probably not of danger to the well-protected fetus. True contact sports involving direct trauma to the abdomen such as boxing or soccer represent potential hazards and should probably be avoided during pregnancy. Downhill-skiing during late pregnancy requires a sense of balance in a body that has a displaced and changing center of gravity; the difficulty of this feat and risk of falling make this activity a poor choice for the average woman in the latter stages of pregnancy. Stretching and strengthening exercises should be beneficial throughout pregnancy. Competition imposes no known risk to a pregnant woman, provided guidelines are followed (performing at the same level of exertion, listening to body signals, and avoiding exhaustion).

While cold weather probably poses no problem for the pregnant athlete, participation during heat and humidity might make her more uncomfortable and more prone to postural hypotension than in the nonpregnant state. High altitude might also pose a problem because of increased oxygen needs. Running uphill feels like harder work than in the nonpregnant state, but represents no greater danger. As long as the pregnant athlete listens to her body signals and trains at a comfortable pace, no harmful effects should be anticipated.

Following an uncomplicated pregnancy and normal vaginal delivery, a women can resume athletic training as soon as her episiotomy has healed. When she can exercise without pain, adequate healing has occurred. If she has had no episiotomy, training can resume with no delay. Swimming and sexual intercourse should be postponed until the cervix has closed (usually by three weeks after delivery), in order to avoid endometritis. After a cesarean section, a patient can safely resume training as soon as she can do so without pain. Pain is a reasonably good indication that healing is incomplete. The same limitations on swimming and coitus apply as after vaginal delivery.

References

1. Erkkola R and Rauramo L: Correlation of maternal physical fitness during pregnancy with maternal and fetal pH and lactic acid at delivery. *Acta Obstet Gynecol Scand* 55:441, 1976

2. Dressendorfer RH: Physical training during pregnancy and lactation, *Phys Sportsmed* 62:74, 1978

3. Emmanouilides GC, Hobel CJ, Yashiro K, et al: Fetal responses to maternal exercise in the sheep. *Am J Obstet Gynecol* 112:130, 1972

4. Morris N, Osborne SB, Wright HP, et al: Effective uterine blood-flow during exercise in normal and pre-eclamptic pregnancies. *Lancet* 2:481, 1956

WOMEN AT THE SERVICE ACADEMIES

John A. Feagin, M.D.

CHAPTER

26

I t was inevitable that women would be admitted to the service academies; women's contributions to the profession of arms, in both peace and war, have been noteworthy. The first class of women, 119 strong, entered West Point on July 7, 1975. Their story, both philosophically and psychologically, is one of which they can be justly proud.

Certain physiologic findings from this sociologic experiment will be reviewed to provide guidance to the athlete and to those who treat her. Although our data come only from the United States Military Academy at West Point, the other academies have made similar findings.

Great credit should be given to the superintendent, the Academic Board, the commandant of cadets, the Department of Physical Education, the Office of Institutional Research, the staff at the U.S. Army Hospital, and the U.S. Army Research Institute of Environmental Medicine for carefully planning the integration of women into a traditionally all-male bastion and for monitoring and documenting their progress.

Preliminary planning

Intense planning for admission of women to West Point began in early 1975. In addition to the obvious initial considerations, Project 60 (using 60 volunteer high school girls) was initiated to evaluate physiologic differences between men and women in this age group, to define what adjustments had to be made in our well-established, all-male physical-education training program, and to search out programs that would provide the optimum physical development and individual improvement.[1] The essential difference between this study and previous ones is that most historical studies have been conducted with Olympic-level athletes, while Project 60 was carried out with an unselected group of female volunteers from the surrounding communities.

Project 60 measured physical, psychological, and anthropometric data over a seven-week period. Body fat, aerobic power and performance, and related variables were compared in a running program and a strength program. Some of the findings of this study can be related to the care and training of female athletes.

Results of training programs

Only certain aspects of the West Point experience will be cited. Anyone who wants in-depth information can obtain it from the Director, Department of Physical Education, U.S. Military Academy, West Point, N.Y. 10996.

In addition to the obvious differences in height, weight, and angular alignment, the female athlete has only 50 per cent of the muscle mass of her male counterpart; also, even though her size is proportionate, she has only about 80 per cent of the ultimate strength of the male. Some of these differences represent social and cultural influences; how much is physiological limitation cannot be answered by currently available data.

No good longitudinal studies are available to determine the effect of prepubertal and postpubertal training on strength development and muscle mass. Without the influence of testosterone, muscle bulk and muscle definition do not occur in the female—even though exercises are muscle-specific. This failure to develop bulk and muscle definition are usually perceived as an advantage by the female athlete.

Body composition: A relative deficiency in lean-muscle mass is unfortunately compensated for in part by a relative increase in body fat. The average untrained female carries a body fat of 24.5 per cent; subsequent training reduces this to 19 per cent (average).

Her male counterpart averages 14 per cent body fat before training; subsequently, his fat may drop to as little as 3 to 5 per cent. An average of 12 per cent difference in body fat is significant and affects performance at every level. There is increased body heat due to increased insulation, and an increased cardiovascular rate, which is necessary for perfusion. The increased weight, which does not enhance performance, also lowers the center of gravity, and the increased rotary mass of the lower extremities increases the moment of inertia. Even with increased cardiovascular fitness, the body fat in the military academy women seldom dropped below 12 per cent.

Cardiorespiratory: Cardiorespiratory fitness of young women entering the service is usually 20 to 25 per cent lower than that of men entering the same program. The aerobic power response to physical training should be approximately the same in both men and women, but firm data are not available. Fundamentally, it is accepted that men have a higher stroke volume, increased vital capacity, increased hemoglobin, and a lower resting and exercise pulse rate. On a similar program, women showed an 8 per cent increase in maximal oxygen utilization, whereas men showed only a 1 per cent increase. The average oxygen utilization for men is 52 ml/kg/min, compared with 43 ml/kg/min for women. This deficit in cardiorespiratory capacity dictates that training programs for men and women should differ, to compensate for the physiological differences between them.

Psychological: There are no comprehensive psychological studies on the effect of training on the woman athlete. In a random group in which a profile of mood-status was determined subsequent to a training program, there was a decreased depression index and decreased anger. The profile also showed decreased physical vigor and decreased eagerness for physical education, which may reflect fatigue and unfamiliarity with an extensive seven-week program.

The lack of knowledge regarding psychological and motivational factors is an important area that warrants research and attention by the sports-medicine specialist.

There are certain other noteworthy observations from Project 60 and Project Summertime (Summertime was an evaluation of the first class of 119 women).[2] Specifically, the attrition rate for women was no higher than for men, although their program was the same (with the exception of minimum physiological differences). The following points are pertinent for those who plan women's sports programs: Upper-body strength was extremely low as compared to the relative high capability for lower-body strength performance. Strength did improve markedly with training, but was not quickly gained. The "fatigue syndrome" was apparent in two ways: There was a 10 per cent decrease in performance of specific muscle-strength activities at the end of seven weeks of training, and there was a higher rate of lower-leg symptoms in women compared with men.

Women had an approximately threefold increase in injuries and lost-duty time compared with men on a similar running program. In addition, lower-extremity fatigue fractures were 10 times more common in women as men. Women on a strength-development program significantly increased their anaerobic capacity and strength. Pre- and post-testing flexibility exercises showed no changes or evidence of inadequacy on the part of the women.

Finally, there is no evidence that menstruation affected performance or physical conditioning; in fact, the symptoms associated with menstruation decreased in a significant percentage of women as a result of this well-designed physical-development program.

Although I've discussed only a small portion of the data obtained, it's clear from our findings that training programs for women must proceed at a different pace and in a different format from those developed for men. The female athlete and her trainer/coach/physician should be aware of the known physiological differences—anthropometric, cardiorespiratory, and psychological—that affect performance. They should also be aware that in-depth data are not now available for many significant areas—the effect of training through puberty on endurance and cardiorespiratory performance; the upper-body strength deficiency; the fatigue syndrome; increased possibility of stress fractures; and psychological differences. Moreover, training programs should be designed for the differences between the sexes. Women's training programs should emphasize increasing cardiovascular fitness, decreasing body fat, increasing upper-body strength, and developing specific mechanical skills, such as running, throwing, changing direction, and the like.

As physicians/coaches/trainers of women athletes, we must seek more in-depth knowledge, and our interest in research should be directed toward a more scientific approach to the training of the woman athlete.

References

1. Peterson JA: Summary Report Project 60. West Point, NY: United States Military Academy, Office of Physical Education, 1976

2. Stauffer, R: Comparison of USMA men and women on selected physical performance measures—Project Summertime. West Point, NY: United States Military Academy, Office of Physical Education, 1976

THE
MATURE
ATHLETE

Christine E. Haycock, M.D.

CHAPTER

27

While most of this book is devoted to the young athlete, we cannot neglect some specific factors relating to the mature participant.

Of the millions of women jogging, swimming, bowling, golfing, and playing tennis, approximately 20 to 25 per cent are older than 50. We have to expect a greater number of medical problems with increasing age, but older women are, nevertheless, being encouraged to participate in athletic activities because of the potential benefits.

Women are now more concerned about their general health; many are dieting, and those who enter exercise programs find it very enjoyable from a social point of view.

My 89-year-old father has been active in sports all his life and continues to play golf. While not indulging in a formal sport, my 85-year-old mother has been a long-walk advocate all her life, even now disdaining cars to go to the supermarket. I am convinced it is this vigorous life-style that is at least partially responsible for my parents' longevity.

While we know that flexibility and strength decrease with age, the process can be slowed by beginning a physical fitness program in youth, and by maintaining it as you age.

The impetus for such programs must come from the family physician. Obesity is often a secondary consequence of psychologically self-imposed inactivity. The individual needs reassurance and encouragement from an authority figure—such as a doctor—to enter an exercise program. In the past, physicians have been reluctant to recommend such programs, in part because of their own inactivity and physical shortcomings.

The mature woman who desires to enter a program after many years of inactivity must take certain precautions. A thorough physical examination—as described earlier in this book—with special emphasis on cardiovascular problems, diabetes, and arthritis is a must.

In addition to the usual cardiograms, stress tests under close medical supervision are required. Blood chemistry profiles—to uncover diabetes or renal disease—are important, as are X-rays to determine if any arthritic problems exist.

If available, preprogram tests to measure muscular fitness, aerobic capacity, and flexibility are also desirable. Dietary counseling, particularly in cases where a loss of weight is desirable, is another valuable adjunct.

Such programs are frequently available at medical centers, at university hospitals, or, in modified form, at local Ys or community centers. The physician should canvass the community to ascertain the availability of such facilities.

Much encouragement for such programs has come from the Federal Government through the President's Council on Physical Fitness, established in 1956 as a youth-fitness program, but expanded in 1963, and reorganized in 1970 to include adult fitness.

Herbert de Vries of the University of Southern California has studied the effects of aging on physical fitness perhaps more than any other investigator in the United States. He has concluded: "In view of the many benefits likely to result from the improvement of physical fitness in the elderly, it seems desirable to begin the implementation of programs in (1) exercise (2) nutrition and (3) stress reduction, or relaxation procedures. However, training of older people in these areas requires instructors with highly specialized preparation and skills."[1] He is concerned that such resources are not currently readily available and is pressing the Government, especially the Subcommittee on Aging, to make funds available for more studies.

As a result of his efforts and those of others interested in gerontology, programs teaching physical fitness for senior citizens are being developed in more and more cities. Such programs generally consist of lectures and discussions on weight control, smoking, and tension reduction.

Exercise routines fall into several categories:

• Relaxation exercises to ease tension by learning to relax different body parts (yoga exercises stress this), visualization techniques, and breathing exercises.

• Aerobic exercises, walking, jogging; folk, square, or aerobic dancing; and even belly dancing.

• Flexibility exercises, including stretching routines, yoga, or simple calisthenics.

• Strength exercises using either isometrics, light isotonics, or weight routines.

In any exercise program the key factor is to start slowly, as aging, flabby muscles are easily injured. It is important that all these programs be graded, starting with very brief routines and gradually increasing as muscle tone improves.

Walking is a relaxing exercise. Increasing the pace to a brisk walk, or to a jog, increases the benefits.

Dancing in its different forms is a method of exercise that most of us have indulged in, and hence it is one that the older citizen can easily be encouraged to participate in again.

Calisthenics, to be successful, must be simple, varied, and fun to do. When performed in a group they are more enjoyable for most than when done alone.

Most older participants should be taught to monitor their heartbeats during exercise by taking their carotid pulse; they should be instructed as to the specific rate (usually about 120 beats per minute) to be maintained. In any event, the pulse rate should never exceed twice the normal rate (rate should be kept below 132 beats per minute). The women should be told to rest if the pulse becomes too rapid.

Hence, we can see that the primary purpose of adult-fitness programs is to improve the physical capacity and vitality of the participants as well as to enhance their ability to deal with tension and frustration.

As a greater portion of the population of the United States enters the over-50 age group, more emphasis on fitness programs will help to limit our rising health-care costs.

Reference

1. de Vries H: Physiology of physical conditioning for the elderly. In *Guide to Fitness After 50* (Harris R and Frankel LJ, eds), pp 47-52. New York: Plenum, 1977

DRUGS AND THE ATHLETE

Louis R. Munch, D.P.E.

CHAPTER

28

With the rise of commercial-professional sports and the increased interest in the Olympic games, both national and international attention is focused on the emotional issue of doping or additive drug use by competitive athletes. It seems that our affluent, consumer-oriented society has produced a breed of athlete with no fear of swallowing or being injected with almost anything if it is given by a physician and if it promises athletic success.[1] However, the actual involvement of the medical profession, in both this country and abroad, can be debated. Some individuals have pointed out that countries such as East Germany and the Soviet Union have highly sophisticated sports-medicine programs in which the use of additive drugs by athletes is very carefully supervised and controlled. They argue that most United States athletes are far behind in the chemical-technology race because Americans are legally forced to experiment on their own, while foreign athletes have the benefits of medical supervision and control. In essence, the specific problem for many athletes is the fierce competitive spiral: "If they're taking it, how can I compete effectively without it?"

Practicing physicians should be aware that restorative drugs may properly be used to therapeutically treat an illness or injury independent of the athletic competition. However, when a specific additive drug is prescribed or artificially used to inflate performance or to allow an athlete to continue performing, then the substance is being abused because it gives rise to unfair advantage.[2] It behooves physicians, coaches, trainers, and athletes to be aware that incidental use as well as purposeful abuse of medications to affect performance can be grounds for disqualification. A classic example occurred in Munich in 1972, when Rick DeMont, Olympic gold medalist in the 400-meter freestyle swimming, had his medal recalled because he was taking small amounts of pseudoephedrine and ephedrine for an asthma condition. In order to prevent a recurrence of the DeMont case in the 1976 Olympics, two drug consultants were hired by the U.S. Olympic Committee. They found that approximately one-third of the Olympic swimming team members had with them in the training camp medications containing banned ingredients that could have caused their disqualification if detected in urine samples.[3]

Another object lesson for sports physicians was the Mandell case. A San Diego psychopharmacologist was put on five years' probation and stripped of his right to prescribe psychoactive drugs by the California Board of Medical Quality Assurance for giving excessive amounts of amphetamines to 11 members of the Chargers football team.[4] Mandell asserted that as a volunteer consultant to that professional team for three years he observed many players taking pregame doses of up to 150 mg of amphetamine to blunt pain and to produce "controlled violence." As his justification, Mandell claimed that the players became desperate when their amphetamine supply was no longer available from the team trainers and that he legally prescribed the amphetamines because he wanted to control the purity of their supply while medically attempting to reduce or stop the players' drug use.[5]

Most of the research literature on the efficacy of various doping agents (amphetamines, caffeine, anabolic steroids, and blood doping) is contradictory and inconclusive. Shinnick summarizes it this way: "A lot of drug information is very contradictory. We have people saying drugs don't help athletes in their athletic performance, yet athletes that I am familiar with are taking drugs and are increasing their performance from sometimes average athletes to world class champions. There is no trust in the medical profession among the athletes."[6]

In educating competitive athletes about the possible medical consequences of additive drugs taken as ergogenic aids, physicians must be careful about their approach and the biases they express, or their credibility will be lost. It is also important to note that a basic principle of pharmacology is that humans are individuals and that even the same person may react differently to the same drug at different times. When we consider this important factor and specific differences in drugs, dosages, methods of administration, time intervals, criterion measures, methods of evaluation (laboratory, clinical, and field), statistical analyses, and supplemental or control considerations, it is not unusual to find differing experimental results.

Anabolic-androgenic steroids

Most sports enthusiasts would probably agree that physical strength and body size are factors that affect the outcome of specific types of athletic activities such as weight lifting, football, wrestling, and various track events. However, the precise role that strength and size play, relative to other physical/psychological/emotional considerations, in the successful outcome of such activities could be debated.

It is interesting that the strength differences between most males and females are usually not apparent until puberty, at which time there is a dramatic increase in the strength of the male's muscles. Ever since it was discovered that testosterone, the main androgen, was responsible for the masculinizing changes that males usually experience, physiologists, coaches, and athletes themselves suspected that high androgen levels might be related to success in athletic competition.[7]

Over the years, a great number of testosterone derivatives—anabolic steroids—were prepared and medically tested in the search for therapeutic compounds that might promote general body growth (favorable nitrogen balance) with fewer androgenic or masculinizing effects than testosterone itself. It must be remembered that all powerful drugs have more than just one effect and that a complete dissociation of anabolic from androgenic effects in these substances has not yet been convincingly achieved.[8] Practicing physicians and others who desire to use such substances to increase the size and strength of athletes should remember that such a use is illegal, medically dangerous, and questionable in outcome. In fact, the Food and Drug Administration has limited these powerful substances to the following conditions: aplastic anemia, disseminated breast cancer, pituitary dwarfism, and serious endocrine disturbances.[9]

Based upon a review of the literature in the fields of medicine, physiology, endocrinology, and physical education, the American College of Sports Medicine has taken this position with regard to anabolic-androgenic steroid use by athletes: "Serious and continuing effort should be made to educate male and female athletes, coaches, physical educators, physicians, trainers, and the general public regarding the inconsistent effects of anabolic-androgenic steroids on improvement of human physical performance and the potential dangers of taking certain forms of these substances, especially in large doses for prolonged periods."[10]

In a reaction to that position statement, Allan Ryan, a noted authority on sports medicine and chief editor of *Physician and Sportsmedicine*, has commented that the statement is "all right," but doesn't go as far as it should. He believes that athletes are not only wasting their money and deluding themselves, but are endangering their health by using anabolic steroids. He asserts: "Myths in sports die hard. Pussyfooting by scientific bodies doesn't help kill them."[11]

Medical authorities have emphasized that any drug sufficiently potent to alter the body's metabolism is also likely to produce a number of possible untoward or undesirable effects. Although these effects are usually dose-dependent and not consistently seen, the best-substantiated hazard in adults is liver damage in the form of intrahepatic cholestasis (interference with bile flow after its formation by liver cells) with the orally active C-17 alkylated steroids.[12] Because the liver is the main organ involved in the deactivation of biochemical substances introduced into the body, it is not unusual to expect some type of hepatic involvement. A second serious pathological liver condition called peliosis hepatis (blood-filled cysts) has been reported in some medical patients receiving androgenic-anabolic steroid therapy.[13] It should be stressed, however, that the main life-threatening concern currently focuses on the suspected link between steroids and liver cancer. To date, primary hepatocellular cancer has been reported in at least 12 medical patients who were given anabolic steroids as part of their therapy.[14-18] These cases strengthen the evidence that exogenous anabolic-androgenic steroids may produce cancerous liver tumors in some individuals.

According to Frasier, the most significant androgen effect in the prepubertal or pubertal athlete is accelerated epiphyseal development and possible premature epiphyseal closure of the long bones. This could chop inches off the child's potential height.[19] Gynecomastia has also been seen in prepubertal children during steroid administration; this is due to the conversion of these agents or a metabolite into estrogens in the body.[20]

In mature men, it is reported that the antigonadotrophic effects of these agents have produced a long list of sex-related dysfunctions, including loss of libido, decreased potency, diminished testicular size, and azoospermia.[19] In women, the following undesirable effects have been reported: masculinization, hirsutism, deepening of the voice, acne, baldness, and clitoral enlargement. It is important to note that under some conditions these effects may not be reversible.[9]

It is clear that the use of anabolic steroids to enhance athletic performance can be medically dangerous and should be strongly discouraged. The medical use of these substances for therapeutic purposes should be reserved for serious life-threatening illnesses, in which case, the risk-benefit ratio warrants their use.

Amphetamines

Because of their strong desire to excel and to break existing records, a number of athletes have resorted to various agents purported to enhance success. As we move closer and closer to the upper limits of physical performance, where it becomes difficult to transcend physical limitations, more athletes are tempted to experiment with these so-called ergogenic aids. (For a comprehensive discussion of the role of ergogenic aids in muscular performance, the reader is referred to the publication edited by Morgan.[21] Those interested in the variety of drugs used in athletic performance are referred to the book by Williams.[22])

Knowledgeable individuals would probably agree that the stimulants most commonly used by athletes are the amphetamines. These substances belong to a class of drugs known as sympathomimetics because they produce effects resembling the stimulation of the sympathetic nervous system. Amphetamines are a close relative of epinephrine, with similar chemical structure and effects. The main effects are thought to be due to cortical and reticular activating system stimulation.[23] The central nervous system stimulation results in increased alertness, elation, euphoria, excitement or irritability, a delay in the onset of fatigue, and anorexia. It is important to remember that fatigue and depression usually follow the central stimulation, which is why somebody said: "'Speed' is like a Christmas package with a time bomb inside."[24]

Medical concerns about the use of amphetamines by athletes have revolved around a number of specific effects that could jeopardize health. For instance, amphetamines tend to produce tolerance in many individuals, so that larger and larger doses become necessary to achieve the same effect. Amphetamines also tend to produce psychological dependence, as the stimulatory effects tend to reinforce their continued use.[25] Some athletes in contact or collision sports such as professional football have used these stimulants to produce hostile or aggressive behavioral changes prior to competition. In some situations, especially at higher dosages, paranoid reactions have been said to occur.[26] Because central stimulation might last longer than initially desired for a particular athletic contest, insomnia or overstimulation might cause some competitors to turn to various sedative-hypnotics such as barbiturates to counter the sympathomimetic effects of the amphetamines.[27]

The use of these substances by athletes could also produce a number of potentially serious and life-threatening situations. First of all, these powerful substances are sometimes used to mask fatigue and to remove the normal physiological and psychological restraints intended to prevent overexertion. It cannot too strongly be emphasized that the combination of high ambient air temperatures, high relative humidity, heavy and long physical activity, and high-dose amphetamine use could result in death from cardiovascular collapse because of impaired temperature regulation. According to Williams, the rationale for this physiological effect is that amphetamines tend to constrict the small blood vessels in the skin and that cutaneous vasodilation is necessary for heat elimination from the body.[22]

It is important to keep in mind that a large number of physiological responses to exercise are magnified by heat. For instance, as hyperthermia develops, one's core and skin temperatures, sweat rate, and heart rate all tend to show a corresponding linear increase. The extent of these physiological changes is contingent upon individual factors, such as one's physical condition, the degree of acclimatization, and one's sex.[28] Nunneley has stated that women are generally less heat-tolerant than men because of their small size, high fat content, low levels of physical fitness, and lack of acclimatization. However, it should be noted that this specific sex response to thermal stress tends to disappear when women athletes are physically conditioned and/or heat acclimatized.[29]

A second life-threatening condition that the amphetamine-using athlete faces is related to the fact that such drugs can seriously complicate the use of surgical anesthesia given on an emergency basis.[30] This poses a special problem in contact or collision sports in which the risk of bodily injury is inherently high.

Because amphetamines mimic the powerful effects of epinephrine, it is not unusual to find hypertension in some young people who have been using these drugs. Moderate to severe hypertension is a fairly common health problem in this country, and the nonmedical use of sympathomimetic drugs by individuals with normally elevated blood pressures could be dangerous. Another life-threatening medical problem is the possibility of developing cardiac arrhythmias. In order to pump the blood needed by the body, the heart muscle functions with a specific rhythm of contractions and relaxations. If this rhythm is disturbed, especially during intense physical exercise, a medical emergency could easily arise. The final serious medical problem, necrotizing angiitis, has been found in a number of amphetamine-users. This disorder is a type of vascular disease characterized by the pathological inflammation and necrosis or death of various cells.[31]

Anti-inflammatory agents and analgesics

It has been said that Joe Namath, former quarterback for the New York Jets, played game after game despite great pain from his battle-scarred knees, and that Willis Reed led the Knicks to victory over the Lakers despite an injured and painful right hip. Because these key players helped their respective teams—despite their personal pain—teammates and fans thought of them as quite courageous. On the other hand, Bill Walton of the Portland Trail Blazers refused to participate in any more basketball games because he didn't want to risk further damage to his injured left foot. As a result of Walton's action, his strength of character was questioned.[32] When one considers the implications of these incidents, an interesting question arises: "When should responsible people prohibit players from playing while injured, and when should responsible people prohibit themselves from playing because of an injury they have sustained?"

Although most people usually consider physical pain to be without redeeming qualities, and something to be avoided, it is important to note that pain serves some useful functions. If we didn't perceive pain when we injured ourselves, serious bodily damage could result. Thus, pain is the means by which our bodies protect us from further injury. With an unmedicated athletic injury, pain produces muscle spasms that tend to splint the injured part; this response acts to prevent further motion or use of the injured area. If anti-inflammatory agents—salicylates, cortisone, phenylbutazone, indomethacin—and analgesics—ethyl chloride spray, procaine, or lidocaine—are introduced, the normal response to painful stimuli would be compromised. The possibility of arthritis in later life from repeated injuries should be of real concern to everyone involved in athletic activities.[33]

It should be kept in mind that a number of undesirable local effects such as collagen necrosis may occur if cortisone is repeatedly injected into an injured joint or tendon. Kennedy and Willis have demonstrated, in their animal experiments, that physiologic doses of local steroids placed directly into a normal tendon can weaken it significantly for up to 14 days following the injection. Because of this finding, they advise patients receiving local steroids to avoid vigorous muscular activity for at least two weeks as a safeguard to prevent spontaneous tendon rupture.[34]

In deciding whether the injured athlete should be allowed to continue participating, the sports physician needs to consider the following: the nature and extent of the injury and the possible consequences; the temperament, motivation, and pain threshold of the athlete; and the game situation and circumstances.[35] It is important for the physician serving young amateur athletes to remember that there is usually a great desire on the part of the injured athlete to return to competition. Because of the typical "do-or-die" school spirit, the sports physician must use sound judgment in order to help protect the injured athlete's health and well-being.

References

1. Power G: Drug scene in sports: Who, what, how and why. *New York Times,* p 2S, Oct 19, 1975

2. Mofenson HC, Greensher J, and Reilly DJ: Drugs in sports. *Clin Pediat* 16:501, 1977

3. Bender KJ and Lockwood DH: Use of medications by U.S. Olympic swimmers. *Phys Sportsmed* 511:63, 1977

4. Amphetamine conferees rally behind psychiatrist. *Medical World News*, pp 40, 45, Oct 16, 1978

5. Mandell AJ: Of football players, amphetamines, and the law. *Medical World News,* p 61, Dec 26, 1977

6. Proper and improper use of drugs by athletes. Hearings before the Subcommittee to Investigate Juvenile Delinquency of the Committee on the Judiciary, United States Senate, Ninety-Third Congress, June 18 and July 12 and 13, 1973. Washington: U.S. Government Printing Office, 1973

7. Lamb DR: Androgens and exercise. *Med Sci Sports* 7:1, 1975

8. Murad F and Gilman AG: Androgens and anabolic steroids. In *Pharmacological Basis of Therapeutics* (Goodman LS and Gilman A, eds), 5th ed, pp 1451-1471. New York: Macmillan, 1975

9. Anabolic steroids for athletes. *Med Let Drugs Ther* 18:120, 1976

10. American College of Sports Medicine: Position statement on the use and abuse of anabolic-androgenic steroids in sports. *Med Sci Sports,* 9:xi, 1977

11. Ryan AJ: Anabolic steroids: The myth dies hard. *Phys Sportsmed* 63:3, 1978

12. Athletes and anabolic steroids. *Drug Ther Bull* 15:43, 1977

13. Bagheri SA and Boyer JL: Peliosis hepatis associated with androgenic-anabolic steroid therapy. *Ann Intern Med* 81:610, 1974

14. Farrell GC, Uren RF, Perkins KW, et al: Androgen-induced hepatoma. *Lancet* 1:430, 1975

15. Johnson FL: Association of oral androgenic-anabolic steroids and life-threatening disease. *Med Sci Sports,* 7:284, 1975

16. Meadows AT, Naiman JL, and Valdes-Dapena M: Hepatoma associated with androgen therapy for aplastic anemia. *J Pediat* 84:109, 1974

17. Committee on Neoplastic Diseases: Is liver cancer induced by treating aplastic anemia with androgenic agents? *Pediatrics* 53:764, 1974

18. Liver tumors and steroid hormones. *Lancet* 2:1481, 1973

19. Frasier SD: Androgens and athletes. *Am J Dis Child* 125:479, 1973

20. Laron Z: Breast development induced by methandrostenolone (Dianabol). *J Clin Endocrin Metab* 22:450, 1962

21. Morgan WP, ed: *Ergogenic Aids and Muscular Performance.* New York: Academic Press, 1972

22. Williams, MH: *Drugs and Athletic Performance.* Springfield, Ill: Thomas, 1974

23. Innes IR and Nickerson M: Norepinephrine, epinephrine, and the sympathomimetic amines. In *Pharmacological Basis of Therapeutics* (Goodman LS and Gilman A, eds), 5th ed, pp 477-513. New York: Macmillan, 1975

24. Sheehy G: *Speed Is of the Essence.* New York: Pocket Books, 1971

25. Edison GR: Amphetamines: A dangerous illusion. *Ann Intern Med* 74:605, 1971

26. Percy EC: Athletic aids: Fact or fiction? *Can Med Assoc* 117:601, 1977

27. Clarke KS, ed: *Drugs and the Coach.* Washington: American Association for Health, Physical Education, and Recreation, 1972

28. Wells CL: Sexual differences in heat stress response. *Phys Sportsmed* 59:78, 1977

29. Nunneley SA: Physiological responses of women to thermal stress: A review. *Med Sci Sports* 10:250, 1978

30. Kostelanetz R: "Nick the knife," or, the life of a football doctor. *New York Times Magazine,* pp 12-27, Dec 19, 1971

31. Grinspoon L and Hedblom P: *Speed Culture: Amphetamine Use and Abuse in America.* Cambridge, Mass: Harvard University Press, 1975

32. Hyland DA: Participation in athletics: Is it worth all the suffering? *New York Times,* p 2S, Nov 26, 1978

33. Simpson GH: Injuries and pain: A former player hurts and regrets. *New York Times,* p 2S, Nov 26, 1978

34. Kennedy JC and Willis RB: Effects of local steroid injections on tendons: A biomechanical and microscopic correlative study. *Am J Sports Med* 4:11, 1976

35. Novich MM and Taylor B: *Training and Conditioning of Athletes.* Philadelphia: Lea & Febiger, 1970

AQUATIC SPORTS

Allen B. Richardson, M.D.

CHAPTER

29

It should be said at the outset that most medical problems occurring in conjunction with aquatic sports can affect both women and men. Competitive swimming and diving have always been popular sports among people of both sexes. Until recently, however, there have been relatively few opportunities, at the college level, for female competition. As collegiate programs develop, and with the advent of women's water polo, we will see more women in aquatic-sports careers.

Although I will deal primarily with competitive swimmers, the material is applicable to most other aquatic sports, including water polo, diving, and long-distance swimming.

Orthopedic problems

Swimmers commonly develop some relatively specific problems related to the shoulder and knee.

Swimmer's shoulder: Shoulder pain is the most common orthopedic affliction of competitive swimmers. Most studies cite an incidence of between 30 and 60 per cent. The cause of the pain is repeated microtrauma of impingement of the head of the humerus (and the attached rotator cuff) on the acromion and the coracoacromial ligament.

Shoulder motion in freestyle, backstroke, and butterfly consists primarily of adduction and internal rotation during the pull-through phase of the arm stroke, and abduction and external rotation during the recovery phase. Body roll of as much as 120° from one stroke to the next allows for maximum reach in freestyle and backstroke; in butterfly, in which body roll is negligible, body lift plays an important part in allowing recovery of the arms.

If one assumes an average daily workout of 10,000 yards, six days per week, an average of 20 strokes per lap, of which 60 per cent is butterfly, freestyle, or backstroke, then each shoulder undergoes 14,400 revolutions per week. As most competitive swimmers train 10 or 11 months per year, each shoulder might sustain 720,000 revolutions a year. Perhaps because of their smaller size, decreased muscle mass, or decreased stroke power, women swimmers tend to take more strokes per lap than men. As expected, among national and world-caliber swimmers, shoulder problems are more common in women. Sixty-eight per cent of the females on the 1978 International Federation of Amateur Swimmers (FINA) World Championship team complained of shoulder problems, compared with only 50 per cent of the men.

As the humeral head repeatedly impinges on the acromion and coracoacromial ligament, the subacromial bursa becomes inflamed and painful. This inflammation eventually spreads to the surrounding rotator cuff and long head of the biceps tendon; the often-made diagnosis of biceps tendinitis is perhaps too narrow a concept, as this is the result, not the cause, of impingement. Once scar tissue has formed and further decreased the space between the acromion and humeral head, the condition may become cyclic and recalcitrant to treatment.

Baseball players are known to develop a very similar condition, again from repeated, forced abduction of the arm during throwing. Although a baseball player's arm does not undergo nearly as many revolutions (perhaps 500 pitches per week) as does a swimmer's, there is considerably greater, more explosive, force applied with each revolution.

The pain is often diffuse and located either anteriorly or anterolaterally about the acromion. The swimmer usually states that the shoulder hurts most during the early and middle season when workouts are longest, and is exacerbated by the use of hand paddles. Most swimmers who have pain are sprinters or middle-distance swimmers (50 yards through 400 yards in competition); this is ironic, as one might expect the distance swimmers—those with the greatest workouts—to experience more pain than others. The painful shoulder is more often than not on the breathing side; most often this is the side of the dominant hand.

The most useful forms of treatment are stretching and warmth prior to practice, followed by ice treatments after practice. Ultrasound therapy is often helpful, with oral anti-inflammatory agents as an adjunct. The judicious use of steroid injections is helpful to the swimmer with persistent symptoms, and surgical intervention should be considered only when these other measures have failed. It should be emphasized that the recuperative period following an operative procedure may be as long as nine months, and returning to full capacity in competitive swimming would be difficult after this long a period of inactivity even if the swimmer had not had medical problems.

With the advent of women's water polo, we expect the same types of shoulder problems seen in male water-polo players. Impingement problems as well as subluxation of the shoulder joint can occur. Impingement or overuse of the shoulder is treated in a similar manner as for swimmers.

Repeated subluxation or complete dislocation of the shoulder is a difficult problem in the athlete who wishes to continue throwing. Most nonsurgical measures do not prevent instability of the shoulder joint, and many operative procedures, although they correct the instability, decrease throwing ability.

Swimmer's knee: Knee problems affect perhaps 25 per cent of competitive swimmers. While knee pain is often thought to be limited to those who swim breaststroke, there are several types of knee problems that affect swimmers.

Chondromalacia refers to a softening of the cartilage, usually the articular surface of the patella. It is a painful condition that may or may not be related to subluxation or dislocation of the patella. In the general population, it is more common in females than males by a ratio of three to two, so it is not surprising that chondromalacia is often the cause of knee pain in female swimmers. It is also most common in the adolescent age group. Because breaststrokers place a large valgus stress on their knees as well as maximum repeated flexion/extension, they tend to exacerbate chondromalacic and subluxation problems.

Chondromalacia-type pain is not, however, limited to breast-strokers. Indeed, it seems that swimmers of all strokes can suffer from this problem. This probably is due to the fact that quadriceps contraction and some flexion/extension are necessary to all types of kicking, and pushing off the wall at the end of each lap requires up to 90° of knee flexion.

Treatment of this very difficult problem is directed toward rest, ice therapy, and anti-inflammatory agents. If patellar malalignment is felt to be the origin of the problem, a surgical realignment can be tried; it often helps. Again, surgical intervention would be advocated only if more conservative measures, especially quadriceps strengthening, had failed.

What is classically known as "breaststroker's knee" is medial collateral ligament strain. It is a result of repeated valgus stress applied to the medial collateral ligament, especially with the breaststroke frog kick. It is also a common condition among water-polo players, the majority of whom employ an "eggbeater" kick to tread water; a combination whip and/or eggbeater kick is also used for quick in-water starts and turns in water polo. The more severe medial collateral ligament strains can lead to effusions and persistent pain, although rarely to instability of the knee.

It is postulated that women demonstrate greater ligamentous laxity than males of the same age and that this may be under the control of the female hormones. While it certainly would lead to increased range of motion of the joint, the increased instability also would tend to cause improper joint function and pain.

Osgood-Schlatter disease is an affliction of the tibial tubercle, also termed tibial apophysitis or football knee, although it is commonly found in other athletes. Because it is relatively common in patients between the ages of five and 15 years, it is not an uncommon condition in competitive swimmers, most of whom begin their careers during this age period.

The Osgood-Schlatter lesion is a result of repeat traction on and subsequent inflammation of the tibial tubercle, which, in this age group, represents a traction apophysis for the attachment of the patellar ligament. In swimming, particularly with the breast-stroke, as well as in water polo, where repeated flexion/extension motions take place, Osgood-Schlatter disease may occur frequently. This may be even more true in divers.

Symptoms vary from individual to individual; however, they nearly always include pain and swelling about the tibial tubercle, particularly with active contraction of the quadriceps muscle. There is often a palpable bony-hard enlargement of the tibial tubercle. Symptoms would be particularly apparent when pushing off the wall, with starts, quick direction changes in the water, or jumping on the diving board.

The cause of this disease is not known. It is slightly more common in males, but this may be a factor of disparate involvement in strenuous sports. In any event, because females tend to develop the lesion at a younger age than males, a coach working with younger athletes may see more of this type of knee pain in female swimmers.

A very closely related cause of knee pain is Sinding-Larsen-Johansson disease. Again, this represents a traction injury to the distal pole of the patella (the other end of the patellar ligament) and can often produce abnormal calcifications that can be visualized on X-rays.

Fortunately, the condition is usually self-limiting and treatment is directed at relieving the irritation and inflammation of the tibial apophysis and, therefore, the pain. Complete avulsion of the patellar ligament is extremely rare. Standard modes of treatment are anti-inflammatory medication, ice packing, short periods of immobilization, and rest. Unfortunately for the female competitive swimmer—who seems to reach the peak of her career at a younger age than the male—the onset of symptoms and disability are likely to occur during this peak. Once a diagnosis of Osgood-Schlatter disease is made, the coach, athlete, and physician should work out a treatment and training program that will allow maximum performance and minimal symptoms.

Miscellaneous orthopedic problems

Triceps tendinitis: This is an inflammation of the insertion of the triceps muscle located at the back of the elbow and is a result of repeated stress to this area. It is found most commonly in divers, particularly platform divers, who subject the triceps tendon to great, sudden stress when they enter the water hands-first. The conservative measures previously cited (particularly rest, ice packs, and oral anti-inflammatory drugs) are the modalities of choice. Injections of cortisone in this area are probably ill advised and should be used only rarely.

Neck and back problems: These are rather common among athletes, including swimmers. Because of constant repeated axial loading, divers seem to be most susceptible to symptoms of muscle strain and spasm. These symptoms can be quite difficult to relieve either by oral medications or training methods. If a specific "point" area of tenderness can be identified, such as is the case with ilio-lumbar ligament strain, an injection of an analgesic and cortisone-like compound might produce lasting relief.

X-rays of the spine should always be obtained in patients with back pain to rule out the possibility of spondylolysis, a small crack or fracture of the vertebrae produced by repeated stress to the spine. With the correct treatment (rest) these common fractures usually heal.

Ankle problems: Pain in the anterior ankle is not uncommon in freestylers, butterflyers, and backstrokers. The vigorous kicking in all three strokes requires maximum plantarflexion of the ankle; simultaneous supination of the foot produces a more efficient kick, but may lead to pain at the anterolateral joint line. These repeated motions lead to stretching and tearing of the capsule that surrounds the ankle joint. As with other athletic injuries, ankle pain may be treated with ice packing after exercise, oral anti-inflammatory agents, and the judicious use of cortisone injections. Taping of the ankle, even in aquatic sports, to prevent maximal plantarflexion while still allowing some kicking, gives the ankle capsule a chance to heal.

Osteonecrosis: Generally, this problem occurs only in divers, both recreational scuba divers and professionals. Osteonecrosis refers to bone death that occurs as a result of the high pressures to which bones are subjected and the expansion of nitrogen gas in the bone-marrow fat. The incidence is highly variable, ranging from 5 to 80 per cent; the average incidence, among reported studies, is 26 per cent.

Osteonecrosis occurs most frequently in the shafts of the femur and humerus; if it occurs near a joint, it can be the cause of premature degenerative arthritis. Unfortunately, bone death is not always associated with symptoms; silent lesions are often seen on the X-rays of otherwise healthy divers. Further, the occurrence of bone necrosis is not necessarily related to a history of the "bends," and the standard Navy Decompression Tables are of little use in preventing bone damage. Because the lesions are irreversible, treatment is directed at the sequela of damage—degenerative arthritis—to bone near the joint.

Nonorthopedic medical problems

Ear infections: This is easily the most common problem among persons who spend four to six hours in the water daily. Symptoms usually begin with a mild, intermittent earache that can rapidly progress to severe pain that is exacerbated by further immersion. Most competitive swimmers, divers, and water-polo players wear neither earplugs nor nose clips, so exacerbation is inevitable. Earplugs are often uncomfortable, and none available today is completely successful in preventing the entry of water into the external ear canal.

The problem stems from the dissolution of protective cerumen in the external ear canal and the subsequent exposure of the tympanic membrane and surrounding tissues to repeated, prolonged irrigation. Pool water, most of which is slightly alkaline, causes maceration of the tissues, erythema, and inflammation, permitting infection by an organism that is not normally pathogenic. The organism most commonly cultured from the ear is one of the Pseudomonas species.

The best treatment in this case is prevention. Because alkaline pool water tends to destroy the normally acidic milieu of the external ear, thorough drying followed by the use of a mild acid is recommended. Solutions of alcohol and boric acid are available under several brand names and probably are equally effective. The alcohol serves as a dehydrating or drying agent, and the boric acid replaces that which has been destroyed. It is appropriate to use these drops after every practice or competition.

Once symptoms are present, treatment consists of decreasing inflammation and treating any infection. Again, many combination drugs are available; they have in common an anti-inflammatory agent and an antibiotic effective against Pseudomonas. Often these combinations include a topical anesthetic as well.

A word of caution to the athlete: Never insert anything hard or sharp, such as hairpins or toothpicks—or even fingers—into the ear. If the ear is painful, the skin is macerated and susceptible to further damage.

A second word of caution: A simple way to tell if it is the outer ear and not the inner ear that is affected is to pull gently on the ear lobe. If this sharply increases the pain, the outer ear is involved. If the pain is not affected by this maneuver, then the middle ear may be affected; this requires a physician's care as soon as possible. Similarly, a physician should be consulted if pain persists in the outer ear for a prolonged period.

Eye problems: Most competitive swimmers now wear goggles, if not all the time, at least during training. Therefore, competitive swimmers rarely develop problems in this area. Long-distance swimmers and "channel" swimmers find goggles almost indispensable to avoid eye damage from prolonged submersion in salt water.

Prior to the use of goggles, chemical conjunctivitis was relatively common. It is still a common problem among participants in the other aquatic sports. Trauma to the eye is not uncommon among water-polo players. A common mechanism of injury is the inadvertent finger in the eye of an opponent immediately after releasing the ball on a hard throw.

Most commonly, the sclera will be contused and develop a hemorrhage that eventually resolves without treatment. Corneal abrasions, however, are quite painful, require special instruments to make the diagnosis, and are usually treated by patching the eye for a short time.

A more serious lesion, usually due to a direct blow, is the hyphema, or hemorrhage into the anterior chamber of the eye. Besides being painful, this can result in significant visual damage; it, too, requires a special instrument for diagnosis, a physician's care, and often hospitalization.

By far the most serious lesion to the eye is a penetrating injury. If an instrument was used and has impaled the orbit, it should not be removed; emergency services at a hospital are immediately required if any vision is to be saved. If the wound to the orbit is open, the eyelid should be closed, if possible, to prevent the loss of the aqueous and vitreous humours from the eye; again, emergency hospital services are immediately required.

Drowning

This is a problem that, as expected, is an extremely rare occurrence among those involved in aquatic sports. However, aquatic athletes should be well versed in resuscitation procedures, precisely because they are around the water so much. The subject of drowning is complicated, and resuscitation depends on practice and experience; I recommend a course in life-saving and water safety, such as that given by the Red Cross.

Drowning is flooding of the lungs with water and rapid fluid and electrolyte imbalance. Consequently, drowning in fresh water is distinct from drowning in seawater. Because of the hypotonicity of fresh water, a rapid increase in the intravascular blood volume occurs as water flows easily across the alveolar walls. The concentrations of sodium, chloride, calcium, hemoglobin, and proteins all decrease by dilution. Massive hemolysis takes place, resulting in increased potassium concentrations. Death occurs secondary to cardiac ventricular fibrillation due to this large electrolyte imbalance.

Seawater is hypertonic and produces the exact opposite effect: Salt rushes into the intravascular spaces, causing elevations of serum sodium and chloride, while water flows into the lungs, causing severe pulmonary edema. Bradycardia, hypotension, and hypovolemia result in death within a few minutes.

Resuscitation of the drowning victim is aimed at restoring electrolyte and fluid balance, postural drainage and suction, and artificial respiration, accompanied by cardiac resuscitation if circulatory collapse has occurred. Once again, the importance of prior instruction in resuscitative measures should be emphasized.

Further reading

American Red Cross: *Life Saving and Water Safety*. Garden City, NY: Doubleday, 1956

Beckman EL and Elliott DH, eds: *Dysbarism-related Osteonecrosis*. Washington: Department of Health, Education, and Welfare, 1974

Counsilman JE: *Competitive Swimming Manual*. Bloomington, Ind: Counsilman Co, 1977

Counsilman JE: *The Science of Swimming*. Englewood Cliffs, NJ: Prentice-Hall, 1968

Eriksson B and Furberg B: *Swimming Medicine IV*. Baltimore: University Park Press, 1978

Kennedy JC, Hawkins R, and Krissoff WB: Orthopedic manifestations of swimming. *Amer J Sports Med* 6:309, 1978

Wintrobe MM, ed: *Principles of Internal Medicine*. New York: McGraw-Hill, 1970

PRACTICAL GUIDELINES

**Mervyn B. Haycock, M.S., and
Christine E. Haycock, M.D.**

CHAPTER

30

E very sport, whether individual or team, pre-
sents its own set of hazards. A knowledge of some of the potential
dangers and methods of prevention may aid the physician in diag-
nosing the patient's problem and provide advice to minimize future
injury.

We cannot deal with every conceivable circumstance, but will
try to highlight some specific areas. Problems covered in other
chapters will be mentioned only briefly here. Our aim is to suggest
what to look for in diagnostic efforts, but not to discuss treatment.
That information is available in other chapters.

Individual sports

Jogging: It is probably true that jogging is the leading individual
sport right now. There is no question that jogging is an excellent
form of exercise and it can, when done correctly, produce excellent
results insofar as cardiovascular fitness is concerned. Jogging can
and should be safe if each individual takes the right precautions.

Be sure of the athlete's general physical and cardiovascular condition by doing a thorough checkup before she begins to jog. If
there is any doubt of her cardiovascular status, or she is older than
35, she should see a qualified cardiac physician for a stress test.

When she jogs, be sure she wears well-fitting clothing that will
not rub or chafe, and running shoes designed to take the pounding

her feet will get. Be sure she does some of the suggested conditioning exercises before she begins, and does not go out and run as if she were in competition. Tell her to run at her own pace and at a distance that she can handle without great exertion. Let her increase her distance as her conditioning improves. Alternate jogging and walking is a good technique for the novice runner.

Where she runs makes a difference: Running on hard surfaces can produce shin splints. This is not especially serious, but it makes running painful. If at all possible, have her run on dirt or grass surfaces and stay away from the edge of the highway. Many joggers have been hit by cars in the early morning or late evening, when drivers did not see them. If she must run at those times, be sure she wears a bright orange-colored jogging suit or puts some kind of reflective band on her running shirt, or even wears it as a head band. She should always run against the traffic so that she can see the oncoming cars and get out of the way.

Do not let her do something foolish like wearing a plastic sweatsuit, unless you are providing close medical supervision. Plastic sweatsuits are intended primarily for weight loss, and if she sweats profusely she will lose both salt and water and upset her electrolyte balance. Most joggers are not trying to lose weight by running; they run because they enjoy it and because they know it maintains their cardiovascular condition.

Jogging has been called probably the best means to help prevent recurrent heart attacks; again, this must be done under careful supervision, and under no circumstances should the jogger exceed the maximum pulse rate that has been set for her by a cardiologist. Many books on jogging are available—Dr. Joan Ulloyt's *Women's Running* (Mountain View, Cal: World Publications, 1979) is a good one for the female athlete.

Ice and roller skating: With proper-fitting skates and a gradual buildup of ankle strength, there is very little that can happen to the normal skater except for occasional spills.

Collisions occur in ice skating because of careless skating, so it is wise for the skater to keep alert and try to stay out of the way of the fast skater if she is a beginner. The beginning skater should skate off to the side or in the center of the rink. It would be wise for her to attend an ice-skating class first. The younger she starts skating, the better.

Instruct the skater that if she slips and begins to fall she should not put her arms out to try to stop the fall; rather, she should fold her arms and hands into the body and fall on the buttocks as she slides across the ice. If she attempts to use her hands to stop her fall or remains in an outstretched position, two things can happen: She may fracture a wrist or arm, or she may be run over by skaters behind her who are not skillful enough to avoid a collision. Skate edges are sharp and can cause severe lacerations.

Roller skates have essentially the same inherent problems as ice skates, and the same precautions apply. Skating out in the street brings the additional hazard of automobiles.

Track and field: There are many track and field events, so we'll discuss them separately.

Sprinting: As in all track events, a proper warm-up is very important. The sprinter must prepare her body for explosive moves, especially in the hamstring and groin muscles. The colder the day, the more stretching and warm-up are required. A sprinter who runs without proper preconditioning and stretching will end up with pulled muscles and perhaps an achilles-tendon rupture. Muscle pulls and strains may put a sprinter out of competition for a considerable time. Sprinters should have a semitight-fitting shoe, and loose-fitting, nonrestrictive clothing.

Distance and cross-country runners: The distance runner has the same problems as the jogger, but because the individual is competing, the fatigue point may be reached and passed. Therefore, it is essential that the runner be in top-notch condition before she does compete.

A runner must also be very careful about her footing, especially off the track, when running cross-country. Stepping in holes or on rocks or on curbs causes more sprains and falls than does running in streets.

Ankle supports and tapes are not recommended unless the runner must always use them. The longer she uses tape to support her ankles, the harder it will be for her to do without the tape; the day she forgets the tape is the day that a slight strain will turn into a major strain or tear.

Proper running form is a must for the distance runner. Once she has good form that is free from excessive movement, the less chance there is of accelerated fatigue. Recent studies have shown that a normal healthy heart cannot be damaged by endurance-running. If the athlete's body did reach a point of total fatigue, she would black out from oxygen reduction before any damage to the heart occurred. The distance runner should never argue with her coach about whether workouts are too long or too demanding. She can probably make it if she persists. The likelihood that she will injure herself is rather remote.

Shoulder stress and pain may also occur in a runner, usually due to oxygen depletion. It can also be attributed to holding the arms up and the wrist and fingers in a rigid rather than a relaxed position as she runs. This shoulder pain and stress may also be just a result of poor conditioning for the distance she is running. If the athlete has conditioned herself to run the half-mile, she should not expect to be able to run two miles with efficiency; her cardiovascular system is just not prepared to handle the oxygen need, and she will suffer muscle fatigue in a much shorter time. Her mind may be willing but her conditioning is weak, and her body will not be able to meet the task.

Hurdling: There are some obvious possibilities for injury in the hurdle race. Hurdles, if hit, should always tip in the same direction the athlete is running. Splintered hurdles or metal hurdles with exposed nuts or bolts can be hazardous. Hurdles should never be placed on cement surfaces, because a fall on cement can be very abrasive. Cinder tracks are another unfortunate choice for the location of hurdling activities, as a fall on cinders can produce some severe abrasions. (Fortunately, there are not too many cinder tracks anymore.) Embedded cinders should be removed as soon as possible and the abrasion washed out thoroughly and treated to prevent infection.

A hurdler should have her steps between each hurdle carefully planned. This won't necessarily make her a better hurdler, but it will avoid many falls due to improper takeoff distance; by using the correct foot to jump each time, she is less apt to hit the hurdle. Hitting the hurdle with the lead foot usually causes the most serious accidents. The trailing foot and the inside leg may hit and tip a hurdle, but as it is falling behind it usually does not cause any injury except a minor abrasion or contusion.

In addition to the usual warm-up prior to running, a hurdler must also do a full routine of stretching exercises for the groin and hamstring areas. If possible, the runner should go down to the track and take a few leisurely jumps before the actual race is run. A muscle pulled during hurdling will be slow to heal and will disable the runner for a considerable length of time, perhaps longer than for the sprinter or distance runner.

Jumping events: All jumping events demand very good preparation by stretching, plus a very slow initial approach to the actual jump. Jumpers should not make an all-out effort without a slow buildup. Most sprains and torn muscles in jumping events occur before the actual competition, or in the first attempt of the competition, because of improperly preparing the body for that explosive move. A long-jumper must work on her steps so she can concentrate on the jump itself. This will also improve the efficiency of her body effort and lessen the possibility of pulled muscles.

Injury to high-jumpers and pole-vaulters has been greatly reduced by the use of air bags and foam-rubber landing pits. Injuries still occur, however, when a partial attempt is made and the athlete misses the landing pit. The sooner an athlete learns to go totally through with the jump attempt, the less likely she is to be injured. A pole-vaulter who faults the jump at the beginning can fall back and land on the hard track, but the jumper who completes the motion—even though she misses the jump—will probably land in the pit and not hurt herself.

It is also important that the jumper learn how to land properly. She should avoid landing on her hands or forearms; it is wise for her to land on her buttocks.

The pole-vaulter must never use a vaulting pole designed for someone lighter than herself. (Most poles have a maximum-weight designation printed on them.) Serious injury can occur if a fiberglass vaulting pole snaps, because it usually occurs during the pull-and-bend part of the vault, and the runner could be impaled.

Heel cups should be worn by triple-jumpers, high-jumpers, and long-jumpers to guard against excessive stress. Sometimes the jumper accidentally lands hard on the heel, causing a bone bruise. Without proper protection, this can be a very painful injury and can put the jumper out of competition.

Throwing events: Women athletes in throwing events may feel they don't have to warm up as much as a jumper or runner; this isn't true. Although the upper part of the body may be most direct-